Color Atlas of Ophthalmic Surgery

Illustrations by Barbara Cousins

21 Contributors

17 92

J.B. LIPPINCOTT COMPANY
Philadelphia

Color Atlas of Ophthalmic Surgery

OCULOPLASTIC SURGERY

David T. Tse, M.D.

Associate Professor, Bascom Palmer Eye Institute, Department of Ophthalmology, University of Miami School of Medicine, Miami, Florida

Kenneth W. Wright, M.D., Editor-in-Chief
Stephen J. Ryan, Jr., M.D., Consultant

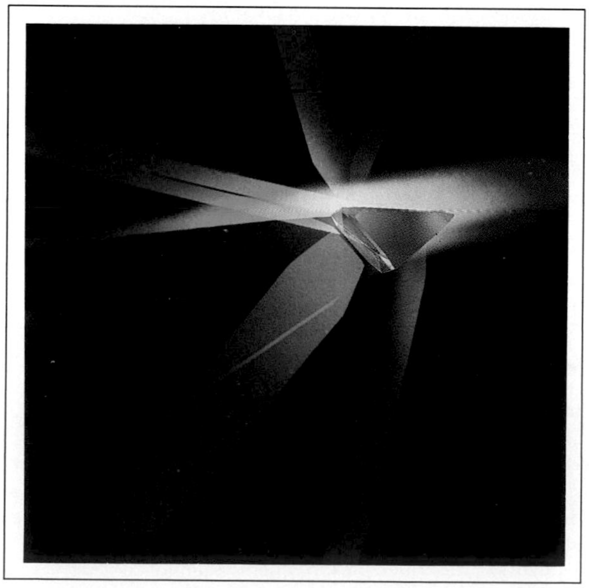

Acquisitions Editor: Lisa McAllister
Editorial Assistant: Emilie J. Moyer
Project Editor: Dina Kamilatos
Indexer: Julia Figures
Designer: Doug Smock
Production Manager: Caren Erlichman
Production Coordinator: Kevin P. Johnson
Compositor: Bi-Comp, Incorporated
Printer/Binder: Arcata Graphics/Kingsport
Cover Photograph: Walter Plotnick

6 5 4 3 2 1

Library of Congress Cataloging-in-Publication Data

Color atlas of ophthalmic surgery : oculoplastic surgery / [edited by]
David T. Tse ; Kenneth W. Wright, editor-in-chief ; 21 contributors.
p. cm.
Includes bibliographical references and index.
ISBN 0-397-51070-5
1. Ophthalmic plastic surgery—Atlases. I. Tse, David T.
II. Wright, Kenneth W. (Kenneth Weston),
[DNLM: 1. Eye—surgery—atlases. 2. Surgery, Plastic—methods—
atlases. WW 17 C7198]
RE87.C65 1992
617.7′1—dc20
DNLM/DLC
for Library of Congress 92-2963
CIP

The authors and publisher have exerted every effort to ensure that drug selection and dosage set forth in this text are in accord with current recommendations and practice at the time of publication. However, in view of ongoing research, changes in government regulations, and the constant flow of information relating to drug therapy and drug reactions, the reader is urged to check the package insert for each drug for any change in indications and dosage and for added warnings and precautions. This is particularly important when the recommended agent is a new or infrequently employed drug.

Dedicated to the memory of my parents;
to my brothers and sisters who encouraged me to pursue a career in medicine;
to my wife, Jean; and my sons, Brian and Jeffrey,
for their love, understanding, and unselfish support.

CONTRIBUTORS

Richard L. Anderson, M.D., F.A.C.S.
Professor of Ophthalmology, Director—Ophthalmic Plastic, Orbital and Reconstructive Surgery, University of Utah, Salt Lake City, Utah

William K. Blaylock, M.D.
Assistant Professor, Department of Ophthalmology, Eastern Virginia Medical School, Medical College of Hampton Roads, Norfolk, Virginia

Delyse R. Buus, M.D.
The Permanente Medical Group, Kaiser Permanente Medical Center, Oakland, California

Marcos T. Doxanas, M.D.
Greater Baltimore Medical Center, Director of Oculoplastic Surgery, Wilmer Institute, Johns Hopkins Hospital, Lecturer in Ophthalmology, Baltimore, Maryland

Steven M. Gilberg, M.D., F.R.C.S.(C)
Fellow, Ophthalmic Plastic and Reconstructive Surgery, Bascom Palmer Eye Institute, University of Miami, Miami, Florida

Russell S. Gonnering, M.D., F.A.C.S.
Assistant Clinical Professor, Department of Ophthalmology, The University of Wisconsin, Milwaukee, Wisconsin

John B. Holds, M.D.
Bethesda Eye Institute, Department of Ophthalmology, St. Louis University Medical School; Assistant Professor, Department of Ophthalmology and Otolaryngology, St. Louis, Missouri

Robert C. Kersten, M.D., F.A.C.S.
Associate Professor of Clinical Ophthalmology, University of Cincinnati College of Medicine, Cincinnati, Ohio

Jan W. Kronish, M.D.
Clinical Assistant Professor of Ophthalmology, Bascom Palmer Eye Institute, Department of Ophthalmology, University of Miami School of Medicine, Miami, Florida

Dwight R. Kulwin, M.D., F.A.C.S.
Associate Professor of Clinical Ophthalmology, University of Cincinnati College of Medicine, Cincinnati, Ohio

Robert E. Levine, M.D.
Clinical Professor of Ophthalmology, University of Southern California, School of Medicine, Los Angeles, California

John V. Linberg, M.D.
Associate Professor, Ophthalmology Department, West Virginia University, Morgantown, West Virginia

Don Liu, M.D.
Associate Professor, Department of Ophthalmology, Doheny Eye Institute, Los Angeles, California

Alfred C. Marrone, M.D.
Associate Clinical Professor, University of Southern California, Estelle Doheny Eye Foundation, Torrance, California

William M. McLeish, M.D.
Assistant Professor, Department of Ophthalmology, Mayo Clinic, Jacksonville, Florida

Thaddeus S. Nowinski, M.D.
Associate Surgeon, Oculoplastic Service, Wills Eye Hospital, Clinical Associate Professor, Thomas Jefferson University, Philadelphia, Pennsylvania

Peter B. Odland, M.D.
Assistant Professor, Department of Medicine (Dermatology), Director, Dermatologic Surgery, University of Washington Medical Center, Seattle, Washington

Kevin R. Scott, M.D.
Ophthalmic Plastic Surgeon, Arlington Eye Associates, Attending Surgeon, Arlington Hospital, Arlington, Virginia

Myron Tanenbaum, M.D., F.A.C.S.
Clinical Assistant Professor of Ophthalmology, Bascom Palmer Eye Institute, Department of Ophthalmology, University of Miami School of Medicine, Miami, Florida

David T. Tse, M.D., F.A.C.S.
Associate Professor, Bascom Palmer Eye Institute, Department of Ophthalmology, University of Miami School of Medicine, Miami, Florida

Duane C. Whitaker, M.D.
Associate Professor of Dermatology, Director, Dermatologic Surgery, The University of Iowa Hospitals and Clinics, Iowa City, Iowa

PREFACE

The field of ophthalmic plastic surgery within the past decade has witnessed a tremendous growth of knowledge in various disease entities, a renewed interest in eyelid and orbital anatomy, and a proliferation of many new surgical procedures based on anatomic principles. It is difficult for a single author to embrace the entire subject of oculoplastic surgery; as a result, a multiauthored text becomes obligatory. The intent of the Oculoplastic Surgery volume of *Color Atlas of Ophthalmic Surgery* is to provide surgeons familiar with surgical anatomy with a broad survey of contemporary oculoplastic surgery. This atlas does not attempt to fill the need for a comprehensive textbook on oculoplastic procedures; rather, it illustrates and provides basic information on surgical techniques that are straightforward and reliable in managing many common oculoplastic conditions that a clinician may encounter in clinical practice. An integrated text, accompanied by color photographs and complementary line drawings, guides the surgeon through each procedure in a step-by-step fashion. Pertinent anatomy, surgical indications, important technical considerations, and complications receive appropriate emphasis in each chapter. Although we have attempted chapter conformity when practical, the individuality of the contributor has been respected. References have purposely not been introduced into the text. Instead, for those who wish to pursue additional information on a particular procedure, a bibliography is provided at the end of the book to serve as a starting point for literature search.

We sincerely hope readers will find this pragmatic text useful in their clinical practice.

David T. Tse, M.D.

ACKNOWLEDGMENTS

The Oculoplastic Surgery volume of *Color Atlas of Ophthalmic Surgery* represents the combined efforts of many distinguished contributors; the editor is profoundly grateful of their patience, cooperation, promptness, and continued interest. The excellence of their individual chapters has made the editorial task light.

I wish to convey special thanks to my secretary, Ms. Kelly "Gucci" Parsons, who typed and retyped many manuscripts, checked references, and kept track of numerous essential details.

I especially like to thank Drs. Delyse Buus, Kevin Scott, and Steve Gilberg for their helpful suggestions and criticisms. Special thanks and appreciation to Dr. Jonathan Macy, who gave generously of his time in reviewing the manuscripts for this volume.

I owe a particular debt to Barbara Cousins, medical illustrator of the volume, for without her expert skill, patience, and forbearance in an arduous task, and the desire to achieve accuracy and effect, this volume could hardly have been made.

I am much indebted to my preceptor and mentor, Richard L. Anderson, who by his exemplary teaching and innovative works, has so greatly influenced and shaped my own treatment philosophy and surgical techniques.

In the course of the two years that this book has been in preparation, many persons on the staff of J.B. Lippincott Company have worked on it. Their able and patient assistance, unfailing courtesy, and consideration are gratefully acknowledged.

CONTENTS

Chapter Twenty-Two
SOCKET RECONSTRUCTION
Jan W. Kronish

Chapter Twenty-Three
ENUCLEATION AND TECHNIQUES OF ORBITAL IMPLANT PLACEMENT
Delyse R. Buus, Jan W. Kronish, and David T. Tse

Chapter Twenty-Four
EVISCERATION
Delyse R. Buus and David T. Tse

Chapter Twenty-Five
EXTENERATION
Delyse R. Buus and David T. Tse

Color Atlas of Ophthalmic Surgery

Chapter One

SURGICAL ANATOMY OF THE EYELIDS AND ORBIT

Marcos T. Doxanas

Appreciation of eyelid and orbital anatomy has dramatically changed our surgical approaches to problems in these areas. No longer are eyelids excised or distorted during attempted surgical repairs. Now, anatomic abnormalities are identified, and attempts are made to alleviate the underlying anatomic aberration. Patients with ptosis, have an exploration of the levator aponeurosis and repair of defects or advancement of the levator. Patients with an ectropion, have lateral tarsal strips created to strengthen the lower eyelid. Patients with entropion may have lower lid retractors reinserted in conjunction with a tarsal strip procedure to stabilize the eyelid.

Jones and Wobig (1976) were among the first authors to appreciate the significance of orbital and eyelid anatomy in surgical concepts. They went on to acknowledge two groups of surgeons of the eyelids.

1. One group are those who might appear to see how much damage they can do to the anatomy of the eyelid and still get good results.
2. The second group are those who try to inflict the least possible injury to the anatomy and also get good results.

It is this second group of surgeons we are attempting to enlighten and train.

OSTEOLOGY

The orbits are paired structures, lying on each side of the sagittal plane of the skull. The orbits are closely related to the paranasal sinuses, with the ethmoid sinuses, nasally; maxillary sinuses, inferiorly; and frontal sinuses, superior nasally. Bony contributions to the orbit are from the calvaria (frontal and sphenoid bones) and the facial bones.

The orbital cavity is pear-shaped, with its widest portion just within the orbital rim, then tapering posteriorly to the orbital apex. The medial walls of the orbits are parallel to one another, whereas the lateral orbital walls are divergent at a 90° angle. The central axes of the orbits, therefore, are directed 45° from one another. The floor of the orbit does not extend to the orbital apex, but terminates approximately at the level of the posterior wall of the maxillary sinus.

The orbital rim is nearly rectangular, with a discontinuity at the inferior nasal margin, which forms the fossa for the lacrimal sac. The orbital margin acts as a buttress to protect the orbit and globe. It is produced by the frontal, zygomatic, and maxillary bones. If the orbit is struck with considerable force, it will produce a fracture at sites of potential weakness, normally the zygomaticofrontal and zygomaticomaxillary sutures. Associated fracture of the zygomatic arch will produce the characteristic trimalar (tripod) fracture.

The superior wall of the orbit is triangular, extending to the orbital apex. The orbital roof is composed primarily of the orbital plate of the frontal bone, with the posterior extent being formed by the lesser wing of the sphenoid. The orbital plate of the frontal bone meets with the ethmoid bone to form the frontoethmoidal suture. The anterior and posterior ethmoidal foramen, with associated arteries and nerves, are located within the frontoethmoidal suture. Care should be taken to identify and, if necessary, clip and ligate the anterior ethmoidal artery when performing surgical approaches to the medial orbit.

The medial wall of the orbit consists primarily of the lamina papyracea of the ethmoid sinus. The frontal process of the maxillary bone and the lacrimal bones contribute to the anterior portion of the medial wall, whereas the sphenoid bone contributes posteriorly. The lamina papyracea is extremely thin and provides a poor anatomic barrier, permitting the extension of infections or tumors from the ethmoid sinuses. The internal septated supporting structure of the ethmoid sinuses provides strength to the medial wall, so it is less commonly involved with blowout fractures of the orbit.

The orbital floor is composed of the maxillary, zygomatic, and palatine bones. The largest portion of the orbital floor is contributed by the orbital plate of the maxillary bone. As noted previously, the orbital floor does not extend to the orbital apex. The inferior orbital sulcus lies within the floor of the orbit and transmits the infraorbital nerve. The central portion of the orbital floor is thin and relatively weak.

The lateral orbital wall is triangular and consists of the zygomatic bone anteriorly and the greater wing of the sphenoid posteriorly. The prominent zygomatic bone will thin before fusing with the greater wing of the sphenoid. A thin bony plate separates the lateral orbit from the temporalis fossa anteriorly and the middle cranial fossa posteriorly.

The sphenoid bone has a pivotal role in orbital osteology. The superior orbital fissure is formed by a gap in the greater and lesser wings of the sphenoid. Structures passing through the superior orbital fissure (from lateral to medial) are the following: lacrimal nerve, frontal nerve, trochlear nerve, superior division of the oculomotor nerve, abducens nerve, nasociliary nerve, and the inferior division of the oculomotor nerve.

The inferior orbital fissure originates at the orbital apex and extends approximately 20 mm toward the central portion of the orbital floor. The fissure transmits the infraorbital nerve and artery and provides a route for the pterygoid plexus. The anterior and posterior alveolar nerves branch from the infraorbital nerve to supply the incisors and canines, and the cuspids, respectively. Damage to these nerves, such as in an orbital floor blowout fracture, may cause numbness in the canine and incisor teeth.

The optic canal connects the middle cranial fossa to the orbital apex. The optic canal is formed by the fusion of two roots of the lesser wing of the sphenoid. The posterior ethmoid sinuses and the sphenoid sinuses are adjacent to the medial wall of the canal. The optic canal transmits the optic nerve, ophthalmic artery, and ocular sympathetic nerves. Within the optic canal, the optic nerve is firmly adherent to the bone by dura. Within the orbit, the dura splits, forming the outer sheath of the optic nerve and the periorbita.

TOPOGRAPHIC ANATOMY

Eyelids

The various surface contours on the mid- and upper face, coupled with varying skin thickness, produce characteristic folds in the periocular area. The palpebral fissure generally ranges from 10 to 12 mm in vertical dimension, and 25 to 30 mm in horizontal dimension. In primary gaze, the upper eyelid margin is generally 1 to 2 mm below the superior limbus. The upper eyelid position gradually lowers as the individual ages. It is important to appreciate that the peak of the upper eyelid margin is nasal to the center of the pupil with the eye in primary gaze. The upper lid contour is extremely important, particularly in ptosis repairs, for which novice surgeons often place the upper eyelid peak at the pupil or even lateral to the pupil. The lower eyelid margin is generally at the inferior edge of the corneal limbus. The lowest portion of the lower eyelid margin is slightly temporal to the pupil.

The upper eyelid crease is horizontally oriented approximately 8 to 12 mm above the eyelashes. It is formed by the subcutaneous insertion of the terminal fibers of the levator aponeurosis. These fibers will firmly adhere to the subcutaneous tissues below the eyelid crease to form the pretarsal portion of the eyelid. The skin overlying the orbital septum has no levator aponeurotic subcutaneous extensions and will fold over the eyelid crease in varying proportions. The lower eyelid has a poorly defined eyelid crease extending to within 2 to 3 mm of the eyelid margin nasally and 5 to 6 mm temporally. The nasojugal fold extends inferior and lateral from the medial canthal angle along the side of the nose. The malar fold extends from the lateral portion of the lower eyelid toward the inferior lateral extent of the nasojugal fold. The nasojugal and malar folds represent the junctions of the thin eyelid skin to the thicker skin of the cheek. In addition, the angular artery and vein will generally be located in the nasojugal fold.

Eyebrow

The eyebrow represents a specialized musculocutaneous plane that is extremely important in facial expression. The eyebrows are best considered an extension of the scalp, or as a cranial appendage. Recently, eyebrow variations have been appreciated in functional and aesthetic surgery in the upper face. In particular, gender variations of the eyebrow contour may influence the planning of cosmetic eyebrow and upper lid surgery.

The anatomy of the eyebrow has been thoroughly described by Lemke and Stasior (1982). These authors described four major layers of the brow: skin, muscle, fat, and aponeurosis. The muscular layer of the brow consists of four muscle groups: frontalis, corrugator superciliaris, procerus, and orbital orbicularis oculi. The frontalis muscle originates from a split in the galea aponeurotica. The frontalis muscle has no bony insertions, which potentiates its contraction and enhances brow mobility. Nasally, the frontalis muscle will interdigitate with the vertically oriented procerus muscle, the obliquely oriented corrugator superciliaris muscles, and the orbital orbicularis muscle. This intermixing of fibers support the brow at this level nasally. The frontalis muscle may not extend to the superior orbital rim laterally, which may contribute to the brow ptosis that is frequently seen clinically in this area.

The frontalis muscle is encapsulated by an anterior and posterior muscular sheath, which is an extension of the galea aponeurotica. The posterior muscular sheath will split as it approaches the periosteum superior orbital rim. The multiple splits in the posterior muscular sheath will produce a potential space for the brow fat pad. The posterior muscular sheath of the frontalis muscle then extends into the eyelid to contribute to the orbital septum. The brow fat greatly enhances brow mobility and is present in varying degrees. Surgical dissections have demonstrated the correlation between the prominence of the pad with the degree of brow ptosis and fullness. The brow fat pad contributes to the sexual variation in brow anatomy; in masculine brows, the brow fat pad is more prominent and extends inferiorly into the eyelid directly anterior to the orbital septum.

Upper Eyelids

Figure 1–1. A sagittal view of normal upper eyelid anatomy. The eyelid has essentially six layers: skin, orbicularis muscle, levator aponeurosis, Mueller's muscle, tarsus, and conjunctiva. However, these layers are variable based on the level of eyelid examined. Near the eyelid margin there are only four layers: skin, orbicularis muscle, tarsus, and conjunctiva. Directly above the tarsal border, five layers of the eyelid are present: skin, orbicularis muscle, levator aponeurosis, Mueller's muscle, and conjunctiva. Care must be taken to identify the level of the eyelid to appreciate its various layers.

The eyelid skin has unique features to enhance its mobility. The epithelial layer is thin and attaches to the orbicularis muscle by a loose connective tissue devoid of dermal-like tissue. In addition, sebaceous glands are not developed extensively in the eyelid, which would anchor the skin to the subcutaneous tissues. These distinguishing features of the eyelid skin account, in part, for its tendency to become redundant and, in exaggerated situations, fold over the eyelid, producing a visual field loss. As an involutional change, this excess skin is called dermatochalasis, but may result from recurrent angioneurotic edema, producing the blepharochalasis syndrome.

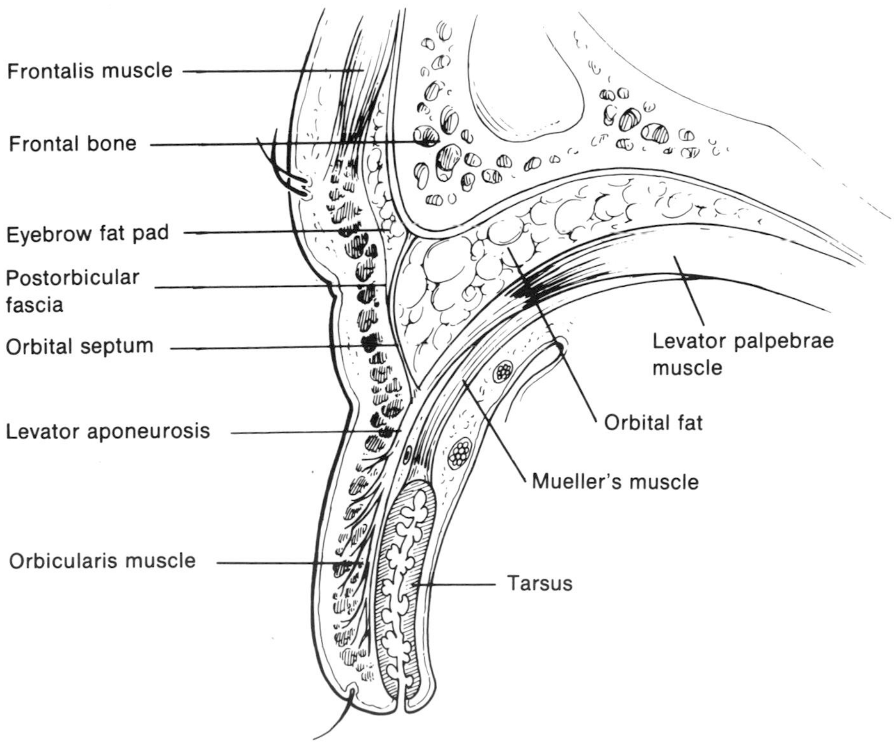

FIGURE 1–1

The orbicularis muscle is the protractor for the eyelids and is under voluntary control from the facial nerve. The concentrically arranged orbicularis muscle is divided into three sections: pretarsal, preseptal, and orbital. The combined pretarsal and preseptal orbicularis muscles form the palpebral portion of the orbicularis and overlie the tarsus and orbital septum, respectively. The orbital orbicularis overlaps the orbital rims, interdigitating with the eyebrow muscles superiorly.

The pretarsal and preseptal orbicularis muscles contribute to the superficial and deep portions of the medial and lateral canthal tendon. The deep extensions of the pretarsal and preseptal orbicularis muscles are referred to as Horner's and Jones' muscles, respectively, and insert on the fascia overlying the lacrimal sac. In addition, the pretarsal orbicularis also contributes to the lateral canthal tendon. Giola and coworkers (1987) identified the pretarsal orbicularis muscle to extend beneath the orbital septum laterally to contribute to the tendinous component of the lateral canthal tendon. Laterally, the preseptal orbicularis muscle joins in the lateral raphe, oriented horizontally in the lateral canthal angle.

The medial canthal tendon (MCT) supports the nasal aspect of the eyelids. The MCT has superficial and deep components that anchor the eyelid nasally and posteriorly against the globe. Anderson (1977) emphasized the role of a superior branch of the MCT extending from the anterior portion of the MCT to insert onto the frontal bone. The superior limb of the MCT anchors the nasal eyelid, preventing dystopias of the medial canthal angle.

The lateral canthal tendon (LCT) has been highlighted in the literature because of a variety of procedures described to correct canthal defects or lid malpositions. Giola and coworkers (1987) have identified both a tendinous and ligamentous component to the LCT. The tendinous portion of the LCT is from the pretarsal orbicularis muscle and inserts on the inner aspect of the lateral orbital rim at the lateral orbital (Whitnall's) tubercle. The ligamentous component of the LCT is a direct extension from the tarsus, which slips posterior to the orbital septum to insert at the lateral orbital tubercle. This deep extension and attachment of the LCT draws the eyelid laterally and posteriorly, approximating the eyelids to the globe. Attempts to surgically reconstruct the LCT must reconstitute the deep posterior extensions of the tendon to maintain lid apposition with the globe (Anderson and Dixon, 1979).

The orbital septum forms the anatomic boundary between the eyelid and the orbit. At one time, the orbital septum was considered a sacred structure, not to be penetrated unless unavoidable. If the structure was violated, it was meticulously closed to reform the anatomic barrier it represented. This impression has changed dramatically.

The orbital septum originates at the arcus marginalis of orbital rim. The orbital septum extends toward the tarsus and fuses with the levator aponeurosis and the lower lid retractors prior to their insertion of the tarsus (Anderson and Beard, 1977). In the upper eyelid, variations in the level of fusion of the orbital septum and levator aponeurosis will produce changes in the level of the eyelid crease and fold. In the Oriental eyelid, the orbital septum fuses with the levator aponeurosis below the tarsal border, thereby eliminating the eyelid crease and producing a prominent lid fold (Doxanas and Anderson, 1984). The preaponeurotic or orbital fat is confined by the orbital septum and forms pockets; however, the multilaminated orbital septum may thin with age, allowing herniation of orbital fat. The nasal fat pockets in the upper and lower eyelids are white, instead of yellow, and should not be overlooked during blepharoplasty surgery. Occasionally, the orbital lobe of the lacrimal gland will prolapse, to produce fullness in the lateral portion of the eyelid. Care must be exercised during blepharoplasty to identify the prolapsed lacrimal gland and distinguish it from orbital fat to prevent its inadvertent excision.

The levator palpebral superioris muscle provides a distinct eyelid retractor. The muscle arises at the orbital apex, directly above the annulus of Zinn. The levator muscle proceeds anteriorly from the orbital apex in the superior orbit adjacent to the periorbita. As the superior orbital rim is approached, the levator fans nasally and temporally.

Figure 1–2. A frontal view of Whitnall's ligament and anterior orbital structures. As the levator muscle extends below the superior orbital

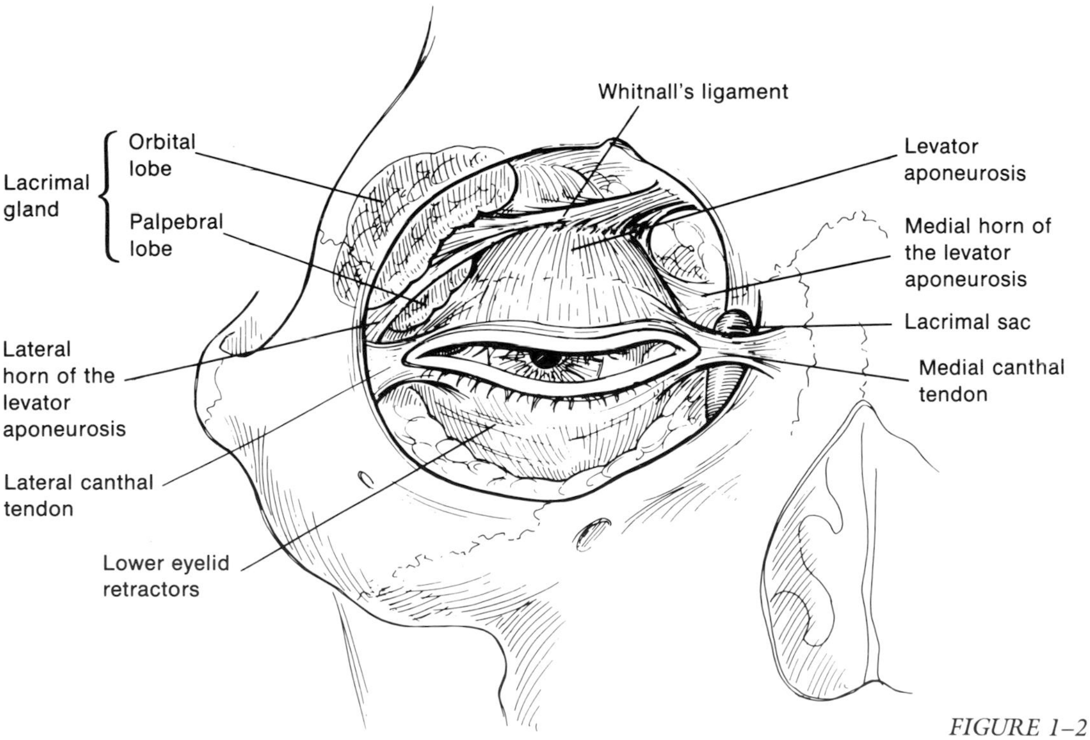

FIGURE 1–2

rim, it is redirected by the superior transverse ligament, also known as Whitnall's ligament. The ligament acts as a fulcrum to redirect the muscle from an anteroposterior to superoinferior direction, enhancing its function. At the level of the superior transverse ligament, the levator muscle starts to transform into its aponeurotic extension. This transformation of the levator muscle to a white shiny structure is complete approximately 10 to 12 mm above the superior border of the tarsus. The aponeurotic fibers diffusely extend anteriorly through the orbicularis muscle overlying the tarsus to insert into the subcutaneous tissues. The superior-most subcutaneous extension of the levator aponeurosis will define the level of the eyelid crease. The posterior portion of the levator aponeurosis attaches to the lower 7 to 8 mm of the tarsus. The superior 2 to 3 mm of the tarsus has loose attachments of the levator aponeurosis, whereas the aponeurosis is most strongly adherent to the tarsus about 3 mm above the eyelid margin. The diffuse extensions of the levator aponeurosis produce a smooth, coordinated movement to the upper eyelid.

Mueller's muscle originates under the surface of the levator muscle, at the level of its transformation to its aponeurosis. Approximately 10-mm above the superior tarsal border, a well-defined smooth muscle is identified. Mueller's muscle attaches to the superior tarsal border in the upper eyelid. In the lower eyelid, Mueller's muscle is not as well defined and generally terminates before reaching the inferior tarsal border. Interruption of the ocular sympathetic nerve fibers will produce Horner's syndrome: ptosis, miosis, apparent enophthalmos, and occasional anhidrosis. Eyelid sympathetics are also implicated in eyelid retraction associated with Graves' disease. Increased adrenergic stimulation to Mueller's muscle may be a contributing factor in the production of upper and lower eyelid retraction.

The tarsal plates provide a firm posterior support or foundation for the eyelids. The tarsus in the upper eyelid is approximately 10 mm at its greatest vertical height, whereas the tarsus in the lower eyelid ranges from 3.2 to 5.0 mm (average 3.7 mm). The tarsus will then taper toward its medial and lateral borders and attaches to the orbital rims by the medial and lateral canthal tendons.

Lower Eyelid

Figure 1–3. A sagittal view of normal lower eyelid anatomy. The upper and lower eyelids are analogous structures. The main distinction is the eyelid retractors. The upper eyelid has a distinct eyelid retractor, the levator muscle, which imparts a high degree of mobility to the eyelid. This is evidenced by the excursion of the upper eyelid, ranging up to 16 mm, between up gaze and down gaze. The lower eyelid does not have a distinct retractor, but instead, a fibrous extension from the inferior rectus muscle. As a result, the relatively immobile lower eyelid

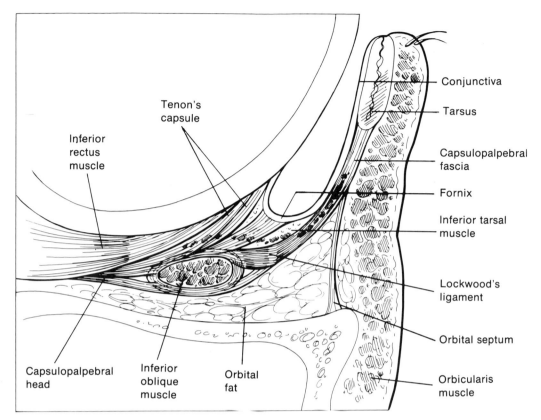

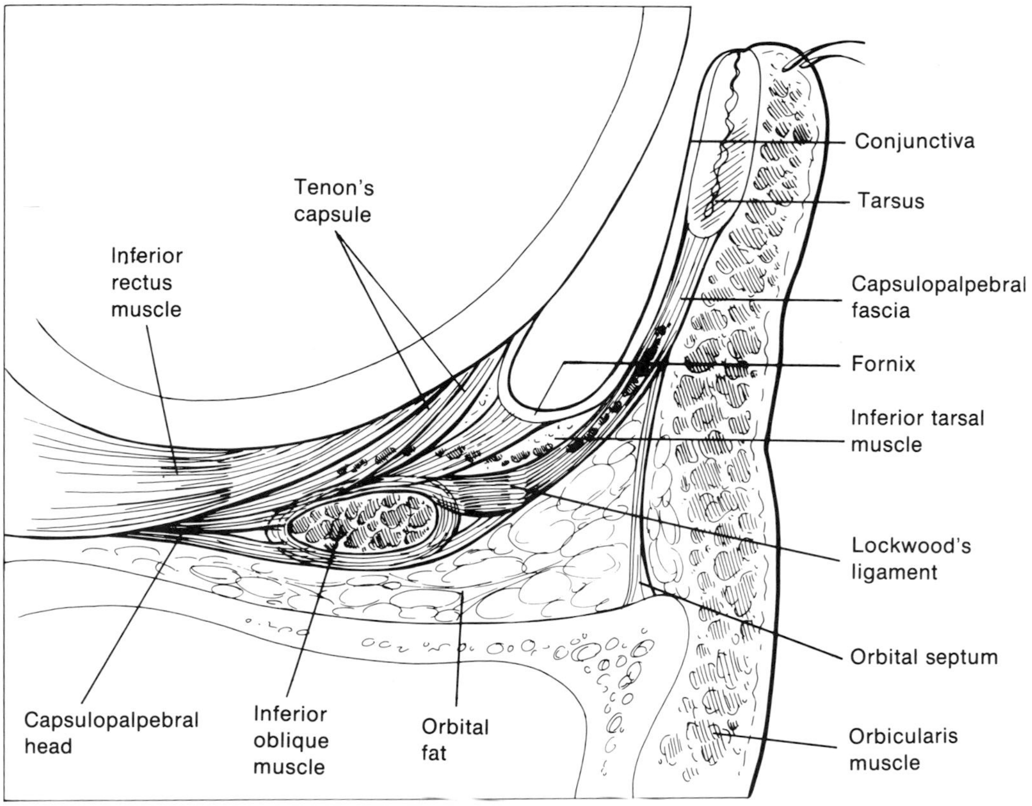

FIGURE 1–3

gains its motion through the action of the inferior rectus muscle. The lower eyelid has a range of motion of only 3 to 5 mm on extreme degrees of excursion from down gaze to up gaze.

The lower eyelid retractor originates from the inferior rectus muscle before its penetration of posterior Tenon's capsule (Hawes and Dortzbach, 1982). The fibrous extension forming the lower lid retractor originates as the capsulopalpebral head of the inferior rectus muscle and splits to encapsulate the inferior oblique muscle. Anterior to the inferior oblique muscle, the fibers reunite to form the capsulopalpebral fascia or aponeurosis. Most of the capsulopalpebral fascia inserts on the inferior tarsal border, although some fibers extend anteriorly through the orbital fat, contributing to the septae dividing the fat pockets. In addition, some fibers extend posteriorly into the inferior fornix (see Figure 1–3). The capsulopalpebral fibers do not extend through the orbicularis muscle to terminate in subcutaneous tissues or extend on the anterior tarsal surface, as does its analogous structure in the upper eyelid, the levator muscle. As a result, the lower eyelid crease is poorly defined.

The orbital septum fuses with the capsulopalpebral fascia before reaching the inferior tarsal border. Conjunctival approaches to the orbital floor will involve this area between the inferior tarsal border and orbital septum as a dissection plane to enter the normal anatomic plane between orbicularis muscle and the orbital septum.

LACRIMAL SYSTEM

The lacrimal system provides for the production, distribution, and drainage of tears. The tear film protects the globe from desiccation and maintains a clear optical surface. The lacrimal excretory system drains tears from the lacus lacrimalis into the inferior meatus. Blockage of the nasolacrimal system or excessive production of tears results in epiphora and produces a diagnostic challenge to identify the cause of and possible site of lacrimal blockage.

The precorneal tear film has three layers: innermost, mucous layer; prominent central aqueous layer; and superficial lipid layer. The mucous layer is produced by the goblet cells of the conjunctival epithelium. The aqueous layer is produced by the main and accessory lacrimal glands. The outermost lipid layer of the tear film is primarily produced by the meibomian glands, with a small component produced by the glands of Zeis and apocrine glands of Moll.

The main and accessory lacrimal glands produce the aqueous portion of the tear film. The main lacrimal gland is located in the superior lateral portion of the anterior orbit. Directly posterior to the orbital rim is a concavity within the orbital plate of the frontal bone that forms the fossa glandular lacrimalis. The main lacrimal gland is divided and supported by the lateral horn of the levator aponeurosis and Whitnall's ligament into an orbital and palpebral lobe. The orbital lobe contains approximately two-thirds of the volume of the lacrimal gland, and the palpebral lobe constitutes the remainder.

The excretory ducts of the lacrimal gland coalesce from the orbital lobe and pass through the palpebral lobe to the conjunctiva. The course of the excretory ducts corresponds to the embryologic path of migration of ectodermal buds from the conjunctiva that forms the lacrimal gland. The 12 to 14 lacrimal excretory ducts primarily open to the palpebral conjunctiva, 4- to 5-mm above the lateral aspect of the superior tarsus. However, some excretory duct orifices may open into the lateral canthal angle. All the excretory ducts pass through the palpebral lobe of the lacrimal gland; consequently, inadvertent excision of this portion of the gland will eliminate all main lacrimal gland secretions.

The accessory lacrimal glands consist of the glands of Wolfring, located at the superior tarsal border, and the glands of Krause, positioned in the conjunctival fornix. These glands consist of small nests of lacrimal glands that drain directly to the conjunctiva. The glands of

Krause number approximately 20 to 40 in the upper fornix and only 6 to 8 in the lower fornix. The glands of Wolfring are less common, numbering approximately 3 at the superior tarsal border and only 1 at the inferior tarsal border. The role of the accessory lacrimal glands is primarily for the maintenance of basic tear secretion.

Figure 1–4. Diagram of the lacrimal drainage system. The lacrimal excretory system consists of the puncta, canaliculus, common canaliculus, lacrimal sac, and the nasolacrimal duct. Tears are allowed to accumulate in the medial canthal angle at the lacus lacrimalis. The tears then enter the lacrimal excretory system at the punctum, or opening of the canaliculus at the posterior eyelid margin. The initial 2 mm of the canaliculus is vertically oriented. The canaliculus then courses horizontally approximately 8 to 10 mm to the lacrimal sac. Before entering the lacrimal sac, the upper and lower canaliculi fuse, forming the common canaliculus. The common canaliculus enters the lacrimal sac at the level of the medial canthal tendon. The lacrimal sac enters the bony nasolacrimal duct and gains entrance into the nose under the inferior turbinate.

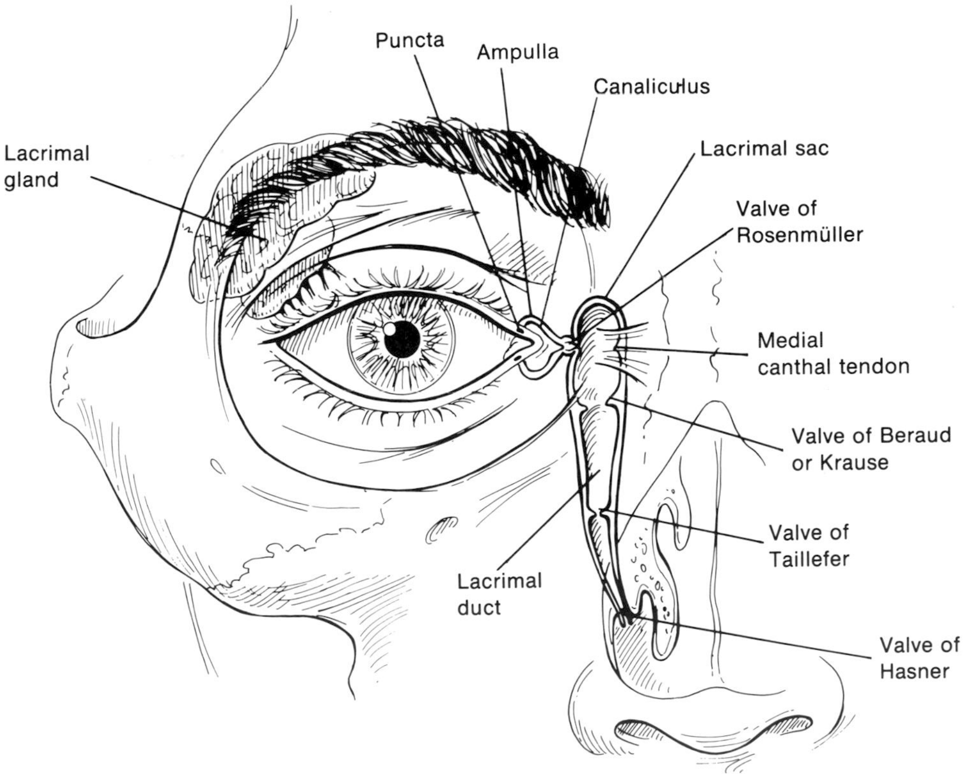

FIGURE 1–4

Multiple valves have been identified in the nasolacrimal system; however, most valves generally represent mucosal folds and are of no functional significance. One valve of importance is the valve of Rösenmuller at the entrance of the common canaliculus into the lacrimal sac. This mucosal fold prevents reflux of the lacrimal sac contents into the canaliculus. Probing of the canalicular system into the lacrimal sac, will render the valve of Rösenmuller incompetent. As a result, blowing of the nose will result in air being regurgitated through the nasolacrimal system onto the globe. The other nasolacrimal valve of significance is the valve of Hasner, which is implicated in congenital nasolacrimal duct obstruction.

ORBITAL CONNECTIVE TISSUE SYSTEM

Diffuse orbital connective systems play a significant role in supporting the globe within the orbit, without restricting ocular motility. Koornneef (1977) has revolutionized the concept of the orbital connective tissue systems by his unique approach to its study. He utilized an operating microscope to dissect the conjunctival fornices and anterior orbit and assessed the posterior orbit by a thick–tissue-sectioning technique, enabling the study of the spatial architecture.

Koornneef identified three distinct connective tissue systems within the orbit. The first, Tenon's capsule, or the bulbar fascia, is the fibrous layer of the connective tissue that encapsulates the globe. Tenon's capsule originates at the limbus as a thin connective tissue layer firmly adherent between conjunctiva and episcleral tissue. As it proceeds posteriorly to the optic nerve, Tenon's capsule is penetrated by the six extraocular muscles. The four rectus muscles penetrate Tenon's capsule posterior to the equator, whereas the obliques penetrate Tenon's capsule anterior to the equator. Posterior to the penetration of the rectus muscles toward the optic nerve, Tenon's capsule is loosely adherent to the globe by fine bands of connective tissue. Tenon's capsule presents a barrier between the globe and retrobulbar adipose tissue. If the posterior Tenon's capsule is violated, the retrobulbar fat may protrude into this area and cause scarring that limits ocular motility.

The second component of the connective tissue system is the anterior orbital connective tissue that supports the globe within the orbit and attaches to the superior oblique tendon, the inferior oblique muscle, and Tenon's capsule. Inferiorly, this connective tissue complex contributes to Lockwood's suspensory ligament, although this structure has a reduced importance in the supporting role of the globe. Koornneef (1977) suggested that the connective tissue septae of the superior orbit provide the primary support for the globe.

The third connective tissue system is derived from the fascial sheaths of the extraocular muscles and forms a characteristic connective tissue framework. They form a nebulous connective tissue septa in the posterior orbit and become better defined anteriorly. In the anterior orbit, the fascial sheaths contribute to the medial and lateral check ligaments. The intermuscular fibrous sheaths extend anteriorly to form a confluent muscle sheath; however, a distinct muscle cone is not recognized in the posterior aspect of the orbit.

The diffuse, well-defined connective tissue systems account for the restricted extraocular motility associated with orbital floor or medial wall fractures. With these fractures, it is unusual to visualize the inferior or medial rectus muscles entrapped within the fracture. More commonly, the check ligaments between the periorbita and the respective rectus muscle will be incarcerated, accounting for the restricted ocular motility.

NERVES OF THE ORBIT

Nerves enter the orbit at its apex to supply the globe and surrounding structures. The optic nerve (cranial nerve II) is actually a direct fiber tract from the brain. The course of the optic nerve is intraocular, intraorbital, intracanalicular, intracranial, chiasmic, optic tract, lateral geniculate body, and finally the optic radiation to the occipital cortex. As the optic nerve exits the globe, it penetrates the sclera to form its intraorbital portion. This is approximately 20 to 30 mm in length, and it takes a sinuous course to the orbital apex. The added length of the optic nerve permits unencumbered ocular movement. The optic nerve is encased in dura, and cerebrospinal fluid bathes the nerve with direct intracranial communications.

The nerves to the extraocular muscles include the oculomotor nerve (cranial nerve III), the trochlear nerve (cranial nerve IV), and the abducens nerve (cranial nerve VI). The oculomotor nerve divides into a superior and inferior branch in the anterior portion of the cavernous sinus. Both divisions enter the orbit through the superior orbital fissure within the annulus of Zinn. The superior branch of the oculomotor nerve extends anteriorly under the surface of the superior rectus muscle, to the levator palpebrae superioris muscle. Oculomotor nerve fibers penetrate these muscles approximately 15 mm from the orbital apex. The inferior division of the oculomotor nerve extends beneath the optic nerve to enter the conal surface in the posterior one-third of the inferior and medial rectus muscles. A disproportionately large branch of the inferior division of the oculomotor nerve extends along the lateral border of the inferior rectus muscle, to innervate the inferior oblique muscle near its midpoint as it crosses the inferior rectus muscle. In the posterior orbit, the nerve to the inferior oblique muscle will supply fine parasympathetic fibers to the ciliary ganglion before proceeding anteriorly.

The trochlear nerve supplies somatic motor fibers to the superior oblique muscle. This nerve has numerous unusual features in its brain stem origin and intracranial course. The trochlear nerve exits on the dorsal surface of the brain stem, necessitating a long intracranial course before entering the cavernous sinus adjacent to the oculomotor nerve. The long intracranial course of the trochlear nerve creates a predisposition to injury with cranial trauma. Once it passes into the orbit through the superior orbital fissure, the trochlear nerve innervates the orbital surface of the superior oblique muscle.

The abducens nerve innervates the lateral rectus muscle. The abducens nerve enters the cavernous sinus adjacent to the internal carotid artery. As it proceeds anteriorly, the abducens nerve moves to the lateral wall of the cavernous sinus to enter the orbit through the superior orbital fissure. The nerve enters the lateral rectus in the posterior one-third of muscle on its conal surface.

The sensory supply to the orbit is from the trigeminal nerve (cranial nerve V). Facial sensation is processed by the ophthalmic and maxillary divisions of the trigeminal nerve. The third (mandibular) division of the trigeminal nerve not only provides sensory innervation overlying the mandible, but also provides motor fibers to the muscles of mastication. The ophthalmic nerve enters the cavernous sinus and divides into its three main branches: lacrimal, frontal, and nasociliary. The lacrimal nerve enters the orbit through the superolateral aspect of the superior orbital fissure and proceeds anteriorly along the superior border of the lateral rectus muscle to reach the lacrimal gland. Before reaching the lacrimal gland, parasympathetic secretomotor fibers, originating from the facial nerve, are provided by the zygomaticotemporal nerve. The lacrimal nerve provides sensation to the lacrimal gland, but predominantly provides cutaneous sensation in the temporal aspect of the conjunctiva, upper eyelid, and eyebrow.

The frontal nerve enters the orbit from the superior orbital fissure, extends anteriorly between the periorbita and levator muscle, and splits into two branches near the orbital rim. The smaller branch, the supratrochlear nerve, supplies cutaneous innervation to the nasal aspect of the upper eyelid and eyebrow. The larger terminal branch of the frontal nerve is the supraorbital nerve, which innervates the forehead and lies directly beneath the frontalis muscle.

The nasociliary nerve has a long complicated orbital route. After the nerve enters the orbit through the apical portion of the superior orbital fissure (through the annulus of Zinn), it crosses over the optic nerve and sends fine branches to the ciliary ganglion. These fibers pass through the ciliary ganglion to form the short ciliary nerves that penetrate the sclera adjacent to the optic nerve. These fibers enter the sclera posteriorly, but extend anteriorly in the horizontal meridian to supply sensory innervation to the iris, ciliary body, and cornea. In addition, sympathetic fibers are delivered to the dilator muscle of the iris from the superior cervical ganglion. The sympathetic contribution to the ophthalmic nerve probably occurs within the cavernous sinus. The nasociliary nerve then passes nasally to the medial wall of the orbit and then branches into the posterior and ethmoidal nerves. The terminal branch of the nasociliary nerve is the infratrochlear nerve, providing sensation to the nasal portion of the eyelids, conjunctiva, lacrimal sac, and caruncle.

The maxillary nerve exits the cranial cavity through the foramen rotundum to enter the sphenopalatine or pterygopalatine fossa. The nerve enters the orbit in the inferior orbital fissure. As the nerve proceeds anteriorly, it enters the infraorbital canal to emerge from the infraorbital foramen approximately 8- to 10-mm below the inferior orbital rim. Within the inferior orbital canal, the anterior superior alveolar nerves provide sensation to the incisor and canine teeth. The infraorbital nerve provides sensation to the lower eyelid, nose, cheek, and upper lip.

The ocular sympathetics innervate the dilator muscle of the pupil and the smooth muscles of the eyelids. These fibers reach the orbit in a three-neuron pathway. The first neuron extends from the posterolateral area of the hypothalamus to terminate at the ciliospinal center of Budge between C-8 and T-1. The second-order neuron departs the spinal cord, to loop inferiorly close to the apex of the lung, and then proceeds superiorly to synapse at the superior cervical ganglion. Postganglionic fibers then follow branches of the internal and external carotid arteries to provide sympathetic innervation to the head and neck. No direct sympathetic nerves have been recognized in the orbit, as these are generally thought to accompany nerves and arteries.

The parasympathetic supply to the orbit is closely related to the oculomotor nerve. Fibers reach the orbit primarily with the inferior division of the oculomotor nerve and synapse at the ciliary ganglion. The ciliary ganglion is embedded in loose connective tissue between the optic nerve and lateral rectus muscle, approximately 1 cm from the orbital apex. Fibers from the ciliary ganglion innervate the ciliary body and iris sphincter muscles.

The pterygopalatine ganglion lies within the superior portion of the sphenopalatine or pterygopalatine fossa. Parasympathetic secretomotor fibers synapse within this ganglion to provide innervation for the lacrimal, submandibular, and sublingual glands.

The facial nerve supplies motor innervation to the muscles of expression, and a smaller portion contains sensory and parasympathetic fibers. This nerve exits the ventrolateral brain stem at the cerebellopontile angle and travels with the nervus intermedius and the acoustic nerve to the internal auditory meatus. The facial nerve enters the fallopian or facial canal in the petreous portion of the temporal bone. It exits from the stylomastoid foramen, emerges posterior to the sternocleidomastoid muscle, and extends through the parotid gland. The facial nerve then divides into an upper (temporofacial) branch and lower (cervicofacial) branch. The upper branch further divides into the temporal and zygomatic extension, and the lower branch divisions include the mandibular and cervical extensions.

ORBITAL VASCULAR SYSTEM

The arterial and venous systems of the orbit are composed of an anastomotic array of superficial and deep components. The arterial system receives deep and superficial contributions through the internal and external carotid arterial systems, respectively. The venous system drains posteriorly, primarily to the cavernous sinus, as well as the pterygoid plexus and anteriorly to the angular vein.

The internal carotid artery extends to the cavernous sinus, yielding its first major branch, the ophthalmic artery, which enters the orbit through the optic canal. Hayreh (1962) has characterized a common branching pattern of the ophthalmic artery as it courses toward the anterior orbit. The topographic classification of branches derived from the ophthalmic artery includes the ocular, orbital, and extraorbital groups. The ocular groups includes the central retinal artery, the ciliary arteries, and the collateral arteries to the optic nerve. The orbital branches of the ophthalmic artery are the muscular, lacrimal, and supraorbital arteries. The extraorbital branches include the posterior ethmoidal, anterior ethmoidal, medial palpebral, and the terminal branches, which include the nasal arteries.

The external carotid artery supplies the superficial arterial system to the orbit. Branches of the external carotid supplying orbital structures are the facial, superficial temporal, and maxillary arteries. The facial artery arises near the angle of the mandible and extends to the medial canthal angle to anastomose with the dorsal nasal artery. The superficial temporal artery is one terminal branch of the external carotid that supplies the lateral portion of the eyelids and forehead. The maxillary artery is the other terminal branch of the external carotid. It gives off numerous branches before reaching the pterygopalatine fossa, and terminates as the infraorbital artery. It gives fine branches to the inferior rectus and oblique muscles and the lacrimal sac before providing arterial supply to the lower eyelid. The superficial and deep arterial systems provide anastomotic network of the eyelids to enhance the vascular supply of the eyelids.

The venous drainage of the orbits is primarily through the superior ophthalmic vein to the cavernous sinus. The superior ophthalmic vein is formed by the union of a superior and an inferior root to extend posteriorly along the medial border of the superior rectus muscle. The vein then passes beneath the superior rectus to enter the superior orbital fissure and cavernous sinus. The inferior ophthalmic vein has a more variable course, starting as a diffuse venous plexus on the floor of the orbit and extending posteriorly to the superior ophthalmic vein or to the pterygoid plexus. In addition, the venous system may drain anteriorly into the facial vein, depending on the pressure gradient of the venous channels.

Chapter Two

FUNDAMENTAL TECHNIQUES IN OPHTHALMIC PLASTIC SURGERY

Marcos T. Doxanas

Fundamental techniques in ophthalmic plastic surgery are similar to those shared by all surgical specialties. The goal of the operative procedure is to alleviate an existing abnormality, with minimal surgical disturbance of the adjacent tissues. This requires the proper orientation of incisions, utilization of anatomic planes to facilitate surgical dissection, and the appropriate closure of incisions. Adherence to these principles, coupled with gentle handling and cauterization of periorbital and orbital structures to minimize tissue necrosis and devitalization, will help to achieve a satisfactory functional and cosmetic result.

ANESTHESIA

Before the initiation of any surgical procedure, appropriate anesthesia is required. Anesthetic options available to the patient are local, local with sedation, and general. Medical or emotional considerations are important factors in determining the anesthetic option, as this decision is individualized for each patient. Those with preexisting medical conditions, especially cardiac abnormalities or hypertension, will benefit from intravenous sedation to reduce anxiety associated with the procedure.

Local anesthetic agents with epinephrine are preferred to enhance vasoconstriction of the highly vascular eyelids; however, these may be contraindicated in patients with hypertension or cardiac arrhythmias. The onset and duration of action of commonly used local anesthetic agents are summarized in Table 2–1.

Lidocaine 2% with epinephrine 1:100,000 is effective for most oculoplastic surgeries. For procedures of longer duration, though, an equal mixture of lidocaine 2% with epinephrine and 0.5% bupivacaine with epinephrine provides prolonged anesthesia. Local anesthetics should be injected subcutaneously with a 30-gauge needle between the thin eyelid skin and orbicularis muscle. One should avoid visible vessels and penetrating the muscle to minimize hematoma formation. The orbicularis muscle and deeper tissues are eventually anesthetized by diffusion of the anesthetic agent. After approximately 10 minutes, the vasoconstricting effects of the epinephrine will help to further reduce bleeding tendencies and hematoma formation. Injection of anesthetics in the periorbital region, excluding the eyelids, should be in the subcutaneous plane. Use of a 25- or 27-gauge needle may facilitate its passage in these thicker tissues.

Regional nerve blocks have a limited role in ophthalmic plastic surgery because the eyelids have an overlapping sensory distribution. Anesthesia obtained by local infiltration of tissues is preferred, given the more reliable results and vasoconstrictive effects of epinephrine-containing agents.

Neuroleptic sedation or analgesia is the preferred method of anesthesia during oculoplastic procedures. The patient has the advantages of being monitored during the procedure to ensure there are no hyper-

TABLE 2–1
Local Anesthetic Agents

AGENT (BRAND NAME)	ONSET	DURATION (min)	TYPE	MAXIMUM CONCENTRATION (mg)	REMARKS
Procaine (Novocain)	Fast	60–90	Ester	1000	Low-potency, short duration
Lidocaine (Xylocaine)	Fast	90–200	Amide	500	Most widely used agent because of rapid onset
Mepivacaine (Carbocaine)	Fast	120–240	Amide	500	Slightly longer duration of action than lidocaine
Bupivacaine (Marcaine)	Slow	180–400	Amide	200	Long duration, mixed with lidocaine to achieve rapid onset

tensive episodes, cardiac arrhythmias, or respiratory problems. Intravenous diazepam or midazolam reduces patient anxiety and is also a potent amnestic agent. Intravenous sedation with thiopental (Pentothal) or methohexital (Brevital) will temporarily sedate the patient, to eliminate recall of the periocular injections. These agents are slowly titrated until the patient achieves an adequate level of anesthesia without respiratory suppression. The specific anesthetic agents to be used are best determined by the preference of the anesthesiologist. When the patient becomes cognizant of his surroundings, the procedure is well underway, and cooperation may be elicited from the patient to monitor eyelid position. With the proper utilization of pharmacologic agents, patients experience little discomfort intraoperatively or postoperatively.

Indications for general anesthesia are diminishing with the improvement of neuroleptic anesthesia. General anesthesia is usually reserved for those patients undergoing more invasive procedures, such as orbital procedures, or in whom cooperation is difficult, such as children. General anesthesia presents minimal risk of long-term morbidity or mortality; however, it involves a more prolonged recovery period compared with alternative anesthetic methods.

HEMOSTASIS

Patients taking aspirin, dipyrimidole (Persantin), or warfarin (Coumadin) will have an increased bleeding tendency. Aspirin inhibits platelet function and should be discontinued 2 weeks before surgery. Patients receiving anticoagulant therapy should consult their internist concerning a short-term discontinuation of its use preoperatively. In this group of patients, the prothrombin time should be obtained before surgery to ensure adequate coagulation control. Patients with a long smoking history may have a greater tendency for more bleeding during surgery, in spite of normal coagulation studies.

Two coagulation modalities currently exist: thermal and electrical. Thermal hot-wire cautery generates heat, far in excess of that necessary to produce cellular destruction and control bleeding. In addition, tissues not directly in contact with the cautery may be devitalized owing to channeling effects. Electrical cautery with unipolar, bipolar, or wet-field modalities is the preferred method to obtain hemostasis. Bipolar cautery destroys less surrounding tissues and produces more effective coagulation. In patients with diffuse oozing from the operative site, bleeding can be controlled with direct pressure or the use of epinephrine-moistened cotton pledgets. Another method includes the application of absorptive agents that promote thrombogenesis such as absorbable gelatin sponge (Gelfoam), oxidized cellulose (Surgicel), and microfibrillar collagen (Avitene). In addition, bone wax is effective in controlling bleeding from bone edges and bony foramen.

BIOPSY TECHNIQUES

Biopsy methods for eyelid lesions include the shave, punch, incisional, excisional, and full-thickness eyelid resection techniques. The tumor size, location, and suspected preoperative diagnosis will determine the biopsy method of choice. Eyelid margin tumors, either a dermal nevus or papilloma, should be treated with a shave biopsy. A diffuse melanotic tumor should have incisional biopsies to determine if dermal extension occurs. Other tumors may lend themselves to excisional biopsy. As such, the biopsy technique is modified to the clinical situation, based on the surgeon's preference and experience.

The punch biopsy is preferred by dermatologists to obtain tissue for pathologic examination. This technique utilizes a 1- to 8-mm punch to obtain a core of tissue including subcutaneous tissues. The round defect is then allowed to granulate. This method is most efficacious in skin with a thick dermal connective tissue layer and not the thinner skin with subcutaneous tissue of the eyelid. The punch biopsy technique should not be used in the eyelids, since a full-thickness eyelid biopsy may inadvertently be obtained.

The shave biopsy is a helpful diagnostic and therapeutic modality for tissue procurement. This technique involves the use of a size 11 Bard–Parker blade or sharp iris scissors to excise a lesion flush with the surface of the surrounding skin. The tissue obtained is generally readily differentiated between a benign or malignant lesion; however, the differentiation of squamous cell carcinoma from benign lesions, such as an inverted follicular keratosis, keratoacanthoma, pseudoepitheliomatous hyperplasis, and actinic keratosis, is not possible, owing to the lack of subcutaneous tissues. As such, the pathologic diagnosis of squamous cell carcinoma should be closely scrutinized following a shave biopsy and warrants further investigation.

Dermal nevi and papillomas have a tendency to occur on the lid margin. Overzealous excision of these tumors can result in lid margin irregularity or trichiasis. The use of the shave biopsy technique will effectively reduce alterations of the eyelid margin. The tumor is removed flush with the lid margin, with a chopping block technique or a sawing motion after the size 11 blade is placed in the center of the lesion. Care should be taken not to violate the eyelashes.

Incisional biopsy is indicated when additional deeper tissue is required to determine dermal extension of an epithelial tumor. This technique is useful for epithelial lesions, such as basal cell carcinoma, squamous cell carcinoma, keratoacanthoma, and acquired melanosis. A wedge from a suspected keratoacanthoma can demonstrate the overall configuration of the tumor, which is helpful in its pathologic evaluation. Areas of a superficial spreading melanotic lesion, which has become raised or indurated, can have a biopsy specimen taken to rule out malignant degeneration.

Figure 2–1. Excisional biopsy is effective for both diagnostic and therapeutic purposes. The tumor is incorporated into an ellipse, which is oriented parallel to normal tissue tension lines. An ellipse oriented perpendicular to these tension lines will amplify scar appearance. Care should be exercised when removing lower eyelid tumors, because excessive skin excision with a horizontally oriented ellipse may produce a postoperative ectropion. If a question exists about a horizontally oriented lower lid excisional biopsy, it should be rotated vertically to prevent the development of postoperative ectropion.

Full-thickness eyelid biopsies should be considered in patients with chronic blepharoconjunctivitis or recurrent chalazion suspected of having a sebaceous gland carcinoma.

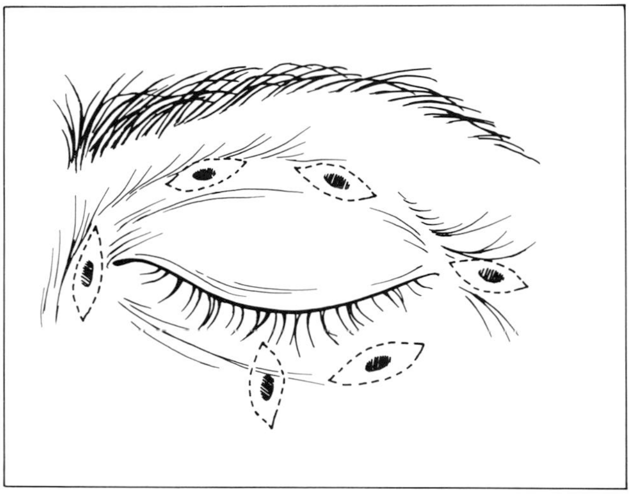

FIGURE 2–1

Figure 2–2. Putterman (1986) has described a method of conjunctival biopsy and mapping to determine the presence and extent of pagetoid spread of the epithelium associated with sebaceous gland carcinoma. This is necessary because pagetoid spread may involve areas of conjunctiva that appear normal. Upper and lower eyelids are everted over Desmarres retractors. Conjunctival biopsies are taken from the superior and inferior temporal, central, and nasal palpebral conjunctiva. The Desmarres retractors are partially released, and temporal, central, and nasal conjunctival specimens are obtained from the tarsal surfaces of the upper and lower eyelids. Additional specimens are obtained from the bulbar conjunctiva, from the superior, nasal, inferior, and temporal quadrants. As such, a total of 16 biopsy specimens are obtained from the conjunctiva.

CLOSURE OF SKIN DEFECTS

Figure 2–3A, B. As noted with excisional biopsies, elliptical skin defects are easiest to close, especially when oriented parallel to lines of relaxed skin tension lines (**A**), with the incision and placement designed to camouflage scar (**B**). The goal of primary skin closure is to oppose skin edges with a minimal amount of tension. If excess surface tension is evident with simple primary approximation of the wound edges, undermining of the skin muscle flaps is indicated. In addition, buried sutures uniting dermal tissue or orbicularis muscle will reduce skin tension. Also, over-tightening of sutures will result in poor wound healing. The surgical dictum for wound closure is to approximate, rather than strangulate tissue.

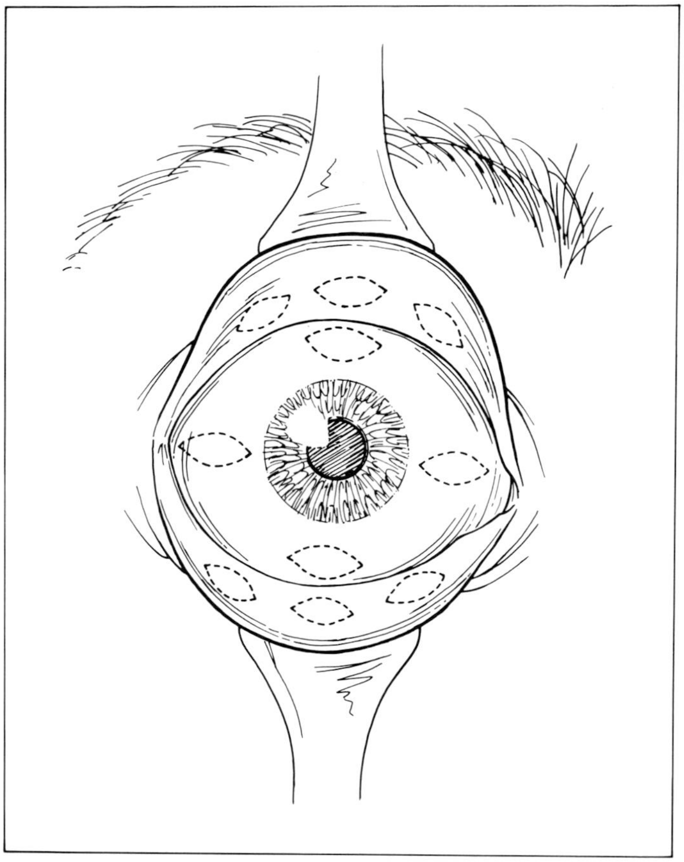

FIGURE 2–2

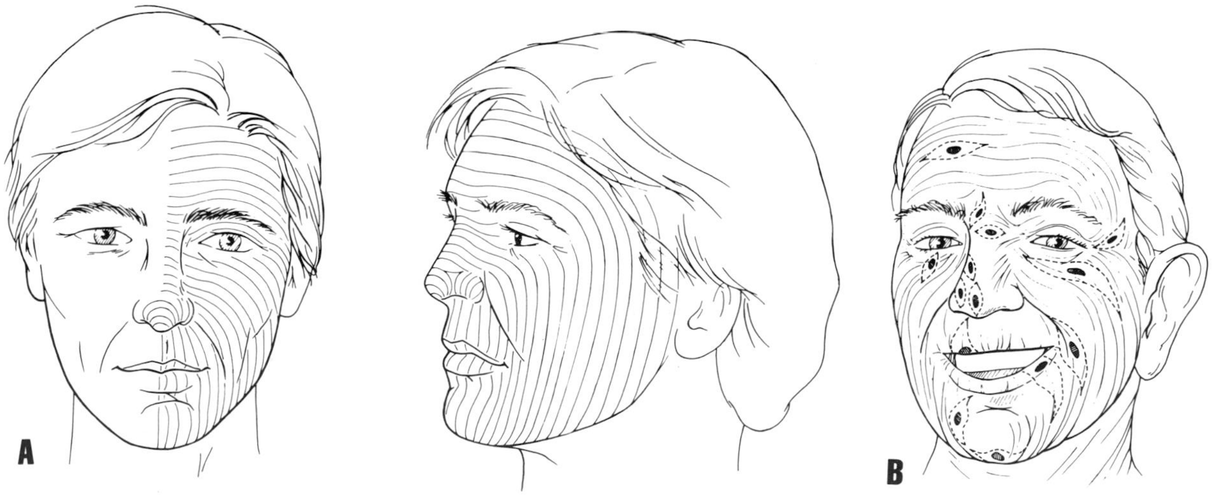

FIGURE 2–3

SCAR REVISION

Certain scars may result in functional problems or cosmetic blemishes that require revision. Techniques of scar revision include dermabrasion, scar excision with dermabrasion, redirection (Z-plasty), and scar excision with dermal platform techniques. It should be emphasized to the patient that scar revision does not eliminate scars, but merely replaces an objectionable scar with one that is less objectionable.

Dermabrasion remains a valuable method to reduce scarring. This is particularly effective with elevated, scarred areas that can be sculpted to produce a smoother surface. After infiltration of a local anesthetic containing epinephrine, a motorized burr is used to eliminate raised areas. Adjacent normal tissue should be abraided of its surface epithelium, so reepithelialization of the area will produce a uniform appearance.

If a scar develops parallel to normal skin tension lines, it can be excised down to the level of the deeper scarred dermis and then reapproximated. If the scar is at oblique angles to normal skin tension lines, redirection techniques are beneficial in camouflaging the scar. The Z-plasty is the most common redirection technique for scar revision. This method involves the transposition of triangular skin flaps to lengthen the tissue parallel to the scar and shorten the skin perpendicular to the scar. Orientation of the two transposition triangles is based on the original scar, which is marked. At each end of the original scar, equal-length marks are drawn at 60° angles to the scar to form a Z configuration (see Chapter 10). The two triangular flaps are adequately undermined, and all underlying bands of scar tissue are excised. If a lesser degree of lengthening is indicated, smaller angles of the end marks to the scar are made. If a long scar requires revision, multiple Z-plasties may be necessary.

GRAFTING

A variety of grafting techniques are essential in the management of eyelid disorders. It is useful to consider the eyelids as a two layered structure, consisting of an anterior and posterior lamella. The anterior lamella consists of the skin and orbicularis muscle; the posterior lamella consists of the tarsus and conjunctiva. Deficiencies of the anterior lamella will result in cicatricial ectropion or lid retraction and often require skin grafting for correction. Deficiencies of the posterior lamella may result from conjunctival shrinkage and may clinically produce cicatricial entropion. Tarsal grafting or mucous membrane grafting is effective in the management of these disorders. Full-thickness eyelid defects are approached by repair of both the anterior and posterior lamella.

Full-thickness skin grafts contain both epidermal and dermal elements. Donor sites include the upper eyelid; retroauricular, preauricular, supraclavicular areas; inner arm; and inner thigh. The donor site should be hairless, to prevent hair growth in the grafted area. Full-thickness grafts have a minimal degree of shrinkage and contracture in the postoperative period.

Once the amount of skin required is determined, a corresponding full-thickness graft is harvested. Because of minimal postoperative contracture, an oversized graft is not required. Care should be taken to excise as little subcutaneous tissue with the graft as possible. After the graft is obtained, additional subcutaneous tissue is removed by everting the graft over the forefinger and debulking the adherent subcutaneous tissue with scissors.

Once adequate hemostasis is obtained, the vascular integrity of the bed is assessed. If a skin graft is to be placed on bare tarsus or the orbital septum, the orbicularis muscle can be mobilized and advanced into the recipient bed to enhance the blood supply of the bed (Doxanas, 1986). The graft is sutured in place with interrupted sutures. Some sutures are tied with long ends to fixate a bolster over the graft. Before placing a Telfa dressing, buttonholes are created in the graft, to prevent the accumulation of blood or serous fluid under the graft. The bolster sutures are tied after the Telfa is covered with acrylon or cotton. The bolster is removed in 5 to 7 days.

Split-thickness grafts consist of epidermal elements only. These grafts are indicated to repair large defects or in instances where a poor vascular bed is anticipated. Split-thickness grafts are also beneficial in lining bone, such as an exenterated socket. Unfortunately, the split-thickness graft heals as a pale, contracted, immobile area and is rarely used in eyelid reconstruction.

Split-thickness grafts are harvested with a mechanical dermatome that shaves the graft from the donor site, most commonly anterior thigh. The standard thickness of split thickness skin grafts is 12/1000 to 18/1000 of an inch (300–450 μm). The thinner the split-thickness skin graft, the more contracture will occur postoperatively. After the graft is sutured into place, Telfa and a bolster dressing are then secured to maintain pressure over the grafted area.

The posterior lamella of the eyelid is reconstructed with free or pedicle (Hughes) tarsal grafts. The tarsal graft has been found to be an excellent donor tissue, resulting in little donor site morbidity (see Chapter 20).

Mucous membrane grafts are beneficial in the reconstruction of the posterior lamella of the eyelid. The oral mucosa is the most readily available source of mucous membrane. The mucous membrane is obtained in a fashion similar to a full-thickness skin graft. The inner surface of the lower lip is the most accessible tissue; however, additional grafts may be obtained from the upper lip or cheek. Care should be exercised to avoid the lips, gums, and Stensen's duct. Since shrinkage of tissue is likely to occur, a graft larger than the defect should be obtained. After injection with an epinephrine-containing anesthetic agent, sharp dissection is used to obtain the full-thickness graft. The graft is placed in an antibiotic solution after it is thinned of its connective tissue. The donor site should have a minimal degree of cauterization, since this enhances postoperative discomfort. Split-thickness mucous membrane grafts, although they may shrink slightly in the postoperative period, can also be used.

Chapter Three

EYELID LACERATION REPAIR

Dwight R. Kulwin
Robert C. Kersten

The first concern when dealing with a lacerated eyelid is to perform a complete eye examination to rule out associated intraocular trauma. Attention should also be paid to the levator function, especially for a transverse laceration of the upper lid. In lacerations of the medial canthal area, the puncta and canaliculi should be inspected for evidence of involvement (see later discussion). Inquiry must be made into the status of the patient's tetanus immunity, and appropriate tetanus prophylaxis should be given if necessary.

Because of the excellent blood supply of the eyelid and periocular tissues, the usual rules for handling wounds do not always apply. Lacerations may be closed well beyond the usual 6-hour "golden period" without risk of infection. Even apparently devitalized tissue need not be debrided, as it will usually survive if attempts are made to reapproximate it.

ANESTHESIA

Lid laceration repair may be carried out with either general anesthesia (for small children), nerve block, or subcutaneous infiltration with local anesthetics. The laceration should be irrigated before infiltration anesthesia. Following infiltration with anesthesia, wounds should be prepared with providone–iodine (Betadine) solution.

FULL-THICKNESS EYELID LACERATION

Tissue debridement is discouraged in eyelid lacerations because of the excellent blood supply that will usually allow preservation of apparently devitalized tissue. Lacerations of the tarsal plate itself are usually fairly linear, but, if extremely irregular, may be trimmed in a pentagonal fashion to allow closure with eversion of the lid margin. Up to one-third of the posterior lamella may be lost and primary closure will still be possible.

The key to satisfactory repair of a full-thickness lid laceration is precise reapproximation along the eyelid margin. Apposition of the tarsal plate is undertaken first. A Westcott scissors is used to separate a plane between the anterior lamella and the posterior lamella. The orbicularis is freed from the underlying tarsus for about 3 mm on either side of the laceration.

Figure 3–1. A 6–0 silk lid margin suture may be passed initially to help align the edges of the tarsus on each side of the defect. The tarsal plate is now apposed with three to four interrupted 7–0 Vicryl sutures on a spatula needle. These sutures are placed at the distal lid margin, the proximal tarsal border, and midway between these two points. The 7–0 Vicryl suture is passed as a lamellar bite of the tarsal plate, taking care to enter on the anterior surface, but not to pass full-thickness through the posterior surface. The anterior lamella is retracted with fine skin hooks to expose the tarsal plate, and the needle enters on the anterior surface approximately 2 to 3 mm from the laceration edge. The needle is passed through the laceration edge, taking care to stay at middepth in the tarsal plate. It is drawn out of the wound and then repassed through the lacerated edge of the opposite side at an identical lamellar depth and again exits the anterior surface of the tarsal plate 2 to 3 mm from the laceration edge.

Figure 3–2. After preplacing three to four lamellar tarsal sutures, the sutures are then clamped with a hemostat. These sutures need not be tied at this point.

Placement of the lid margin suture is performed next. This is perhaps the most important suture to place in preventing postoperative lid notching.

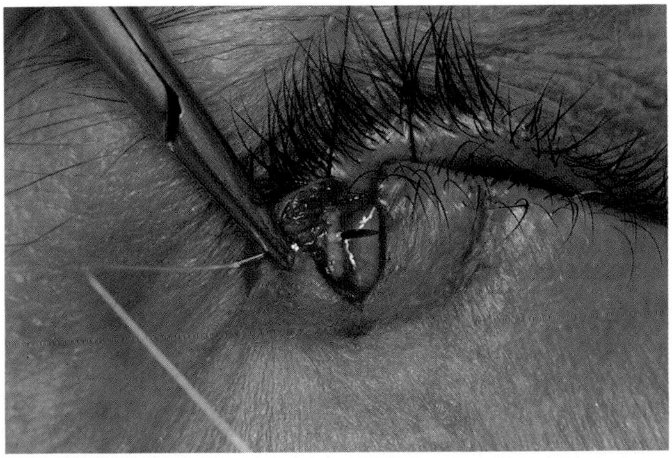

FIGURE 3–1

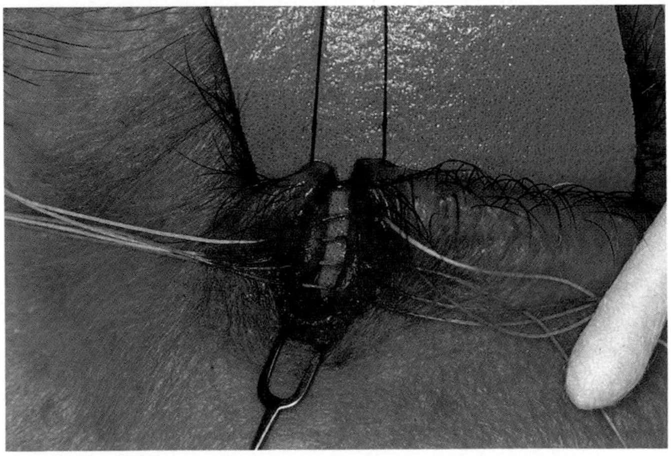

FIGURE 3–2

Figure 3–3. A 6–0 silk suture is passed in a vertical mattress fashion through the tarsal plate. The needle point is passed through a meibomian gland orifice, approximately 2 mm from the laceration edge, and exits from the cut edge of the tarsal plate, 3 to 4 mm from the margin. The needle is then inserted at a similar point 3 to 4 mm from the margin on the opposing lacerated tarsal edge, emerging through a meibomian gland orifice 2 mm from the cut edge. The needle is then passed back through the lid margin in a "near-to-near" fashion, taking care to again enter through the meibomian gland orifice, but now passing about 1 mm from the lacerated edge. The needle should again exit the lid margin and enter the opposing lid margin at similar levels (see Figure 3–2). This suture is not tied, but left long until the previously placed Vicryl sutures on the tarsal plate are tied. The lamellar tarsal sutures are then tied, drawing the tarsal edges into firm apposition. The suture ends are cut on the knots. The 6–0 vertical mattress silk suture is tied at the lid margin. These sutures are left long. A second 6–0 silk suture is passed in an interrupted fashion through the lash follicles, entering and exiting 2 mm from the lacerated edge. The long ends of the lid margin suture are then draped over and tied into the lash follicle suture. Once the long ends of the suture have been tied within the lash follicle stitch, the ends of the lash follicle stitch may be cut short.

Figure 3–4. Skin and orbicularis are closed with a single layer of 6–0 nylon sutures. The long end of the 6–0 silk lid margin suture is incorporated in the first two skin sutures to prevent the ends from turning back in and abrading the cornea. At the end of lid margin closure, a slight eversion of the wound margin is desirable as scar contraction will flatten the lid margin with time.

Antibiotic ointment is instilled and a patch may be applied. The skin sutures are removed after 1 week, and the lid margin suture is removed at 2 weeks.

CANALICULUS LACERATION

Any laceration in the medial portion of the upper or lower eyelid should be presumed to involve the lacrimal canaliculi, until proved otherwise. Because the dense fibrous tissue of the tarsal plate is significantly stronger than the medial canthal tendon, an avulsing force placed anywhere along the lid margin will preferentially tear the medial soft tissue, causing disruption of the lacrimal canaliculus. Because the canaliculus adjacent to the punctum is very superficial in the lid, even minor lacerations in this area must be carefully examined for canalicular involvement. It is not uncommon for a medial laceration that appears to involve only one eyelid to extend through the opposing cana-

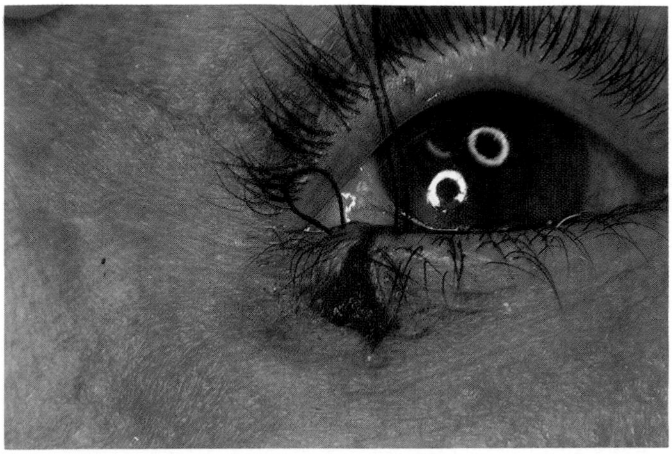

FIGURE 3–3

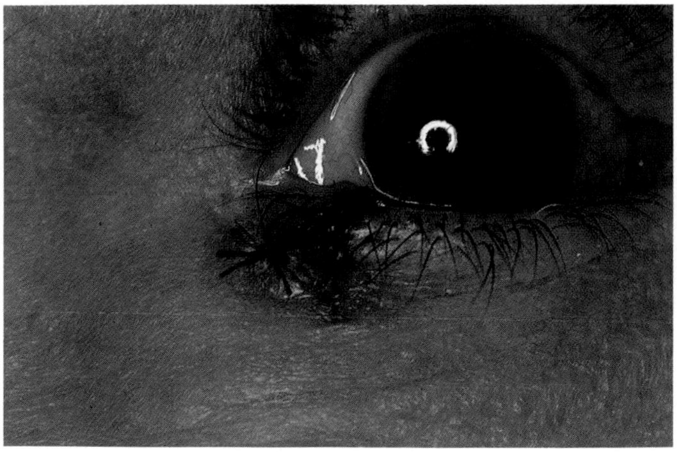

FIGURE 3–4

liculus as well. These injuries can be particularly easy to overlook, and if the opportunity for early repair is lost, more difficult, and less successful procedures will be required to relieve epiphora. Although it is true that patients may be largely asymptomatic with a single intact canaliculus, those patients cannot always be accurately identified initially. Therefore, all canalicular lacerations should be repaired.

The key to satisfactory repair of a canalicular laceration is the identification of the proximal (medial) cut end of the canaliculus. The lacerated canaliculus is bridged with a temporary silicone stent that is passed through both the superior and inferior canaliculus; down through the nasolacrimal duct into the nose; and tied to form a continuous loop.

General anesthesia is preferred. It prevents patient discomfort during manipulation to the nasolacrimal system and nose. In addition, it obviates the need for injection with local anesthetic, which may distort the tissues and obscure the proximal cut end of the canaliculus.

We prefer to use a Catalano silicone stent to bridge the laceration. This has a malleable metal tip, which minimizes damage to the canaliculi, reduces the chance of false passage through the nasal lacrimal duct, and is less traumatic to the nasal mucosa during retrieval from the nose. With good exposure, a dry operative field, and magnification of an operating microscope, it is almost always possible for the surgeon to locate the proximal cut end of the canaliculus. It may be helpful to pass the Catalano stent through the punctum and distal cut edge of the laceration so that one may use the course of the stent tip to anticipate the location of the proximal cut end. If the proximal cut end can still not be identified after meticulous examination, it may be helpful to slowly inject hyaluronate sodium (Healon), which has been stained with fluorescein, through the opposing intact canaliculus. This will allow a small bubble of the fluorescein-tinged hyaluronate to present at the proximal cut end. Irrigation with aqueous solution, such as sterile milk or fluorescein, is usually of little benefit. Once the proximal cut end has been identified, the Catalano stent, which has previously been passed through the punctum and distal segment of the canaliculus, is introduced through the proximal cut end under microscopic control. It is advanced through the internal common punctum to abut the medial wall of the lacrimal sac. While maintaining pressure against the lacrimal fossa, the stent is then rotated superiorly and directed down through the nasolacrimal duct to exit into the inferior meatus beneath the inferior turbinate. (For a detailed description of the silicone intubation technique, see Chapter 6.) The opposite end of the Catalano stent is passed through the intact canaliculus in the same fashion.

Once the laceration has been bridged with the silicone stent, attention is directed toward closure of the canalicular epithelium and reformation of the lacerated medial canthal tendon structures. Although much emphasis is placed upon the importance of microscopic reanastomosis of the canaliculus, it is of greater importance to exactly reapproximate the medial canthal tendon structures, such that the punctum is returned to its normal position in contact with the lacrimal lake. This is particularly important when one is dealing with the deeper, more medial laceration in which the severed ends of the canaliculus are oftentimes significantly distracted. Consequently, reanastomosis of the canaliculus differs between the more distal, less distracted lacerations, and in the more proximal, greatly distracted lacerations. In distal lacerations that lie close to the punctum, in which the medial canthal tendon structures are still intact, closure of the canaliculus is carried out around the silicone stent using three interrupted 8–0 Prolene (isotactic polypropylene) sutures. These are passed in an interrupted fashion superiorly, anteriorly, and inferiorly around the canaliculus to reanastomose the cut epithelial ends, under microscopic control. Once the canalicular ends have been reunited, closure of the overlying skin and orbicularis can be carried out with interrupted sutures. In more proximal, deeper lacerations, it is frequently difficult to identify the epithelium of the lacerated canaliculus, as it is oftentimes obscured by its "deep in a hole" position. In this circumstance, reapproximation of the soft tissues overlying the canaliculus is of greater importance, since by bringing these tissues into approximation, one will necessarily bring the canalicular ends together around the indwelling silicone stent. This ensures that compression of the overlying tissues will result in approximation of the canalicular epithelium. For repair of the medial canthal tendon, we use a double-armed 5–0 Vicryl suture. This is passed in a horizontal mattress fashion using microscopic control. An initial horizontal bite of orbicularis and soft tissue immediately anterior to the distal cut end of the canaliculus is taken. Then, using the microscope to identify the proximal lumen (now intubated with the silicone stent), the horizontal mattress suture is completed at a similar depth. Once this is drawn up and found to properly reapproximate, one may then leave this suture untied while the 8–0 Prolene sutures are passed through the canalicular epithelium. Once the Prolene sutures have been passed, it is necessary to tie the 5–0 Vicryl suture first to bring the tissues close together so that the 8–0 Prolene sutures can be tied without "cheese wiring" through the canalicular epithelium. This can be quite cumbersome, as there can then be six free suture ends projecting through the wound after the Vicryl suture has been tied. It is helpful to use bulldog clamps to keep each of the three pairs of 8–0 Prolene suture identified. Some very medial and deep lacerations cannot be adequately reapproximated with the horizontal mattress 5–0 Vicryl suture. In these cases, the double-armed 5–0 Vicryl suture can be passed through the soft tissues overlying the distal cut end, as previously described. However, to properly reapproximate to the medial cut end, it may be preferable to pass each arm of the double-armed suture separately, entering the orbicularis and soft tissue adjacent to the cut edge of the canaliculus and then passing superficially up to exit through the skin surface. If both arms are passed in this fashion (one superior to and the other inferior to the cut end of the canaliculus) the two ends can be tied together with the knot on the surface of the skin. It is no problem to leave the Vicryl suture exposed for 2 weeks time. Once sufficient wound strength has developed to unite the medial canthal tissues, the suture can be cut flush with the skin. After reapproximating the canaliculus and the medial canthal tendon structures, the skin can be closed with interrupted fine sutures.

At the completion of the procedure, the ends of the Catalano stent are tied to one another in the inferior meatus. First, pass the two ends of the Catalano stent through a small block of silicone so that traction to the stent in the medial canthal region will not pull the knot through the inferior meatus and lodge in the nasolacrimal duct or sac. We use a 7- to 8-mm section of a No. 20 scleral buckle. A 20-gauge needle can be used to poke two holes in the silicone, through which the stent ends pass, before being tied to one another. The silicone stent is usually left in place a minimum of 6 weeks. With a more proximal, deeper, laceration, we prefer to leave them in place for 6 months.

TRAUMATIC PTOSIS

A transverse laceration in the upper lid may completely sever the levator aponeurosis and Mueller's muscle from their attachment to the tarsal plate. In these cases, there is usually a profound ptosis, with minimal levator function. Over time, the upper lid retractors may scar down and retract to result in some improvement of ptosis. When the laceration defect is incomplete, ptosis with retention of lid excursion may result. Ideally, one should do the following procedure under local anesthesia so that the levator function can be assessed intraoperatively.

In all cases of transverse upper lid laceration with acute ptosis, inspection should be carried out through the wound under local anesthesia. In most patients, the septum usually has also been violated; if not, it should be opened and orbital fat allowed to prolapse forward. Proper identification of orbital fat is essential, as it is the key anatomic landmark to the underlying traumatized levator aponeurosis. If fat does not spontaneously prolapse, slight posterior pressure on the globe may force it forward into view.

Fat is retracted superiorly and the underlying aponeurosis is identified. This is seen as a white, translucent sheet beneath the orbital fat. If surgery is being performed under local anesthesia (preferable in all adults), then asking the patient to look up and down will confirm identification of the aponeurosis by its corresponding movement.

The aponeurosis is reapproximated to its distal cut edge or to the tarsal plate, with interrupted 5–0 Vicryl sutures, passed in a horizontal mattress fashion. Lacerated skin edges are reapposed with 7–0 nylon sutures. No attempt is made to close the orbital septum, since it scars down nicely if left undisturbed, whereas closure may induce lid retraction and lagophthalmos.

Chapter Four

ORBITAL BLOWOUT FRACTURES

Robert C. Kersten
Dwight R. Kulwin

DEFINITION

The term *blowout fracture of the orbit* refers to a fracture of an orbital wall, typically the orbital floor or medial wall, or both, with an intact bony orbital rim. This was felt to be caused by an isolated blow to the eye, displacing it posteriorly, and thereby, hydraulically increasing orbital pressure to the thin bony orbital walls, rupturing them outward. Recent evidence has suggested that this fracture may also result from a blow directed to the orbital rims, causing them to bend without fracturing, resulting in buckling of the thinner bone of the orbital walls.

These fractures may occur after any blunt frontal trauma to the globe or orbital rims and may occur even in the absence of sufficient force to cause a "black eye."

DIAGNOSIS

Signs and symptoms suggestive of an orbital blowout fracture should be sought in all patients who have sustained blunt periorbital trauma. These include eyelid ecchymosis, limitation of extraocular muscle excursion, subcutaneous emphysema, and enophthalmos or hypo-ophthalmos. A pathognomonic sign of an orbital floor fracture is the finding of hypesthesia of the ipsilateral cheek, upper teeth, or tip of the nose. This occurs because the fracture usually extends through the infraorbital groove and canal along the floor of the orbit, injuring the infraorbital neurovascular bundle.

Radiographs may show disruption of the orbital floor and opacification of the maxillary sinus. However, some fractures will not be evident on plain films, and if one's index of suspicion is high, coronal and sagittal computed tomography (CT) scans are indicated to definitively examine the orbital walls.

INITIAL MANAGEMENT

At the time of the initial consultation, a thorough ocular examination should be performed. Significant ocular injuries have been reported to occur in 10% to 30% of patients. Any limitation of extraocular excursion should be quantitated and, if the degree of swelling allows, forced duction testing should be performed to distinguish restrictive from paretic motility dysfunction. Exophthalmometry should also be performed.

The patient is instructed to refrain from taking any anticoagulants and advised not to blow the nose. If there are no contraindications, oral prednisone, 1 mg/kg daily may be given for 1 week. Prednisone reduces long-term motility dysfunction as well as more rapidly delineates those patients who will require surgery. Fractures involving the medial wall have a greater incidence of orbital cellulitis, and some authors have recommended broad-spectrum antibiotic prophylaxis for 5 days in this subgroup.

SURGICAL INDICATIONS

Fewer than 50% of patients with orbital wall fractures will require surgical intervention. Orbital blowout fractures likely to require treatment fall into two categories: small fractures, which are more likely to result in tissue entrapment and motility dysfunction; and large fractures, which are more likely to cause ocular displacement owing to a substantial increase in bony orbital volume. One should observe the patient every few days during the first 2 weeks after the injury, looking for change in extraocular motility dysfunction and forced duction testing as well as to assess any early enophthalmos.

Surgery is indicated in those patients with persistent entrapment, as evidenced by restrictive motility and positive forced duction; significant enophthalmos; and significantly displaced fracture in which eventual enophthalmos seems likely to occur.

One should obtain direct coronal and sagittal orbital CT scans of all patients before surgery. This scanning will demonstrate significant displacement of the orbital walls (greater than 5-mm displacement or more than 50% of an orbital wall) and may also demonstrate extraocular muscle entrapment within the fracture site.

TIMING OF SURGERY

Surgery is best performed between 10 and 20 days following injury. Before this time, it is not possible to reliably separate those patients requiring surgery from those who will spontaneously improve. Beyond 20 days, scar formation makes dissection more difficult. One should attempt to operate on all patients who have a mechanical restriction of gaze within this period.

If a patient has normal motility and a "borderline" large fracture, the patient should be reexamined frequently. If enophthalmos develops, surgical intervention can be performed at that time.

GOALS AND PRINCIPLES OF SURGERY

Orbital blowout fracture repair is performed on those patients with persistent tissue entrapment, resulting in a mechanical restriction of ocular movement, enophthalmos, or a large fracture. The goal is to elevate orbital contents out of the fracture site and then to resurface the orbital floor with either an alloplastic implant or an autogenous graft.

Patient Preparation

General anesthesia is used. A broad-spectrum antibiotic and 12 mg of dexamethasone are given intravenously at the start of the procedure. Before the surgical scrub, local anesthetic with epinephrine is infiltrated across the width of the lid, so that 10 to 15 minutes will have elapsed before the incision is made, allowing maximal vasoconstriction. A full-face preparation is performed. When draping the patient, both eyes should be left exposed so that forced ductions can be made and compared intraoperatively.

Selection of Approach

Figure 4–1. Several different approaches can be used to access the orbital floor. One can perform either an anterior approach through a lower lid crease incision or a posterior approach through the conjunctiva, in conjunction with a lateral canthotomy and inferior cantholysis. Either approach allows entry into the plane between orbital septum and orbicularis muscle. Dissection is then performed within this plane, down to the infraorbital rim.

The percutaneous approach is a simpler procedure without the need to disrupt the lateral canthus. The disadvantages are that it leaves a facial scar (although usually almost imperceptible) and, especially in younger patients, it may cause contracture of the skin–muscle flap postoperatively, resulting in lower lid retraction. The advantages of the conjunctival approach are the lack of a visible scar and reduced risk of lid retraction. The disadvantages are that disinsertion of the lateral canthal tendon is required and medial exposure is more limited. More extensive canthotomy and incision of orbicularis muscle laterally are required to fully expose medial wall fractures.

Lid Crease Approach

The lower lid crease is marked across the width of the lid, and forced ductions of each eye are performed and compared, to establish a baseline. An incision of the lower lid crease is made with a size 15 Bard–Parker blade or straight iris scissors. This begins medially at the punctum and extends laterally to a point at or just beyond the lateral canthus. A bipolar cautery is preferred for maintenance of hemostasis in blowout fracture repair and other orbital surgery, as a unipolar cautery may be preferentially conducted along orbital nerves. After the skin is incised, scissors are used to snip full-thickness through the orbicularis muscle to expose the postorbicular fascia. This is a thin layer of connective tissue on the surface of the tarsus and septum. Dissection is then carried inferiorly between the orbicularis muscle and the orbital septum. Scissors are quite helpful in separating the orbicularis fibers from the underlying orbital septum, and Guthrie skin hooks are used to place anterior traction on the skin–muscle flap to keep the plane of dissection well defined. Dissection is carried down to the infraorbital rim in this fashion.

Transconjunctival Approach

Figure 4–2. At the start of the procedure, a lateral canthotomy is carried out, with a scissors directed horizontally, extending 3 to 5 mm in length. The scissors are then rotated 90° inferiorly, and insinuated between skin and conjunctiva, cutting all the tissues of the lateral retinaculum in between. Several snips are required to cut through the lateral canthal tendon and the overlying orbicularis muscle until the lateral edge of the lid can be completely distracted from the orbital rim.

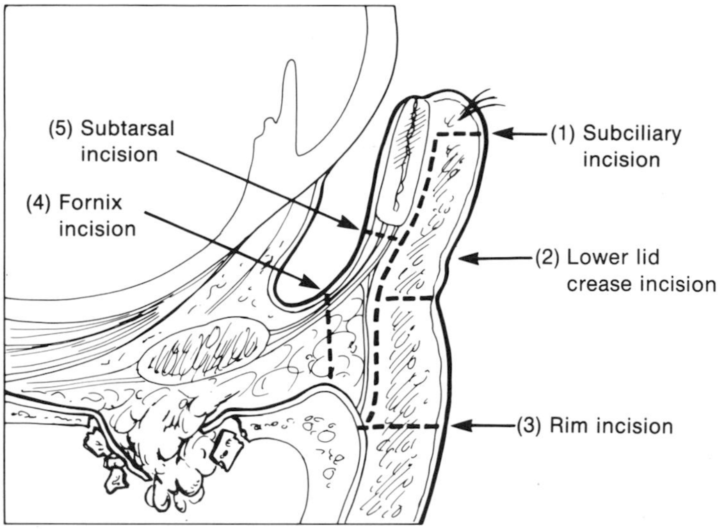

FIGURE 4–1

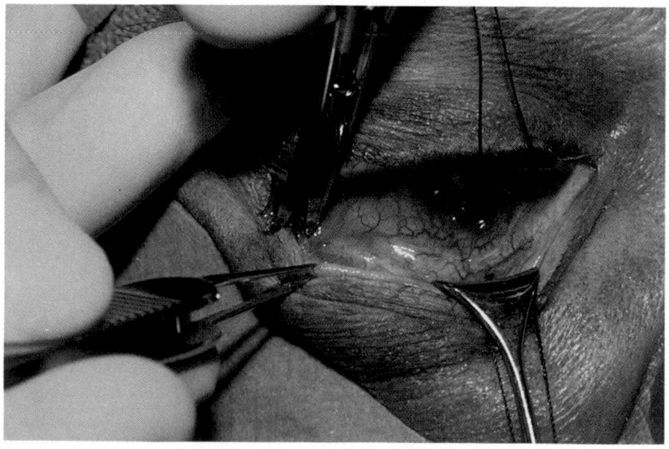

FIGURE 4–2

Figure 4–3. The lid margin is then grasped by the assistant and retracted, while scissors are used to separate the fused edge of conjunctiva and retractors from the inferior margin of tarsal plate. This incision is begun at the lateral canthotomy and carried medially to the punctum.

Figure 4–4. A silk suture is passed through the cut edge of conjunctiva and retractors, drawn superiorly, and clamped to the drapes. This maneuver facilitates the plane of dissection between conjunctiva and retractors posteriorly and orbicularis anteriorly, and also affords protection of the cornea.

Exposure of Infraorbital Rim

The plane of dissection is the same whether the percutaneous or transconjunctival approach is used. The only difference is that the plane is entered from the posterior surface if the transconjunctival approach is used. Scissors are used to dissect inferiorly between the orbicularis muscle anteriorly and the septum posteriorly, down to the level of the infraorbital rim. During dissection, it is important to maintain traction on the lid margin to prevent folding of the skin and orbicularis. Otherwise, the plane of dissection may be obscured, which can result in full-thickness "buttonholing" through the anterior lamella. Bipolar cautery is helpful to maintain hemostasis, but is generally unnecessary if dissection is maintained in this avascular plane between septum and orbicularis. Dissection performed within this plane also keeps the septum intact and prevents orbital fat from prolapsing into the field.

Dissection down to the infraorbital rim is aided by frequent finger palpation to keep the position of the rim clearly in mind. Once the dissection has reached the rim, a Desmarres retractor can be used to retract the skin–muscle flap inferiorly. Soft tissue overlying the rim can be bluntly dissected with Stevens scissors until the periosteum is exposed.

Figure 4–5. While using a finger to palpate the rim, the periosteum is then incised with a scalpel blade. Incision is begun medially at the level of the punctum and carried across the rim, ending just below the lateral orbital tubercle. The incision is placed just below the rim on the anterior face of the maxilla, but care must be taken to avoid straying too inferiorly with the knife blade, damaging the infraorbital nerve. The posterior edge of the periorbita is elevated across the width of the rim with a periosteal elevator (Joseph or Freer), and a suture may be placed through the free edge of the periorbita to allow later identification.

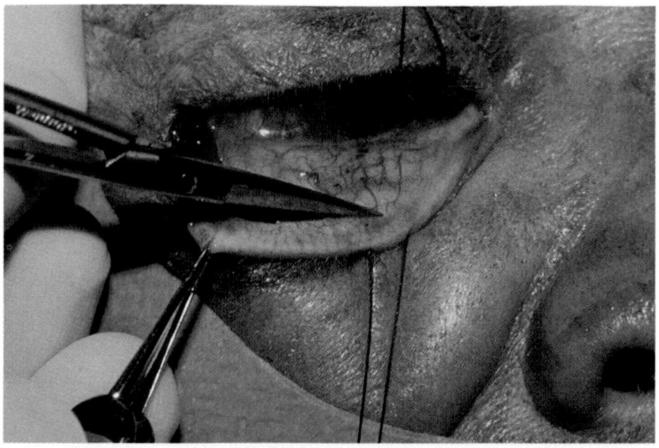

FIGURE 4–3

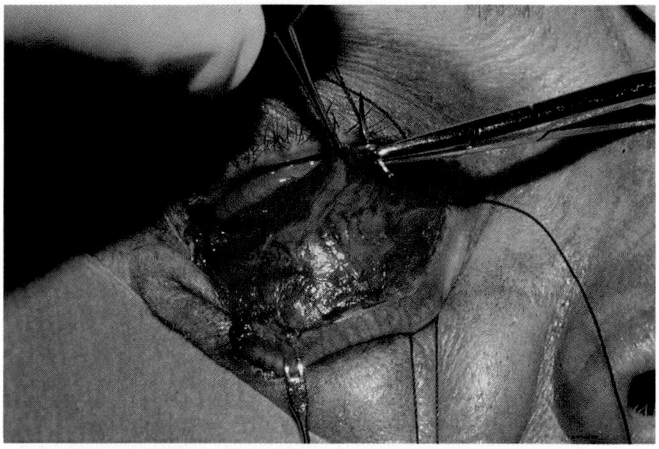

FIGURE 4–4

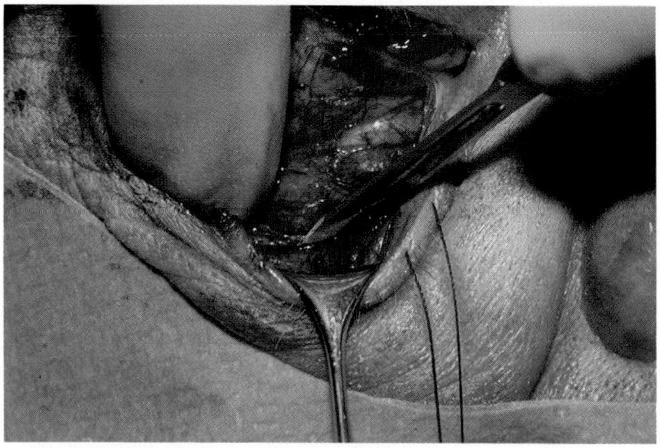

FIGURE 4–5

Exploring the Floor

Once the periorbita has been elevated across the width of the rim, the blunt edge of a Freer periosteal elevator is used to gently elevate the periorbita posteriorly along the floor. Periorbita over the floor is easily elevated, except where it is entrapped by the fracture. The orbital fracture will usually be encountered 5- to 10-mm behind the rim, just medial to the infraorbital neurovascular bundle. The fracture is usually occluded by orbital soft tissue prolapsing through the lacerated periorbita. Before attempting to directly elevate the orbital contents out of the fracture, dissection is carried medially and laterally around the fracture. Elevation of the orbital contents is necessary to allow visualization and can be achieved with malleable retractors or right-angle (Sewell) orbital retractors. One should try to identify intact bone behind the fracture, but this may be difficult because the visualization is obscured by prolapsing tissues. Care must be taken to relax retraction of orbital contents every few minutes to prevent ischemia of the orbital tissue or globe.

Reduction of Prolapsed Tissues

The most tedious and difficult portion of the procedure involves the elevation and disimpaction of periorbital tissues from the fracture site. The periosteal elevator is insinuated between the orbital tissue and fracture and used to pry the soft tissue from the fracture site. Two orbital retractors are helpful in lifting the prolapsed tissues in a "hand-over-hand" fashion. This is usually a frustrating and repetitive procedure, as orbital contents tend to continually spill-around the retractors and back into the fracture. If the tissues are tightly impacted in the fracture, it may be helpful to enlarge the fracture with Kerrison rongeurs to facilitate release of the tissues. In more adherent cases, or in older fractures, it may be necessary to grasp prolapsed orbital fat and fibrous tissue with a hemostat to apply traction superiorly.

Figure 4–6. There are three tissue layers that must be distinguished during the disincarceration of prolapsed orbital tissues: (1) orbital contents, superiorly; (2) maxillary sinus mucosa, inferiorly; and (3) sandwiched between these two, the infraorbital neurovascular bundle. In long-standing fractures, it can be very difficult to identify the infraorbital nerve, as the sinus mucosa and orbital contents may be adherent to it. Cautious sharp dissection with Westcott scissors may, on occasion, be necessary to free the nerve from adjacent scar tissue.

Identification of the infraorbital foramen, on the face of the maxilla beneath the rim, will locate the anterior extent of the nerve. Its course along the floor can then be extrapolated as it runs posteriorly and medially to join the infraorbital fissure. The infraorbital canal may be seen as a ridge on the anterior orbital floor, perpendicular to the rim.

The goal during this stage of surgery is to completely separate the orbital contents from the underlying infraorbital nerve and sinus mucosa. Although it is preferable to keep the sinus mucosa intact, it may have been lacerated by the displaced bony fragments during the initial trauma, and maneuvers to reposition orbital contents may further enlarge these rents. It is important, however, not to incarcerate any sinus mucosa within the orbit because an epithelial-lined cyst may develop.

The end point in this stage is to free all adhesions between orbital tissue and the fracture and to completely elevate the orbital contents above the plane of the fracture. This can be confirmed by direct observation of the entire floor defect and by forced duction testing, comparing with the contralateral side. Once this is achieved, attention is directed toward resurfacing the orbital floor to cover the fracture and to maintain support of the orbital contents.

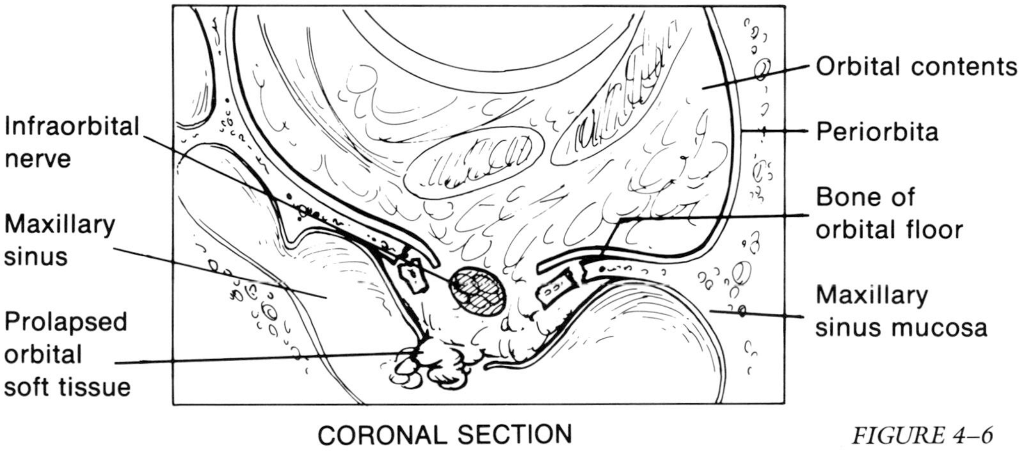

FIGURE 4–6

Choice of Floor Implant

Orbital implants can be either alloplastic (Teflon, Supramid, silicone sheet) or autogenous (split cranial bone, iliac crest bone, or temporalis fascia). The harvesting of autogenous bone or fascia grafts involves an additional operative site, additional morbidity, and usually offers very little advantage over alloplastic materials. One exception is the presence of a total floor defect in which there is no bony buttress at the periphery of the fracture to support the implant. In this situation, split calvarial bone grafts may be used and are fixated anteriorly to the infraorbital rim with miniplates. This has provided good restoration of orbital volume and floor support.

However, almost all fractures can be managed with alloplastic implants. Teflon implants, which come in three preformed sizes, for the left or right orbit may be selected. These contour nicely to the orbital floor, engender minimal fibrosis, and have an extremely low infection or extrusion rate. Although preformed, the implants often need to be trimmed with large scissors to match contour with the orbital floor.

Placement of Floor Implant

The implant is slid beneath the retracted orbital contents to cover the floor defect. The implant must be seated behind the orbital rim, without impinging posteriorly on the infraorbital fissure. It may be necessary to trim the posterior extent of the implant, while leaving its medial and lateral extensions intact. Once the implant has been seated and is resting in the concavity just posterior to the infraorbital rim, forced ductions are again repeated. If there is residual restriction, the implant must be closely inspected around its entire periphery. It must be ascertained whether it completely covers the fracture and whether tissue is trapped between the fracture and the implant.

Fixation of Implant

Some surgeons prefer to fixate the implant to the infraorbital rim by wiring, by titanium miniplate fixation, or with cyanoacrylate (Super Glue). Occasionally, this may be appropriate for very large fractures in which there is inadequate floor support. However, for the vast majority of orbital floor fractures, no implant fixation is necessary. To achieve implant stability, be sure the implant is large enough to completely cover the defect so that the contents will not prolapse down into the maxillary sinus, and yet, be certain the implant is small enough so there is no tendency for displacement forward. If the implant is properly sized, the infraorbital rim has a natural lip that will prevent forward migration.

Figure 4–7A. After the implant has been properly sized and placed along the floor, and if forced duction are satisfactory, the periorbita is sutured to the periosteum along the infraorbital rim with several interrupted 5–0 Vicryl sutures. Suturing of these tissues can be difficult because the periosteum may be friable. If the implant is properly sized, periosteal closure is probably not essential; however, it should be attempted.

Figure 4–7B. If it is impossible to suture the periosteum over the face of the maxilla, then the suture can be passed through the orbicularis muscle directly overlying the periosteal edge. This will reposition the periorbita so that it will scar into satisfactory position. After periorbital closure, forced ductions are again performed. If they show residual restriction, the periosteal suture should be released and the floor implant inspected again to ensure that it has not shifted position.

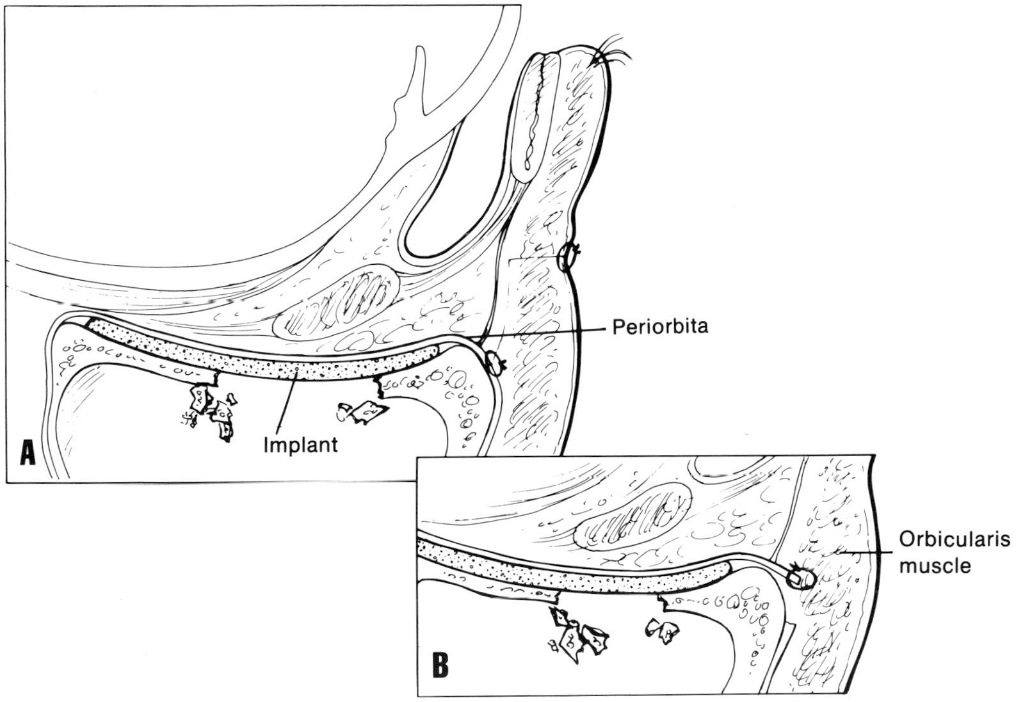

FIGURE 4–7

Incision Closure

Closure of the infraciliary or transconjunctival incision is then carried out. If a percutaneous approach has been used, the skin–muscle flap is merely draped over the septum, and the cut edges placed into apposition. The skin is closed with 6–0 nylon suture. A layered closure is not desirable, as it will tend to shorten the orbicularis layer and result in postoperative lower lid retraction. If interrupted sutures are used, only three or four sutures are required.

If a transconjunctival approach is used, conjunctiva and retractors are sewn to the inferior border of the tarsus using a running 6–0 chromic suture. This is begun medially. It is not necessary to bury the knot beneath the punctum, for this is sufficiently medial to the cornea that it is not irritating. No attempt is made to close the retractors separately because they are intimately contiguous with conjunctiva and will be brought into satisfactory position by the conjunctival closure.

Figure 4–8. An additional step is required in the transconjunctival approach to reapproximate the lateral canthal tendon to the tarsus. This is done with the remnant of 5–0 Vicryl suture from the periosteal closure. A horizontal mattress suture is passed first from inferior to superior through the cut edge of the inferior crus of the lateral canthal tendon at the medial margin of the cantholysis. This is then carried through the superior crus of the lateral canthal tendon, entering just inside the canthotomy. The suture exits the superior crus adjacent to the orbital rim and is passed through the orbital cut edge of the inferior crus. The sutures are then tied. It is not necessary to reattach the tendon directly to periosteum, unless the patient has significant lowered lid laxity. In that event, reattachment in a fashion identical with that of a lateral tarsal strip can be performed (see Chapter 10). The canthotomy is then closed with one or two interrupted 6–0 chromic sutures.

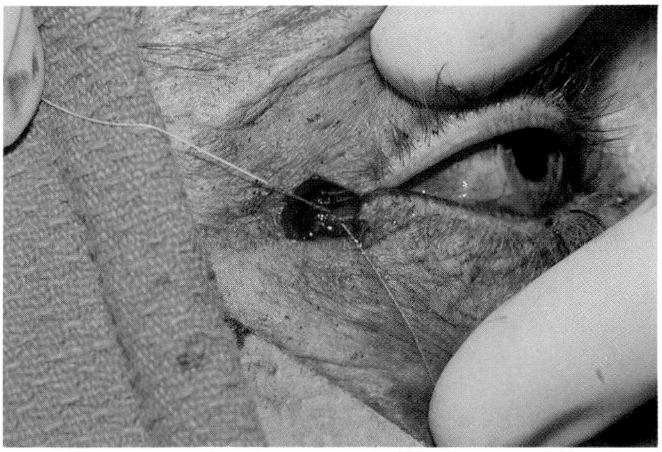

FIGURE 4–8

POSTOPERATIVE MANAGEMENT

All patients are hospitalized following surgery to allow frequent vision and motility examinations in the first 24 hours after surgery. This also allows intravenous antibiotics and steroids to be continued. The patient's head is kept elevated at 45° to 60°. Ice packs are applied to the orbit intermittently for the first 48 hours.

Visual acuity and pupillary checks are carried out by the nursing staff every 2 hours to allow early detection of orbital hemorrhage.

The patient is instructed to refrain from blowing his nose for 2 weeks postoperatively. Oral antibiotics are continued for 3 to 5 days postoperatively. Topical antibiotic ointment is applied at the end of the procedure and may be repeated postoperatively as desired by the surgeon.

The patient is counseled preoperatively that diplopia may actually be worse in the immediate postoperative period because of swelling and manipulation of the orbital contents. Motility usually improves within the first 7 to 10 days after surgery. However, large series have shown that up to 20% of patients may still have significant residual diplopia. This is probably related to fibrosis of the inferior rectus muscle caused by the initial trauma. If this fails to resolve within 3 months, vertical extraocular muscle surgery may be required.

Infraorbital hypesthesia may also be exacerbated immediately postoperatively, especially if surgery is performed on "old" fractures in which significant adhesions to the infraorbital nerve existed. Sensation almost invariably returns, but may take several months.

Some degree of enophthalmos may persist once the postoperative swelling resolves. This is more likely if combined floor and medial wall fractures were present. Nonetheless, the medial wall component of the fracture is usually not addressed, unless marked prolapse of soft tissues or entrapment is present. In extensive cases with enophthalmos, one may consider bone grafting the medial defect through an external frontoethmoidal incision or bicoronal flap exposure.

Chapter Five

PUNCTOPLASTY

Steven M. Gilberg, William McLeish, and David T. Tse

Acquired epiphora is a common complaint that requires a logical clinical and anatomic approach to both its understanding and management. Tearing is due to either excessive tear production or inadequate tear drainage. The surgeon must determine which of these two situations exists before intervention can be initiated.

OVERPRODUCTION

Excessive tear secretion leads to epiphora by overwhelming a normal lacrimal drainage system. The most common causes of increased tear production include environmental irritants, allergens, central nervous system or emotional disturbances, cholinergic agents, ocular inflammatory disorders, and frequently paradoxic tear hypersecretion related to aqueous tear deficiency. Identification and elimination of these factors may lead to resolution of the patient's epiphora.

LACRIMAL DRAINAGE SYSTEM OBSTRUCTION

Once tear overproduction has been eliminated as a causative factor, the surgeon is effectively left with diagnosing and managing an anatomic disorder causing a relative or absolute outflow obstruction. The evaluation of the lacrimal drainage system begins with the external and slit-lamp examinations seeking to answer the following questions: Is the patient's blink adequate? Are the puncta positioned properly? Are the puncta open or closed? Is the lacrimal sac palpable or can material be expressed from the puncta with digital pressure over the sac? In answering these questions, one can begin to determine whether the obstruction lies in the upper or lower lacrimal system.

Upper Lacrimal System Obstruction

The lacrimal pump mechanism relies on the frequent contracture of the pretarsal and preseptal orbicularis muscle during blinking for proper functioning. Patients with generalized facial akinesia, such as Parkinson's disease or progressive supranuclear palsy, may manifest epiphora on the basis of an ineffective lacrimal pump. In seventh nerve palsies, paralytic lower lid ectropion, along with poor orbicularis tone, contributes to the symptom of epiphora.

Normal lid contour, with proper anatomic positioning of the punctae within the tear meniscus, is required for adequate tear drainage. Displacement of the punctum from its normal position is most frequently the result of lower eyelid ectropion. Evaluation and appropriate surgical correction of eyelid malpositions should be completed before undertaking any lacrimal drainage system repair. When punctal stenosis is a secondary phenomenon, caused by chronic punctal eversion, simple correction of the underlying eyelid malposition along with punctal dilation may be sufficient to reestablish drainage.

In addition to external and slit-lamp examinations, the likely site of obstruction within the lacrimal drainage system can be identified by the following series of functional tests.

Fluorescein Dye Disappearance Test

The fluorescein dye disappearance test is a rapid, semiquantitative screening method for the presence of lacrimal drainage system obstruction. The test is best performed by simultaneously instilling a single drop of concentrated 2% fluorescein solution into each inferior fornix. Five minutes after instillation, the degree of fluorescein clearance is grossly quantified. Observing the patient at a distance with the cobalt blue light of the slit lamp may be of aid in detecting subtle differences. Any asymmetry between eyes or an obvious delay in the clearance of dye from both eyes can be easily appreciated. Symmetric delays are more difficult to diagnose and require detailed study with the primary and secondary Jones dye tests.

If the fluorescein dye disappearance test documents a functional delay in the presence of a stenotic punctum, a review of possible etiologic factors should first be conducted. Punctal stenosis may be caused by trauma, such as that induced by repeated canalicular probings; chronic use of topical cholinesterase inhibitors or antiviral agents; ocular pemphigoid; infections, such as herpes zoster; and the presence of a congenital punctal membrane.

With the elimination of etiologic factors and verification of the functional block, punctal stenosis is managed by means of a punctoplasty procedure. Attempts to repeatedly dilate the punctum frequently lead to restenosis and risk possible iatrogenic trauma and creation of false passageways. The technique of punctoplasty will be discussed later.

Lower Lacrimal System Obstruction

If the puncta have been evaluated and considered normal, attention is turned to the lacrimal sac and nasolacrimal duct. In the normal individual, the lacrimal sac is never palpable. Should the initial examination of a patient complaining of epiphora demonstrate a distended lacrimal sac, a nasolacrimal duct obstruction is almost certainly present. Likewise, expression of purulent discharge with gentle pressure over the lacrimal sac is all but pathognomonic for nasolacrimal duct obstruction. If neither punctal stenosis nor distension of the sac is present, then Jones I and II dye tests are needed to further localize the site of obstruction.

Jones I Test

The primary Jones test is a second method of establishing the overall patency of the lacrimal drainage system and corroborates the results of the dye disappearance test. First, the nasal mucosa is anesthetized with aerosolized 4% cocaine. The fluorescein solution previously instilled into the fornix for the dye disappearance test will be searched for under the inferior turbinate. While spreading the external naris with a nasal speculum, a calcium alginate swab is inserted under the inferior turbinate. The applicator tip is examined for evidence of fluorescein dye.

The presence of dye is described as a positive test, which indicates a patent drainage system and obviates the need for further testing. The absence of dye, or a negative test, is suggestive of two possibilities. First, fluorescein dye failed to enter the sac due to an upper system (i.e., punctum, canaliculus, or common punctum) obstruction. In this situation, a delay in dye clearance during the dye disappearance test should corroborate this finding. Second, fluorescein dye was able to enter into the sac, but could not be recovered under the inferior turbinate due to either a partial or complete nasolacrimal duct obstruction. In both circumstances, dye clearance would also be delayed. To further localize the site of obstruction, or to differentiate a partial from a complete nasolacrimal duct obstruction, a Jones II test is performed.

Jones II Test

Following a negative Jones I test, the fornices are irrigated free of remaining fluorescein. A lacrimal irrigation cannula (23 to 27 gauge) on a saline-filled 3-ml syringe is inserted through the lower punctum and into the canaliculus. While the patient's head is tilted forward and the nose positioned over a metal basin, saline is gently irrigated into the sac. There are three potential outcomes:

1. **Recovery of dye-tinged fluid** from the nose indicates a patent canalicular system, but a partial nasolacrimal duct obstruction. The dye is able to enter

into the sac, but cannot be passively recovered in the nose; hence, a negative Jones I test, because of resistance at the level of nasolacrimal duct. However, in this instance, the resistance is overcome by the pressure of the irrigating fluid.

2. **Recovery of only clear fluid** from the nose indicates a relative stenosis of the upper canalicular system, usually at the level of punctum or common canaliculus. In this situation, dye is not able to enter into the sac; hence, no dye is recovered in the nose with active irrigation of the sac. A delay in dye clearance (on dye disappearance test), coupled with the detection of canalicular stricture on probing should be confirmatory.
3. **No fluid recovered** from the nose, with fluid reflux out of the canaliculi. Three possible scenarios may occur in this particular circumstance:
   - Reflux of clear fluid around the irrigation cannula, without distension of the lacrimal sac. This is indicative of a severe canalicular stricture, involving the canaliculus intubated with the irrigation cannula.
   - Reflux of clear fluid out of the unintubated canaliculus, without distension of the lacrimal sac. Occasionally, a jet stream of fluid may be seen refluxing out of the upper canaliculus upon irrigation. This is indicative of a complete stricture at the level of common canaliculus.
   - Reflux of clear or dye-tinged fluid, with distension of the lacrimal sac. This is suggestive of a complete nasolacrimal duct obstruction. The presence of dye in the fluid refluxing out indicates that the dye was able to enter into the sac through a patent upper system, but became stagnant within the sac because of an outlet obstruction.

Based on the outcome of these functional tests, one can identify a likely point of obstruction and initiate appropriate treatment. In this chapter, surgical treatment of isolated punctal stenosis will be discussed. Management of partial or complete nasolacrimal duct obstructions will be reviewed in subsequent chapters.

PUNCTOPLASTY

Several punctoplasty procedures have been described in the past. In the *one-snip* procedure, a single vertical incision into the ampulla is made through the posterior wall of the punctum with a sharp Westcott scissors. In most instances, such a slit will close soon after the procedure. The second variation, a Jones *two-snip* punctoplasty is performed by creating a 2-mm high, V-shaped opening posteriorly. Even with excision of a wedge of punctal tissue, appositional closure of the punctum can occur. To reduce the incidence of postoperative closure, we have had the most success with a *three-snip* punctoplasty followed by placement of a circular silicone stent within the canalicular system. The rationale for the placement of a silicone stent here is analogous to stent placement to ensure patency of the internal ostium following a dacryocystorhinostomy (DCR). The silicone stent not only prevents appositional closure secondary to the healing process, but also mechanically dilates the stenotic canaliculi.

Three-Snip Punctoplasty Procedure

After application of topical anesthetic, peripunctal infiltration of the inferior punctum is carried out with 2% lidocaine with epinephrine. The punctum is dilated with a punctal dilator.

Figure 5–1. The posterior rim of the punctum is grasped with a 0.12-mm forceps and one blade of a sharp Westcott scissors is inserted into the ampulla. A vertical snip incision is made at the lateral aspect of the posterior rim.

Figure 5–2. A second vertical snip incision is made at the medial aspect of the punctum while grasping the posterior edge of the punctum with 0.12-mm forceps.

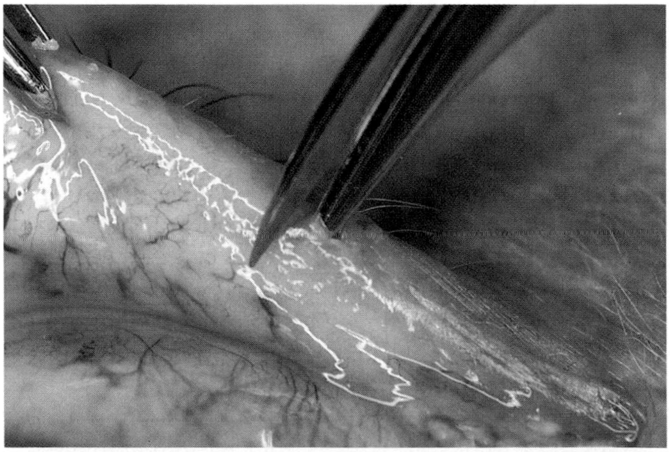

FIGURE 5–1

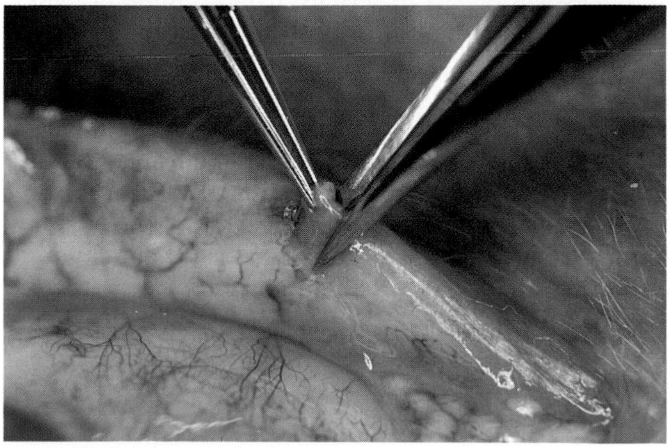

FIGURE 5–2

Figure 5–3. This posterior flap of tissue is grasped with a 0.12-mm forceps and excised by a horizontal third snip joining the inferior margins of the first two cuts. The wedge of tissue excised is made within the ampulla and not in the horizontal portion of the canaliculus, as has been previously described in another variation of the three-snip punctoplasty. It is important to visualize the epithelial lining of the ampulla.

Figure 5–4. The newly formed opening is a defect in the posterior wall of the ampulla, properly positioned to serve as an opening for tear drainage. Light bipolar cautery may be applied to control bleeding. A circular "doughnut" silicone stent is then placed in the upper system to ensure patency.

Pigtail Probe and the Circular Doughnut Silicone Stent Placement

Doughnut silicone intubation describes the shape of the stent once it is intubated into the upper lacrimal system and encircles it for 360°. The stent passes from one punctum through its corresponding canaliculus, into the opposite canaliculus and exits the other punctum, forming a complete circle. The Worst round, eyed pigtail probe is used. It is important to avoid the use of the crocheted probe as iatrogenic canalicular damage is common. The use of the Worst pigtail probe requires a thorough knowledge of the anatomy of the upper lacrimal drainage system. In most patients (90%), the canaliculi join to form the common canaliculus before entering the lacrimal sac. In the remaining 10%, the canaliculi gain entrance into the lacrimal sac independently and, thus, the smooth, continuous drainage system that facilitates introduction of the probe is not present. This latter group can be difficult, or impossible, to intubate using the pigtail probe.

The eyed pigtail probe is introduced into the upper punctum and gently rotated through the canalicular system after peripunctal anesthetic infiltration. Excessive force is not necessary, and difficulty intubating the system may indicate stenosis or obstruction of the canaliculi. If resistance is met, it is worthwhile to attempt to intubate the system from the inferior canaliculus. One should never try to force the probe into the canalicular system. Once the tip of the pigtail probe enters the canaliculus, the shaft is digitally rotated to advance the tip toward the sac. The spiral portion of the probe should be kept in the same plane as the canaliculi. It is important to recall that the common canaliculus lies immediately posterior to the medial canthal tendon. A slight posteriorly directed probe rotation should facilitate its passage. If the probe cannot be retrieved through the opposite canaliculus after multiple attempts, this procedure should be aborted to minimize trauma to the canalicular system.

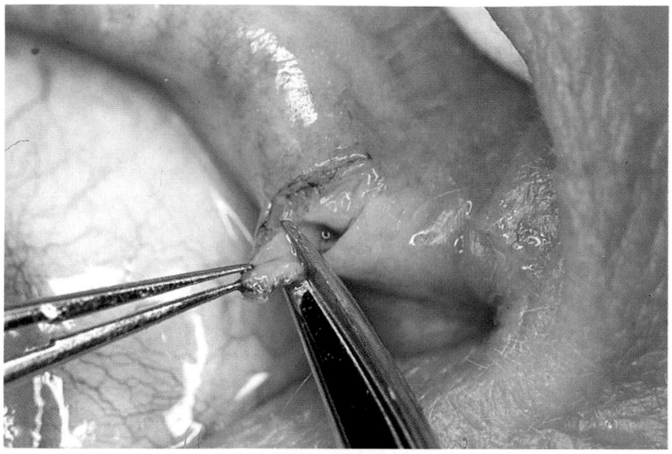

FIGURE 5–3

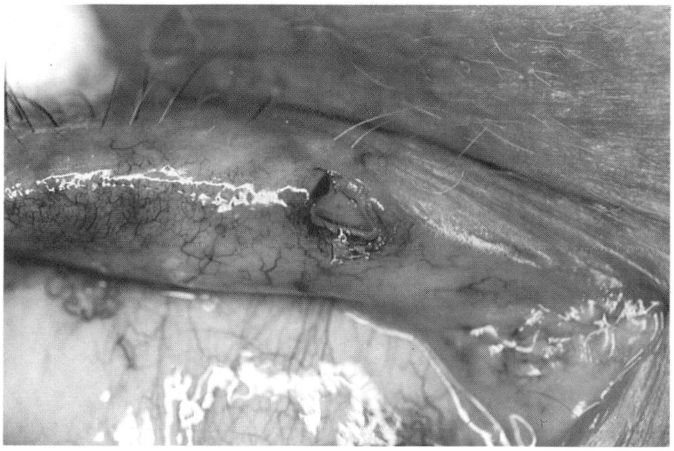

FIGURE 5–4

Figure 5–5. Continued rotation of the probe allows the tip to exit the opposite punctum. A 5–0 Prolene suture is threaded through the eyehole.

Figure 5–6. The pigtail probe is then gently rotated in a retrograde fashion, pulling the Prolene suture through the canalicular system. Sterile ophthalmic antibiotic ointment is applied to one end of the Prolene suture as lubricant and a 25-mm piece of silicone tubing (0.6-mm outside diameter) is threaded onto the Prolene suture. To prevent inadvertent removal of the suture, the two ends of the Prolene suture are secured with a hemostat.

Figure 5–7. A gentle continuous pull of the Prolene suture exiting one punctum, while advancing the stent through the opposite punctum, leads to rotation of the silicone stent into the canalicular system.

After intubation of the system, approximately 2.0 mm of stent should protrude from each punctum. Excess may be removed by cutting partially through the tubing (without cutting the suture within), then grasping the surplus with toothed forceps and avulsing it from the remainder of the stent. The hemostat is then momentarily released and the excess tubing removed. Care should be taken not to inadvertently pull the suture out.

Figure 5–8A. The Prolene suture is then tied with four single throws, thus uniting the ends of the stent to form a circular configuration. The suture is cut close to the knot.

Figure 5–8B. The knot retracts partially into the lumen of the tubing.

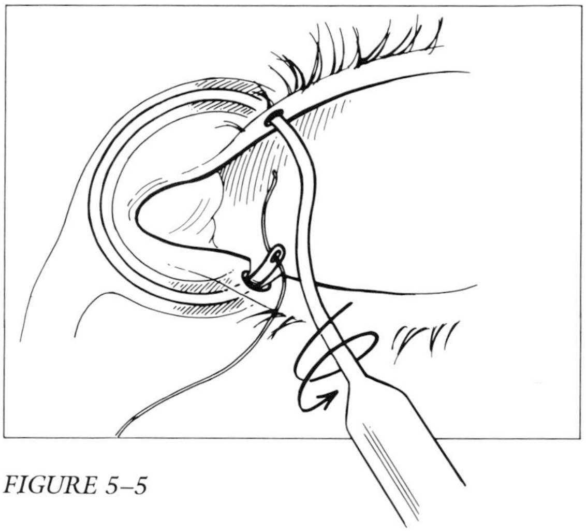

FIGURE 5–5

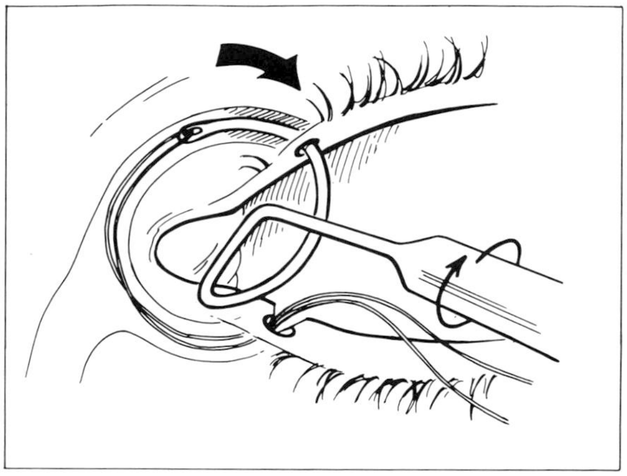

FIGURE 5–6

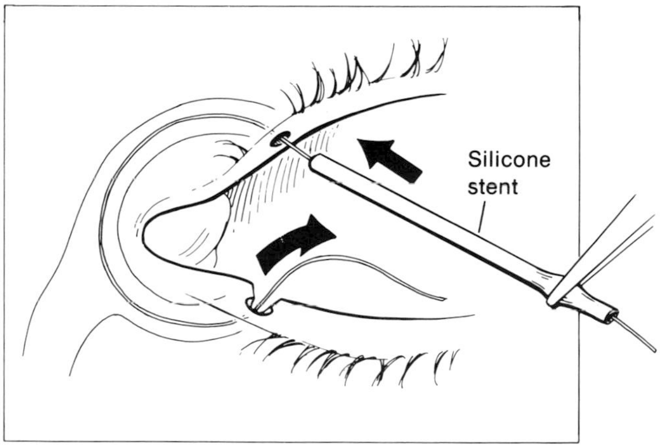

FIGURE 5–7

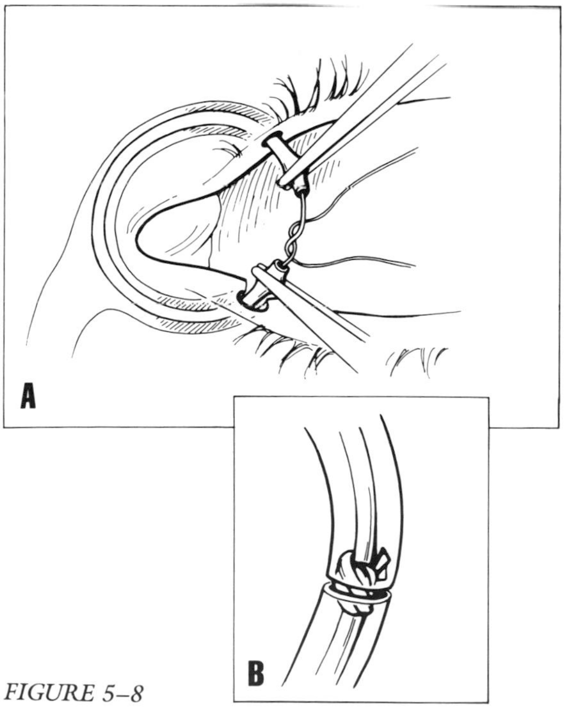

FIGURE 5–8

Figure 5–9. The doughnut stent is rotated 180° to position the anastomosis in the region of the common canaliculus. This rotation prevents erosion of the punctum and irritation of the conjunctiva should the ends of the sutures become exposed.

The silicone stent is removed in 8 to 12 weeks. On removal, the stent is rotated to expose the knot and the ends of the tubing. The suture is then cut, allowing the suture and the tubing to be pulled out as a single unit.

Finally, the silicone stent intubation technique detailed in this chapter is also useful in repairing traumatic canalicular lacerations. The pigtail probe allows rapid identification and intubation of the transected proximal canaliculus. The silicone stent is intended to reduce constriction at the site of the canalicular anastomosis.

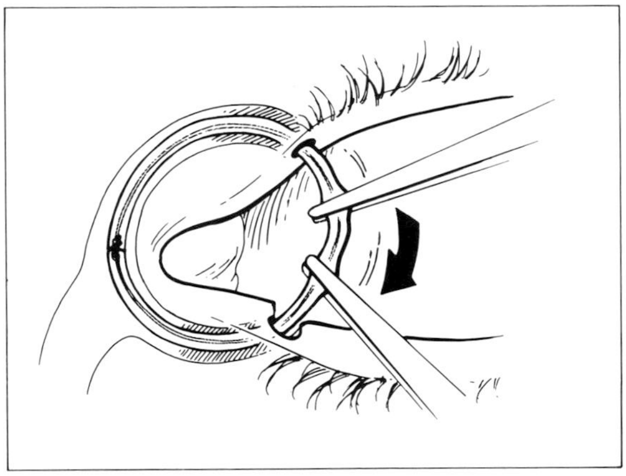

FIGURE 5–9

Chapter Six

NASOLACRIMAL DUCT PROBING AND INTUBATION

Kevin R. Scott
David T. Tse

Embryologically, the nasolacrimal drainage system develops from an invagination of surface ectoderm, which originates in the naso-optic fissure. Canalization occurs first in the central portion of the nasolacrimal passageways and then proceeds segmentally in both directions. Normally, the process of canalization is completed by the end of the 9-month gestational period. This system may fail to open anywhere throughout its course; however, the distal end of the nasolacrimal duct (NLD) is the most common site of obstruction. The blockage of tear drainage results from a thin membrane, at the level of the valve of Hasner, failing to perforate at birth. Additionally, there are a multitude of other less common anatomic variations within this system that can cause obstruction, including impaction of the inferior turbinate or a complete bony obstruction of the nasolacrimal duct.

The incidence of symptomatic congenital nasolacrimal duct obstruction ranges from 1% to 6%, of which one-fourth to one-third are bilateral. The incidence of obstruction in premature infants is much higher. Since the ability to produce tears is present at birth, stagnation of tears within the nasolacrimal sac frequently results in tearing and mattering of the lashes within the first few weeks of life.

PREOPERATIVE EVALUATION

The proper workup of a child with epiphora should begin with a careful history. It is important to establish the onset, duration, and severity of tearing, as well as a history of ocular infection or facial trauma. It is also incumbent on the ophthalmologist to rule out the more visually threatening causes for tearing, before concluding it is related to an obstruction of the nasolacrimal system. For instance, congenital glaucoma may have tearing as the initial presenting symptom. A detailed history and examination may reveal additional symptoms and signs of glaucoma: photophobia, blepharospasm, breaks in Descemet's membrane, an increased diameter, or clouding of the cornea. Additionally, careful examination can help to eliminate the following: entropion, ectropion, trichiasis, distichiasis, epiblepharon, punctal atresia, conjunctivitis, foreign bodies, and more rare disorders such as crocodile tears in association with Duane's retraction syndrome.

For adequate evaluation of a tearing neonate or young child, either loupes or, in a cooperative child, a slit lamp is required. A systematic approach to the examination will aid in eliminating these additional causes of tearing. The key components of the ocular examination include determination of eyelid and lash position and documenting punctal patency, corneal clarity, and corneal diameter.

In cases of nasolacrimal duct obstruction, inspection alone may reveal an increased tear lake, epiphora, mattering of the lashes, or a distended lacrimal sac. Gentle pressure over the lacrimal sac will frequently result in regurgitation of the stagnant material from within the sac. When possible, document if the discharge refluxes from the upper, lower, or both puncta. This is an indirect verification of the patency of the canalicular system.

A thorough evaluation of the lacrimal drainage system in neonates and young children is often limited. Therefore, the ophthalmologist must rely primarily on the history and external examination. The modified fluorescein dye disappearance test, as described by Katowitz and Welsh (1987), however, is a simple and useful method in assessing the integrity of the outflow system. In this test, a drop of 0.5% proparacaine is first instilled into the fornix, followed by 1 to 2 drops of 2% fluorescein solution. In a patent outflow system, the fluorescein is normally cleared from the tear lake within 10 minutes. The qualitative comparison of the rate of fluorescein egress from both sides is determined by directing a slit-lamp cobalt blue light at the eyes of the patient from several feet away. This should be done in a partially darkened room. From this distance, the light should illuminate the entire face of the child and is generally nonthreatening. Since a crying child precludes proper interpretation of this test, the parent should remain with the child throughout the test. A delay in fluorescein clearance is suggestive of an outflow obstruction.

MEDICAL MANAGEMENT

There is general agreement that the best initial management of a NLD obstruction is a combination of nasolacrimal sac massage and topical antibiotics to reduce the amount of mucopurulent discharge. Massage of the nasolacrimal sac has been shown to be effective in increasing the rate of spontaneous resolution of a distal membranous nasolacrimal duct obstruction.

Proper massage technique involves the parent placing his or her index finger over the medial canthal tendon and applying pressure in a nasal and downward direction to increase the hydrostatic pressure within the lacrimal sac. The parents are instructed to keep their fingernails trimmed to avoid trauma to the skin and ocular tissues. Massage should be performed four times a day with 10 to 15 repetitions each time. Following the massage, topical sulfacetamide, 10% solution, is instilled four times daily.

TIMING OF INITIAL PROBING

Controversy exists about the timing of initial probing in a patient with congenital nasolacrimal duct obstruction. This controversy results primarily because a high percentage will spontaneously resolve with conservative medical management alone. Katowitz and Welsh (1987) reported 54% of congenital nasolacrimal duct observations resolved spontaneously by 6 months, and only an additional 17% resolved by 13 months. Peterson and Robb (1978), reported similar results, with 54% resolving within 6 months, and only an additional 14% spontaneously resolving by 13 months. Katowitz and Welsh (1987) also reported that delaying initial probing beyond 13 months of age resulted in decreasing success as well as increasing complexity of therapy required to achieve success.

In patients with persistent symptoms of NLD obstruction, despite an optimal course of medical therapy, consideration for probing should be given. We recommend that the initial probing be performed between 6 months and 1 year of age. This will allow most patients to resolve spontaneously, yet maintain the maximum response to a first probing.

LOCATION OF THE INITIAL PROBING

Additional controversy exists over whether to perform the initial probing in the office with a papoose restraint or under general anesthesia. Our individual preference is to perform probing under general anesthesia because it permits a more controlled, gentle, and complete evaluation of the nasolacrimal system. Additionally, this approach to NLD probing allows a comprehensive examination under anesthesia, as well as a controlled infracturing of the inferior turbinate.

Since there is no consensus on timing and location of probing, the parents need to be fully informed of the possibility for spontaneous resolution, balanced against the ocular discomfort for the child and inconvenience for them with continued medical management. They should also be informed of the reduced success rate if probing is performed after 13 months of age. Exceptions to the 6- to 12-month rule arise in cases of acute purulent dacryocystitis or a dacryocystocele (amniotocele). Treatment of these cases will be outlined later.

NASOLACRIMAL DUCT PROBING

Operative Procedure

On arrival to the operating room, endotracheal anesthesia is delivered by the anesthesiologist and intravenous access is obtained.

Figure 6–1. The instruments needed for probing include cotton gauze, nasal speculum, bayonet forceps, Freer periosteal elevator, assorted Bowman probes, punctal dilator, clear suction catheter, 2% fluorescein dye, irrigation cannula, 3 mm syringe, nasal atomizer, and 4% cocaine solution. The nose is then sprayed with 4% cocaine solution on the involved side. With use of a fiberoptic headlight, loupes, nasal speculum, and bayonet forceps, the nose is packed under and around the inferior turbinate with a strip of cotton gauze moistened with 4% cocaine. The solution should be squeezed out of the gauze before packing the nose to avoid toxicity. One to two percent cocaine solution can be used in very young or frail children. The anesthesiologist should be informed of the use of cocaine, and a dose of 3 mg/kg must not be exceeded.

After 5 minutes, the packing is removed and the nasal cavity inspected.

Figure 6–2. If the inferior turbinate is hypertrophic and impacted against the lateral wall, the blunt end of a Freer periosteal elevator is used to gently infracture the turbinate toward the septum. The tip of the periosteal elevator is inserted under the inferior turbinate and gentle pressure is applied to the turbinate until a slight crack is felt. This maneuver is performed using both hands to allow a slow, steady movement, which guards against inadvertent injury to the nasal septum.

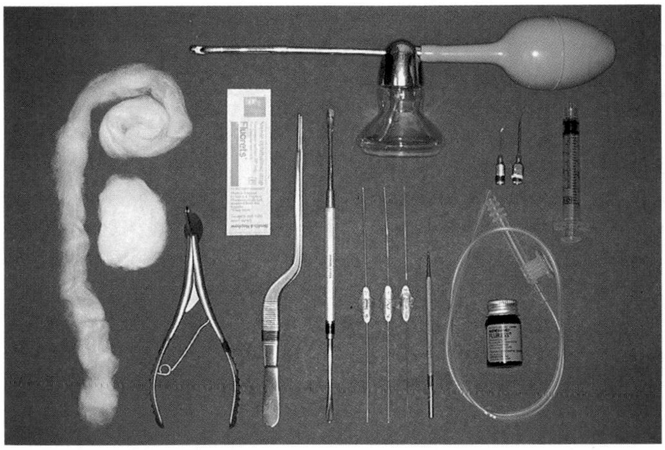

FIGURE 6–1

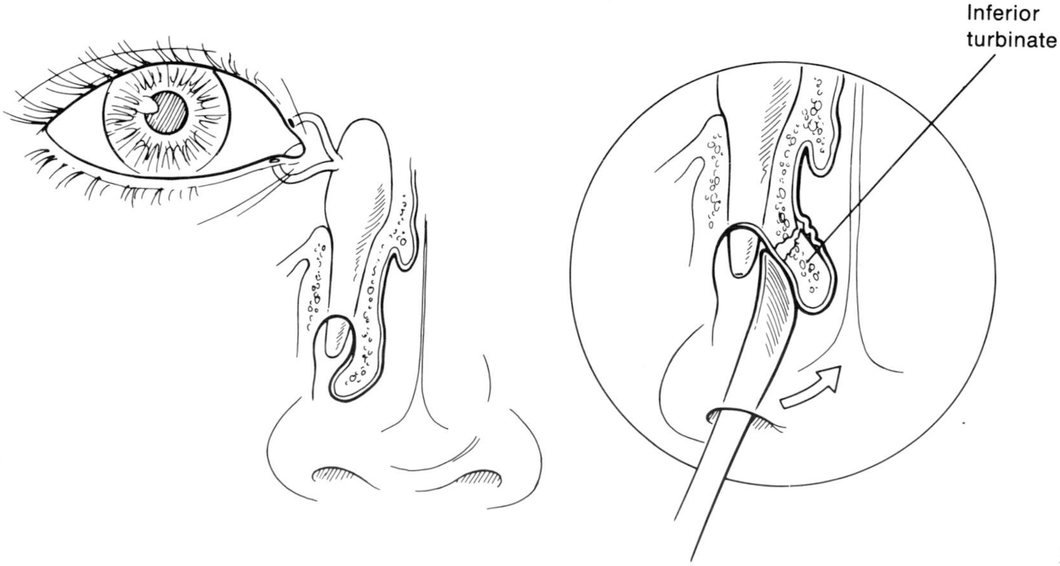

FIGURE 6–2

Figure 6–3A. The superior punctum is dilated with a punctal dilator. A size zero Bowman probe is bent slightly to create a smooth curvature, which facilitates passage down the nasolacrimal duct. The probe is introduced into the punctum for approximately 1½ to 2 mm in a vertical direction and rotated laterally to parallel the lid margin.

Figure 6–3B. As the probe is advanced toward the lacrimal sac, lateral traction on the upper lid is applied. This traction avoids the formation of accordion folds in the canaliculus (inset). A soft stop encountered while advancing the probe may represent a stricture or membranous blockage within the canaliculus or the common internal punctum. After reaching the nasolacrimal sac, a "hard" stop is felt against the bony lacrimal sac fossa. If there is any question whether the sac has been reached, relax the traction on the lid and attempt to advance the probe medially. If this results in movement of the eyelid toward the nose, then the tip of the probe is still in the canaliculus.

Figure 6–3C. The tip of the probe should remain in contact with the bone while the probe is pivoted 90° superiorly and advanced inferiorly in a slightly posteriolateral direction. The direction of the probe is in vertical alignment with the second incisor. The probe is gently pushed downward until the membranous obstruction is reached. A slight inferior pressure will result in a "give," allowing the probe to enter the inferior meatus. A nasal speculum is inserted into the external naris in an attempt to directly visualize the probe. The nasal speculum should be inserted so the blades separate vertically to avoid damaging the septum.

Figure 6–3D. If the probe cannot be visualized, a size 3 Bowman probe can be used to make a metal-on-metal contact with it. Not advancing the probe far enough or false passage of the probe in a submucosal plane, are common causes for not being able to make contact with the probe.

Following confirmation, the probe is removed and an irrigating cannula on a 3-ml syringe is inserted through the superior canaliculus into the lacrimal sac. Two percent fluorescein solution is gently irrigated through the system. Yellow-green-tinged fluid should easily be retrieved with a clear suction cannula positioned under the inferior turbinate. If the fluorescein solution regurgitates out of the opposite canaliculus and no fluorescein is recovered from the nasopharynx, then stenosis of the NLD should be suspected. Additionally, a scraping sensation felt when passing the probe may signify a marked stenosis of the duct. These findings should be reviewed with the parents and are helpful in explaining why additional procedures may be necessary in the future, should probing fail.

When a bilateral obstruction exists, the same procedure is repeated on the contralateral side. To avoid confusion when irrigating the second side, all residual fluorescein from the first side must be suctioned from the nasopharynx.

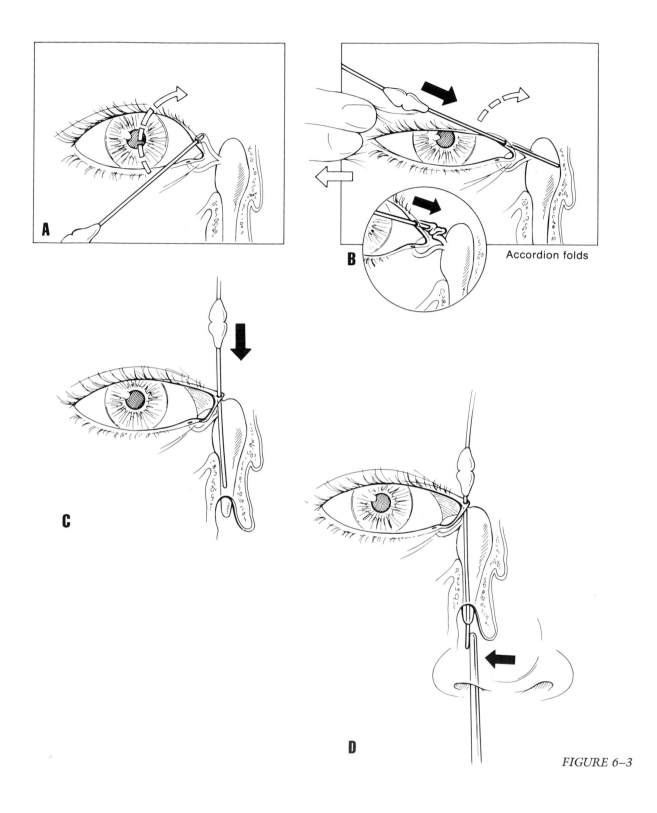

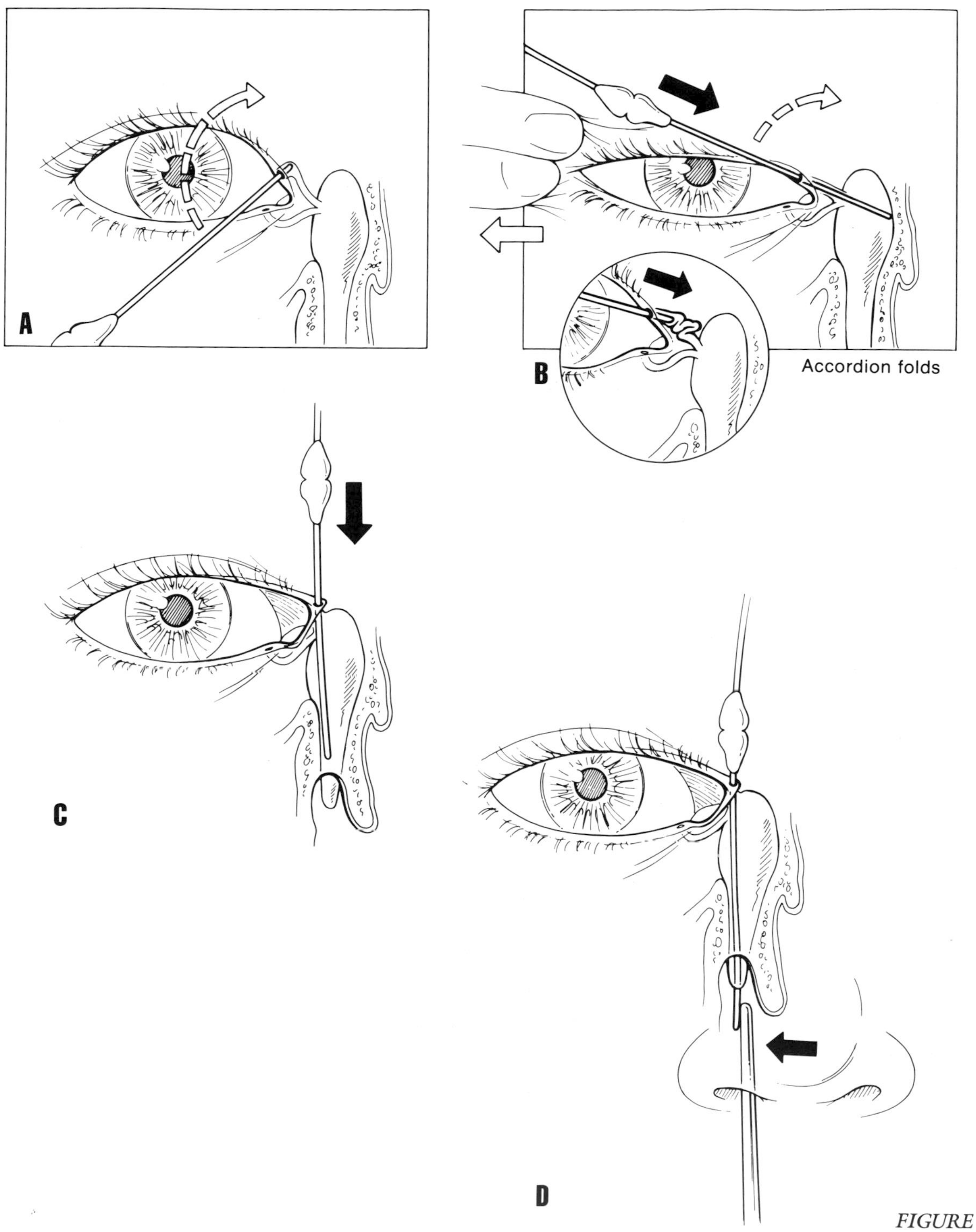

FIGURE 6–3

Postoperative Management

After the nasolacrimal system has been probed and patency established, the patient is started on a regimen of sulfacetamide, 10% solution, four times daily for 1 week. The patient is seen in 3 weeks, and the fluorescein dye disappearance test is repeated. If the patient is still symptomatic, and the dye disappearance test is delayed, a trial of massage and antibiotics is initiated for 4 to 6 weeks. After this period, persistent epiphora and mattering should be treated with a repeat probing, along with silicone intubation.

NASOLACRIMAL INTUBATION

Silicone intubation is indicated for patients who have had a seemingly adequate initial probing, but still remain symptomatic. Frequently, it has been noted that the patients who required silicone intubation were those with a tight probe passage through the nasolacrimal duct on initial probing, or those for whom there was an inability to irrigate into the nose, despite confirmation of the probe in the proper location.

Katowitz and Welsh (1987) reported 63 patients with congenital nasolacrimal duct obstruction who had an initial NLD probing at or after 24 months of age. A third of these patients responded to a first probing. In 71% of those patients who had failed the initial probing, symptoms resolved following nasolacrimal intubation. Therefore, if during the initial probing of a child older than 24 months there is a suggestion of a tight NLD, we convert to a primary nasolacrimal intubation.

Operative Procedure

Endotracheal anesthesia is used in all silicone intubation procedures. The technique and precautions are the same as those outlined previously for the nasolacrimal probing. After several minutes, the packing is removed, and the nasal cavity is inspected. The inferior turbinate is then infractured, as previously described (see Figure 6–2).

The Crawford silicone stent, with a stainless steel probe and an olive tip, is our preferred intubation set. The newest modification of the original Crawford silicone stent has the added advantage of a suture within the tubing. Before using the stent, the stainless steel probe is bent slightly or curved for easier advancement into the nose.

The superior punctum is gently enlarged with a punctal dilator.

Figure 6–4A. The Crawford probe is introduced into the superior punctum and advanced through the nasolacrimal system in the same fashion as that outlined for nasolacrimal probing. Once the probe is in the nasal cavity, metal-on-metal verification of its proper placement is made with a modified groove director inserted into the inferior meatus.

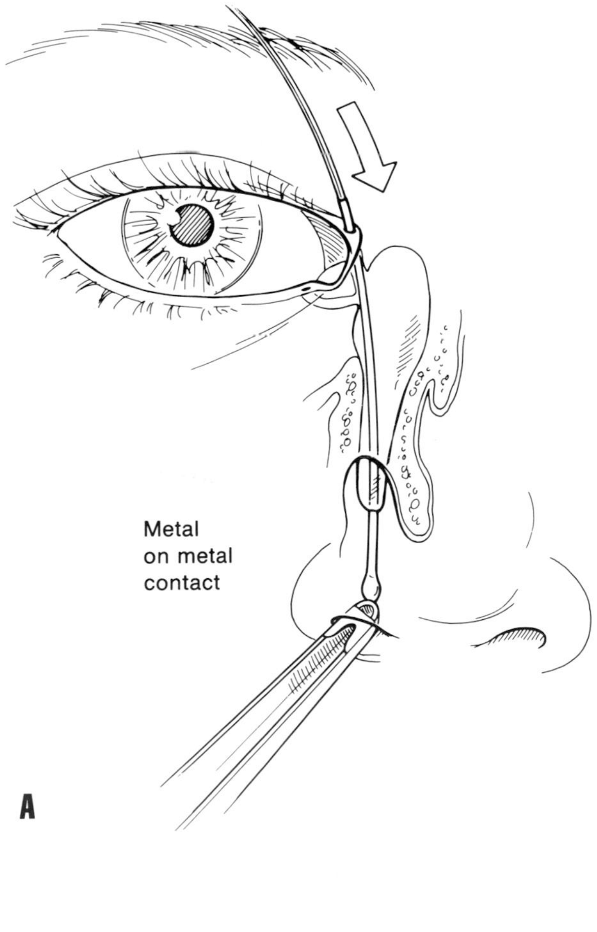

FIGURE 6–4

Figure 6–4B. Once contact is made, the probe is pulled superiorly several millimeters to allow the groove director to be advanced underneath the inferior turbinate and against the lateral nasal wall.

Figure 6–4C. The probe is advanced into the groove, and the olive tip is engaged by the keyhole groove at the end of the director.

Figure 6–4D. The groove director is then withdrawn from the nose, while the probe is pulled in the opposite direction to avoid disengagement. The second stainless steel probe is similarly passed through the inferior canaliculus and retrieved from the inferior meatus. The advantages of this retrieval method are as follows: (1) it avoids the use of a hook to fish for the probe, thereby minimizing trauma to the nasal mucosa; (2) the groove director protects the floor of the nose because the tip of the lacrimal probe does not come in contact with the nasal mucosa during the entire procedure, thereby further reducing trauma to tissues; (3) the groove director traps the lacrimal probe if it directs itself posteriorly; and (4) retrieval is easy because the groove director guides the olive tip into the keyhole, ensuring capture.

Figure 6–4E. The difference between the end of a modified groove director and a Crawford hook is shown (from top to bottom, modified groove director, Crawford stainless steel probe, Crawford hook).

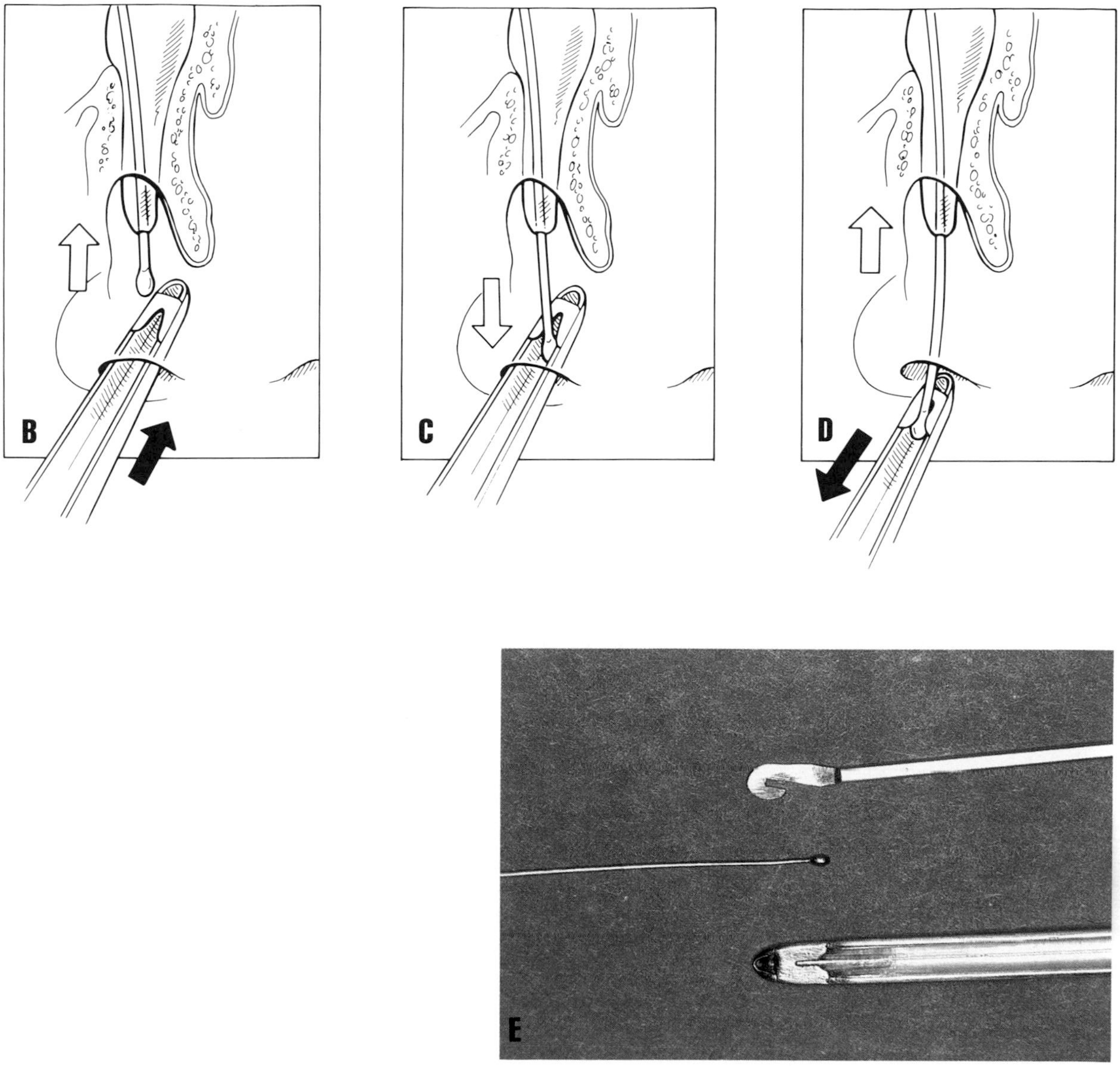

FIGURE 6–4 (Continued)

Figure 6–4F. The two ends of the Crawford silicone stent are pulled from the nose until the tubing forms a small loop between the two punctum. A muscle hook is used to engage the tubing between the two punctum, while the silicone tubing is pulled from the nose inferiorly under slight tension. A Castroviejo locking needle holder is used to grasp the tubing just at the level of the external naris. The Crawford tube is cut at the attachment site to the stainless steel probes.

Figure 6–4G. When using the Crawford silicone stent with a suture within the tubing, a Crawford stripper is used to remove the silicone from both ends, without cutting the suture inside. The suture is then tied in four single square knots and cut close to the knots. Before releasing the nasal end of the tubing, the tension of the silicone tubing between the punctum should be checked and approximately 3 to 4 mm of temporal slack is needed to avoid "cheese-wiring." After this is confirmed, the muscle hook is removed before releasing the knots.

Figure 6–4H. The tubing is then released to hang loosely under the inferior turbinate. If desired, a 5–0 Prolene suture can be placed just within the nasal vestibule on the lateral wall to fixate the stent, thereby reducing the chance for displacement into the nasolacrimal sac. If the intubation is performed utilizing a silicone stent without an internal suture, then the silicone tubing is tied to itself in a similar fashion with four knots. The use of four single throws will keep the total knot size small, which allows for easy passage out of the canalicular system should the knots become inadvertently pulled into the lacrimal sac. In an attempt to avoid displacement of the silicone stent into the nasolacrimal sac, a 5–0 Prolene suture can be placed just within the nasal vestibule on the lateral wall to fixate the silicone stent.

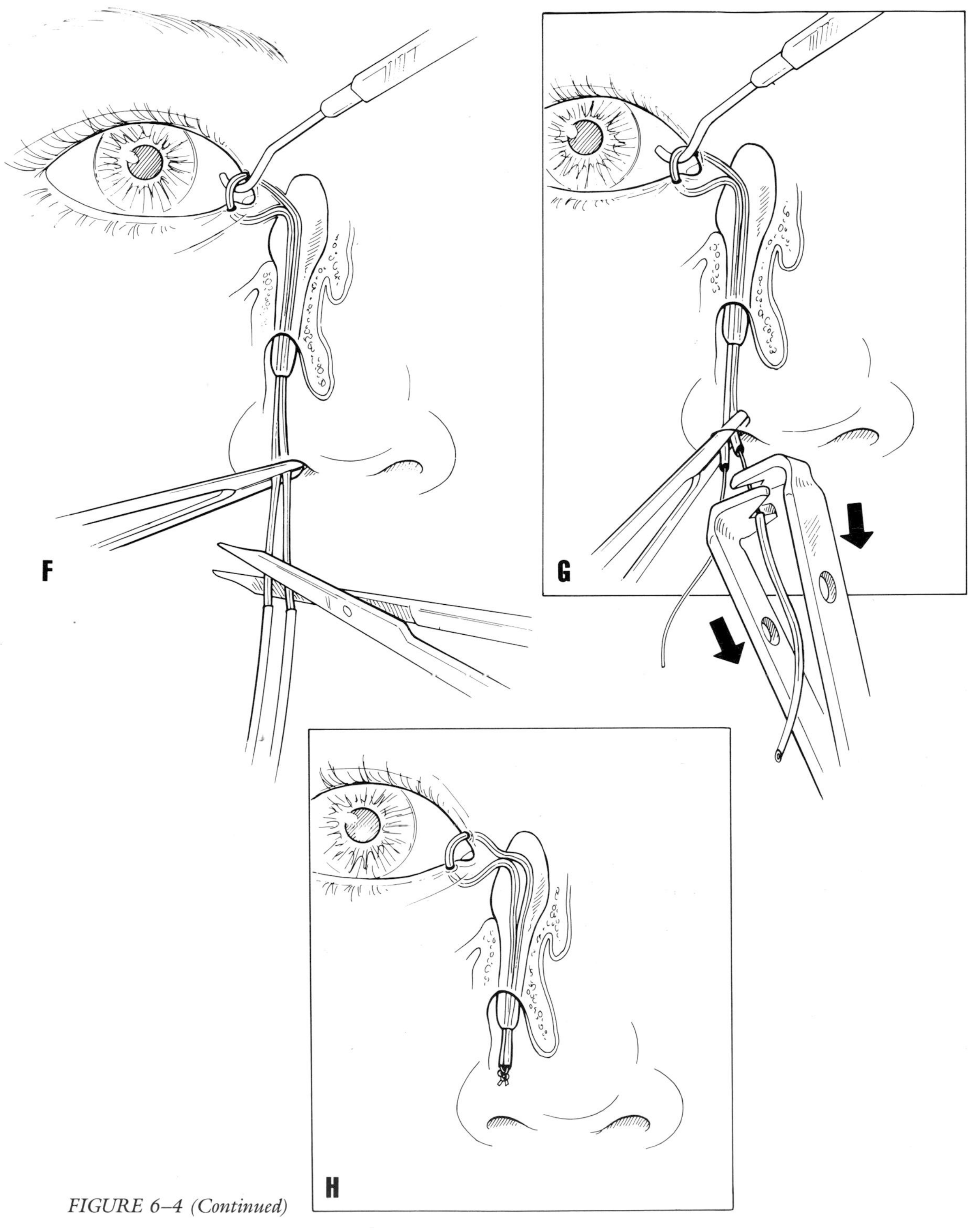

FIGURE 6–4 (Continued)

POSTOPERATIVE MANAGEMENT

Following silicone stent intubation, the patient is started on a steroid-antibiotic solution four times a day for one week. The patient is reevaluated at one week following silicone stent placement. If the patient is without any stent related problems or evidence of persistent dacryocystitis, the stent is kept in place for six months to a year.

COMPLICATIONS OF SILICONE INTUBATION

Silicone tubing within the nasolacrimal system is generally well tolerated. Problems can occur, however, if the tubing is tied too tightly with "cheese-wiring" through the punctum and canaliculus. Because of this possibility, the punctum needs to be checked on each postoperative visit and the tubing removed if cheese-wiring is noted. A slight enlargement of the punctum is common and does not necessitate removal. A pyogenic granuloma can form near the punctum and should be excised with light cautery applied to the base. If the tubing has already been in place for several months and the patient is asymptomatic, the tubing, along with the pyogenic granuloma, should be removed.

Occasionally, the tubing may cause conjunctival and corneal irritation secondary to persistent contact during adduction of the eye. If the keratoconjunctivitis is not relieved by topical lubricating ointments at bedtime, then the tubing should be removed.

Prolapse of the tubes, with the knots dislodged into the lacrimal sac is a common problem associated with silicone intubation. To avoid this problem, fixation within the naris may be considered. Additionally, various authors have described the use of a silicone button, retinal sponge material, and ventricular shunt tubing attached to the intranasal portion of the silicone to guard against retraction of the knots into the lacrimal sac. Should the knots prolapse into the nasolacrimal sac, the silicone tubing can be removed through the superior canaliculus, provided not too many knots were placed originally. Avoid cutting the silicone stent until the knots are externalized.

On rare occasions, dacryocystitis may persist or recur with the silicone stent in proper position, which necessitates removal of the stent and subsequent dacryocystorhinostomy (DCR).

Silicone Stent Removal

In general, the silicone stent can be removed in the office, without the need for general anesthesia. In a small and uncooperative child, a papoose restraint may be necessary. The nostril is sprayed with a 4% cocaine solution, particularly under the inferior turbinate. With the head stabilized, the silicone tubing is visualized under the inferior turbinate or at its fixation point within the naris. The tubing is then grasped with an alligator forceps and pulled from the nose, after cutting the loop at the medial canthus. If unable to locate the stent within the nose, the loop at the medial canthus is grasped with a forceps and the knots are pulled into the sac. The knots are then rotated out of the superior canaliculus and the stent cut with a scissors. In a very uncooperative child, inhalation anesthesia, using a face mask, may be necessary for the removal of a silicone stent.

Postoperative Management

The patient is seen 3 weeks after stent removal and a modified fluorescein dye disappearance test is repeated to document the patency of the system. If tearing symptoms persist and the fluorescein dye disappearance is delayed, a DCR procedure along with silicone stent placement should be considered.

SPECIAL CASES

A *dacryocystocele* (amniotocele) is a distention of the nasolacrimal sac in the neonate. This condition presents as a cystic-appearing bluish mass in the area of the nasolacrimal sac below the medial canthal tendon. The lesion typically enlarges secondary to a ball-valve effect at the level of the common internal punctum, in conjunction with an NLD obstruction. Amniotic fluid, mucus, or tears accumulate within the sac and may become secondarily infected. Our preference is to initially treat a dacryocystocele conservatively with massage and topical sulfacetamide, 10% solution, four times a day. If there is no improvement after several weeks on medical management alone, an in-office nasolacrimal probing can be performed to the level of the lacrimal sac to prevent the development of dacryocystitis. Typically, this is all that is needed to decompress the sac, and the child can then be treated for a typical nasolacrimal duct obstruction with massage and topical antibiotics. A full probing in a neonate is discouraged.

This condition must be differentiated from a capillary hemangioma and a meningoencephalocele. Capillary hemangiomas tend to have a more reddish and solid appearance, with moderate to high internal reflectivity by ultrasound. Additionally, capillary hemangiomas can develop above or below the medial canthal tendon. A meningoencephalocele tends to be pulsatile, occurring mainly above the medial canthal tendon and has a cystic appearance by ultrasound.

Acute dacryocystitis during the neonatal period usually presents with distention of the lacrimal sac, purulent ocular discharge, and surrounding erythema. Since this condition may rapidly progress to periocular cellulitis, intravenous antibiotics and warm compresses are the mainstay of treatment. If the distended sac begins to point on the skin surface, drainage with a small-gauge needle is indicated to decompress the sac. The aspirate is sent for cultures and Gram stain to guide the initial antibiotic therapy. Once the acute swelling and inflammatory changes have subsided, a nasolacrimal duct probing should be considered to prevent recurrences.

Chapter Seven

DACRYOCYSTO-RHINOSTOMY

David T. Tse

Dacryocystorhinostomy (DCR) is a drainage procedure designed to bypass the site of nasolacrimal duct obstruction by forming a fistula between the lacrimal sac and the nasal cavity. This procedure is performed in adults who have chronic epiphora or dacryocystitis secondary to complete or partial obstruction of the nasolacrimal duct, and in children who have recurrent dacryocystitis or have failed previous probings and silicone intubations. This procedure is indicated for these conditions when the upper and lower canaliculus are patent. A DCR procedure is contraindicated when malignancy of the lacrimal sac is suspected. Additionally, a DCR should not be performed on a patient with acute dacryocystitis. One should wait until the infection has been cleared with systemic antibiotics and for an opportunity to reassess the patient's symptoms and patency of the lacrimal drainage system by appropriate diagnostic tests.

PREOPERATIVE EVALUATION

Before surgery, a thorough nasal speculum examination of the nostrils should be performed. The surgeon needs to rule out any nasal abnormalities, such as deviated nasal septum, polyps, or tumors, that could compromise the success of the procedure. It is also necessary to assure that there is adequate space adjacent to the planned internal ostium.

To avoid bleeding, the patient is advised to refrain from taking aspirin, aspirin-containing products such as Alka-Seltzer, and anti-inflammatory agents for at least 2 weeks before surgery. In patients with systemic hypertension, good blood pressure control before surgery is mandatory, since cocaine and epinephrine are used during this procedure. Patients with discharge from the sac are instructed to massage the sac and to use topical antibiotics for several days before surgery.

SURGICAL TECHNIQUE

Anesthesia and Skin Marking

A DCR procedure can be performed under either general or local anesthesia. However, local anesthesia combined with mild sedation is preferred because it has the advantages of superior hemostasis, fewer postoperative side effects, and wider patient acceptance. Even when using general anesthesia, nasal packing with cocaine-moistened cotton strips, coupled with external subcutaneous injection of a lidocaine solution that contains epinephrine, should be given to facilitate hemostasis. Improved visualization of anatomy from meticulous control of hemostasis is the key to the success of this procedure.

Upon arrival in the operating room, the patient's nasal cavity on the involved side is sprayed with 5% cocaine solution. The cocaine solution will vasoconstrict the vascular mucosa and provide mucosal anesthesia to minimize discomfort during subsequent packing. The maximum recommended dosage of cocaine is 3 mg/kg. Five minutes later, the anterosuperior nasal cavity adjacent to the lacrimal fossa is packed with a strip of cotton gauze moistened with 5% cocaine solution. Nasal packing should be performed with the aid of a fiberoptic headlight, nasal speculum, and bayonet forceps.

Figure 7–1. The bayonet forceps should be directed toward the medial canthus, placing the packing in the middle meatus, between the head of the middle turbinate and inferior turbinate. Proper placement of the packing within the nasal cavity is important since it serves not only to vasoconstrict and anesthetize the mucosa, but it also acts as a barrier to prevent inadvertent laceration of the nasal septum when the mucosa is incised. It must also be emphasized that excessive upward packing force be avoided to prevent perforation of the cribriform plate. Another strip of cotton gauze is inserted into the posterior nasal cavity to catch any oozing that may run toward the oropharynx. This is useful while operating on an awake patient.

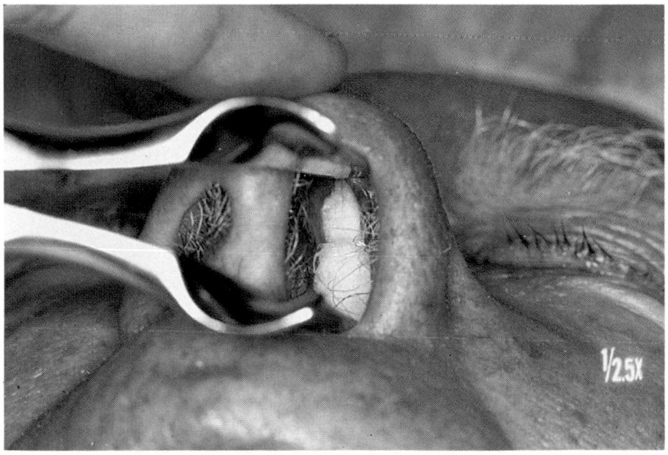

FIGURE 7–1

Figure 7–2A, B. After the nostril has been packed with the cotton gauze, a marking pen is used to mark the proposed incision site. The proposed linear skin incision is located midway between the medial canthal angle and the dorsum of the nose (*asterisk*). A line is drawn 10- to 12-mm medial to the medial canthal angle, beginning at the level of the inferior edge of the medial canthal tendon, extending downward and laterally in a straight line toward the nasal alar fold for a distance of 1.5 cm. This incision is parallel to the angular vessels and lies within the thicker nasal skin. Do not curve the incision to involve the thinner eyelid skin because postoperative cicatricial contracture will result in a bowstring scar.

Local anesthesia is obtained by subcutaneous infiltration of lidocaine 2% with 1:100,000 dilution of epinephrine into the operative site and in the region of the infratrochlear nerve above the medial canthal tendon. Subcutaneous injections along the anterior lacrimal crest and into the lacrimal fossa are also given. A 30-gauge 1½-in. (3.75-cm) needle with a 5-ml syringe is used, and no more than 3 to 4 ml of anesthetic is needed. Anterior ethmoidal nerve block is frequently unnecessary. Subcutaneous injection along with nasal packing should be completed 10 to 15 minutes before surgery, so that adequate vasoconstriction and anesthesia will have been achieved before incision.

The patient is then prepared and draped while the surgeon scrubs. The nose and face are left open so that there is access to the nose for nasal inspection and silicone stent retrieval during surgery.

Skin Incision

Skin incision over the preplaced marking is made with a size 15 Bard–Parker blade. The incision should be no deeper than the subcutaneous fascia. If the area has been infiltrated 10 minutes before the operation with the lidocaine–epinephrine mixture, bleeding is minimal. With the skin edges tented up by forceps, the remaining strands of superficial fascia are cut with Stevens scissors. All bleeding points and subcutaneous vessels are cauterized with a wet-field bipolar cautery.

Figure 7–3. Frequently, the angular vessels (*arrow*) can be readily identified and retracted away with a rake retractor. If the angular vessels are severed inadvertently, it is best managed by ligating or cauterizing each end of the cut vessel.

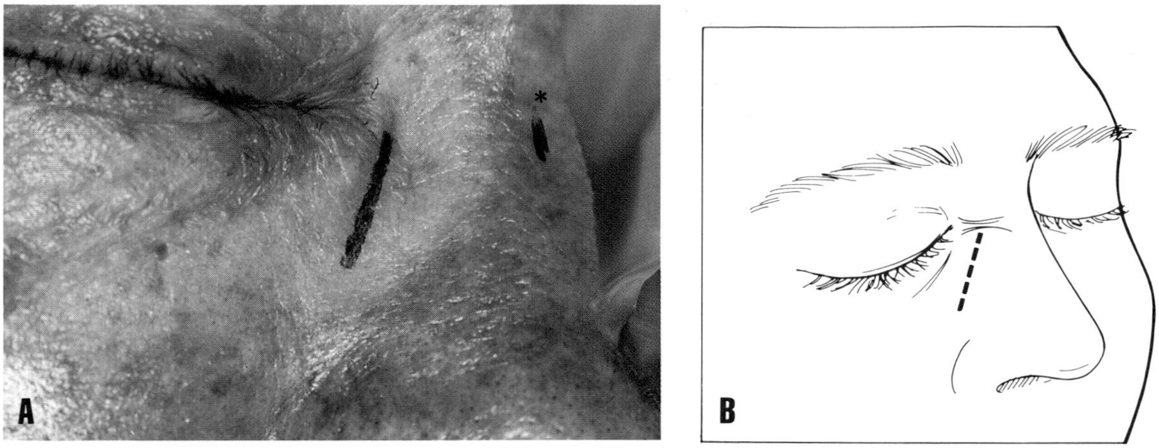

FIGURE 7–2

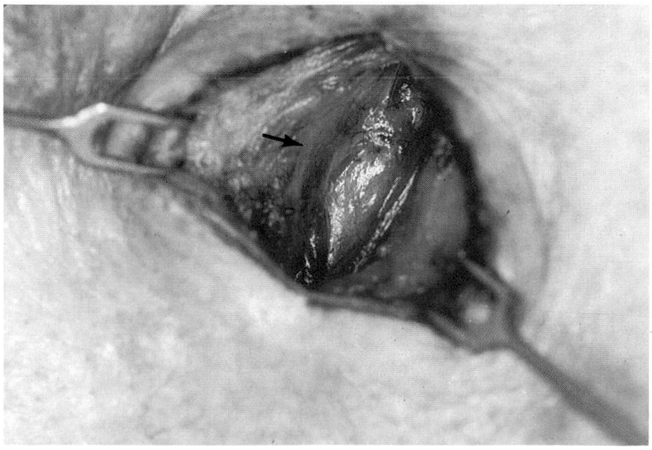

FIGURE 7–3

Figure 7–4. A curved Stevens scissors penetrates the orbicularis muscle fibers just nasal to the anterior lacrimal crest, and the blades are spread vertically to expose the periosteum of the frontal process of the maxilla.

Figure 7–5. With the blunt rake retractors spreading the incision, the periosteum is incised (edges outlined by *arrowheads*) 3 to 4 mm anterior and parallel to the crest with the sharp end of a Freer elevator. The periosteal incision extends from just below the medial canthal tendon to the inferior orbital rim.

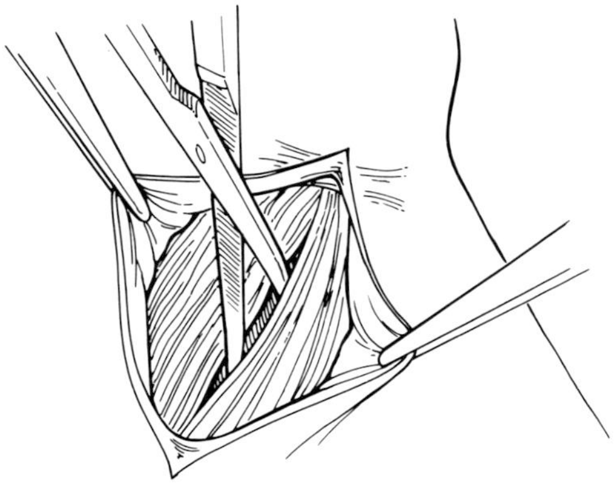

FIGURE 7–4

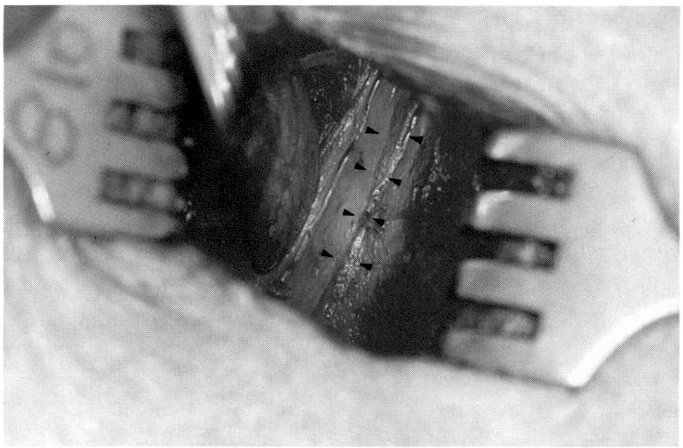

FIGURE 7–5

Figure 7–6. As the periosteum is reflected toward the anterior lacrimal crest (*arrowheads*), bone bleeding from the sutura notha (*asterisk*) is frequently encountered. Sutura notha, a small vascular groove situated 1 to 2 mm from the anterior lacrimal crest, is often mistaken by surgeons for the edge of the crest, and they will incorrectly begin rounding for the lacrimal fossa. Bone bleeding from this indentation can be stopped with bone wax. Once the anterior lacrimal crest is reached, the surgeon should be cautious in rounding the edge. One should be gentle not to push the elevator against the sac too hard or without control. The tip can lacerate the sac, causing bleeding and making flap anastomosis difficult later in the procedure. The periosteum posterior to the crest is loosely adherent and the blunt end of the Freer elevator is used to reflect the lacrimal sac laterally, with its periosteal lining.

Figure 7–7A. As the lacrimal sac and proximal nasolacrimal duct are reflected laterally to expose the full dimension of the lacrimal fossa, the suture line between the lacrimal bone and maxillary bone in the middle of the fossa can be identified. The periosteum anterior to its line of incision is also elevated for a few millimeters so that it will not be excised during bone removal.

Osteotomy

Figure 7–7B. The tip of a small, curved hemostat is placed over the suture line and the thin bone is ruptured with a gentle push. One has to be careful not to push the tip of the hemostat too deeply to perforate the mucosa, thereby causing bleeding to obscure the surgical site. The bony opening can be enlarged by spreading the hemostat blades.

Figure 7–8. A 90° Hardy–Sella punch is then introduced through the bony opening to begin bone removal. The heel of the Hardy–Sella punch is used to push away the mucosa (*asterisk*) while engaging the bony edge (*arrowheads*). This is to ensure that the nasal mucosa will not be damaged with each bite of the instrument. The bone removed includes the anterior lacrimal crest down to the nasolacrimal duct, and the superior nasal wall of the nasolacrimal canal.

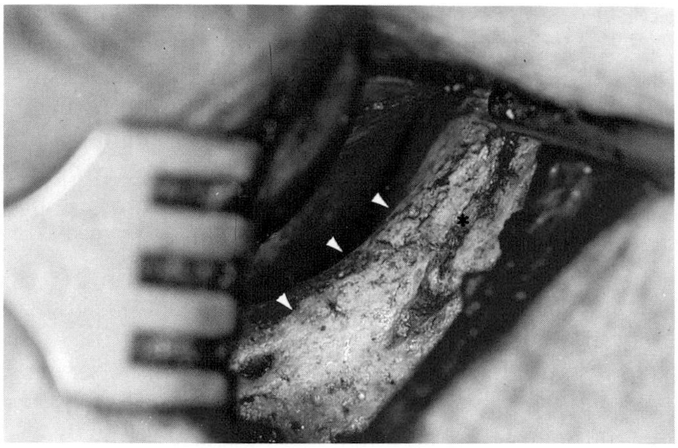

FIGURE 7–6

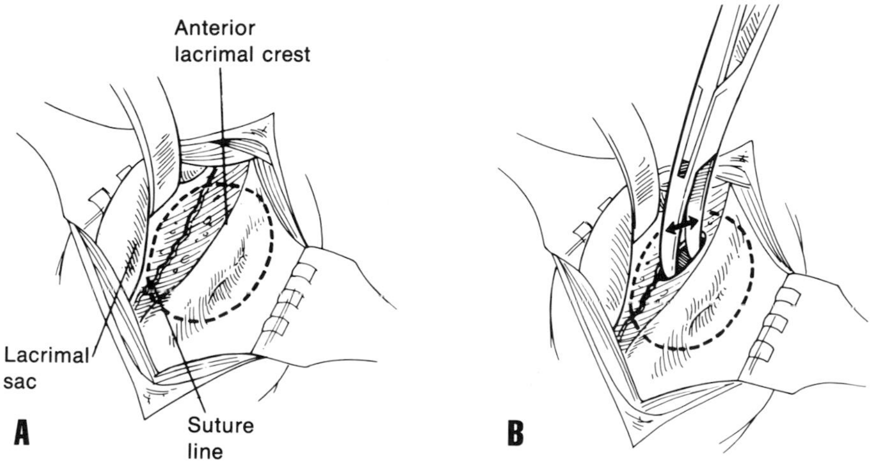

FIGURE 7–7

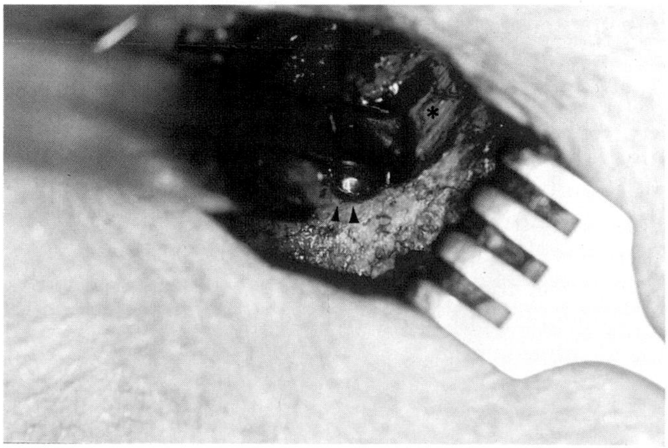

FIGURE 7–8

Figure 7–9. The nasal (medial) wall of the bony nasolacrimal canal is the most difficult, yet the most important piece of bone to remove. A flat tipped, front-biting rongeur is used to break the thick anterior attachment of the canal from the maxilla. Removal of this osseous ridge facilitates communication of the nasal cavity with the membranous nasolacrimal duct and lacrimal sac. When removing bone from the superoposterior aspect of the nasal window, rotation or rocking of the rongeur while engaging the bone should be avoided. This is to prevent an inadvertent bony fracture extending into the adjacent cribriform plate, resulting in cerebrospinal fluid leakage. The area of bone removal will vary widely in adults, depending on the anatomy of the lacrimal drainage system and nose. In general, the osteotomy opening is about 15 × 15 mm, with the boundaries extending anteriorly to about 5 mm anterior to the anterior lacrimal crest, posteriorly to the posterior lacrimal crest, superiorly to the medial canthal tendon, and inferiorly to the inferior orbital rim. Once osteotomy has been completed, bleeding from bone can be stopped by sealing the edges with bone wax. If mucosal bleeding is encountered, a small amount of lidocaine 2% with epinephrine (1:100,000), can be injected into the mucosa with a 30-gauge needle to provide hemostasis. A cotton pledget soaked in 5% cocaine can also be placed against the mucosal surface for hemostasis.

Incision Into the Sac

Complete hemostasis should be obtained before opening the lacrimal sac.

Figure 7–10A, B. A 00 Bowman probe is inserted through the superior canaliculus into the lacrimal sac, tenting up the medial wall of the sac. A size 66 Beaver blade is used to cut over the probe until the tip of the probe protrudes from the sac, thus verifying a full-thickness incision through both the periosteal and mucosal layers of the lacrimal sac. One blade of a Westcott scissors is then inserted through the lacrimal sac opening, and the incision is enlarged in a superoinferior direction, extending from the top of the fundus to the nasolacrimal duct. Following sac opening, the interior of the sac is carefully examined for tumor or dacryolith. A probe should also be inserted into the sac and the tissue surrounding the internal ostium inspected. If there is evidence of common canalicular stenosis or scarring in preventing smooth passage of the probe, the internal ostium can be resected with a Westcott scissors. A silicone stent must then be inserted to prevent stricture or complete closure.

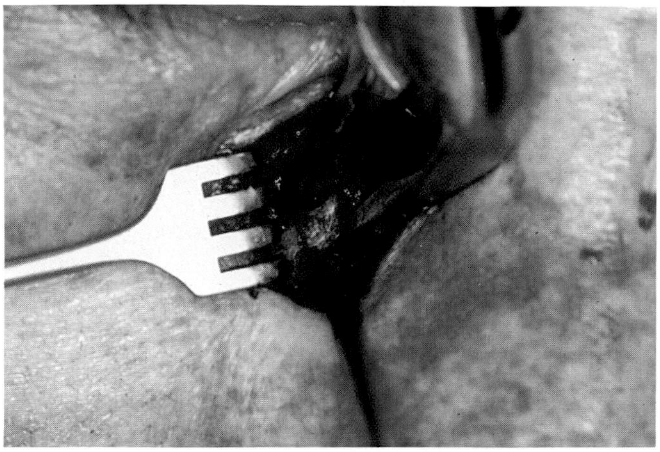

FIGURE 7–9

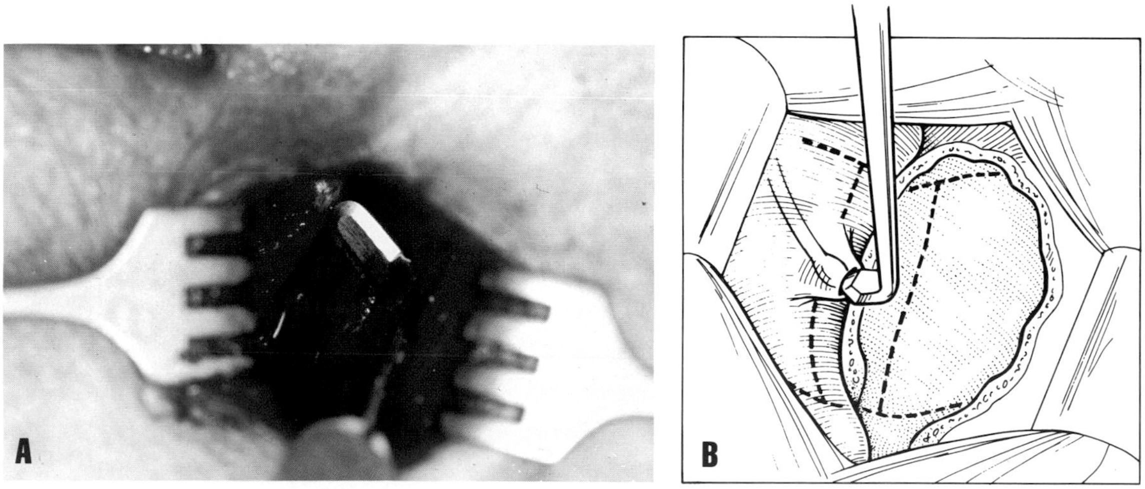

FIGURE 7–10

Incision of Mucosa

An H-shaped incision is designed (see Figure 7–10A), and the mucosa is incised with a size 66 Beaver blade at the point where the Bowman probe protrudes from the lacrimal sac and hits the nasal mucosa. The horizontal incision should be made along a line directly opposite the lacrimal sac incision. Westcott scissors can extend the mucosal incision superiorly and inferiorly to provide anterior and posterior flaps with dimensions similar to those of the lacrimal sac flaps.

Figure 7–11. Through the mucosal incision, the preplaced nasal packing can be seen, thus verifying the proper positioning of the mucosal incision. The nasal packing helps to insulate the nasal septum and middle turbinate from injury while the mucosa is being incised. Additionally, the packing in the nostril would prevent mucosal bleeding from running toward the oropharynx. Mucosal bleeding from the edges of the incision is then cauterized.

Figure 7–12A, B. Once hemostasis has been assured, the packing is removed from the nostril with a bayonet forceps. To avoid wound contamination, never pull the packing out through the osteotomy site; it should always be removed through the external naris.

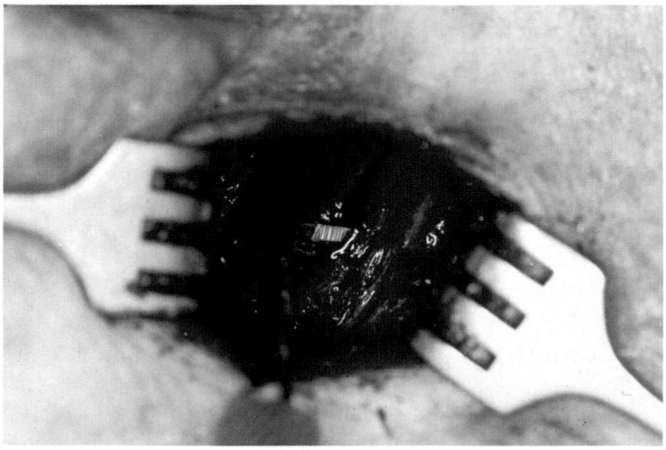

FIGURE 7–11

FIGURE 7–12

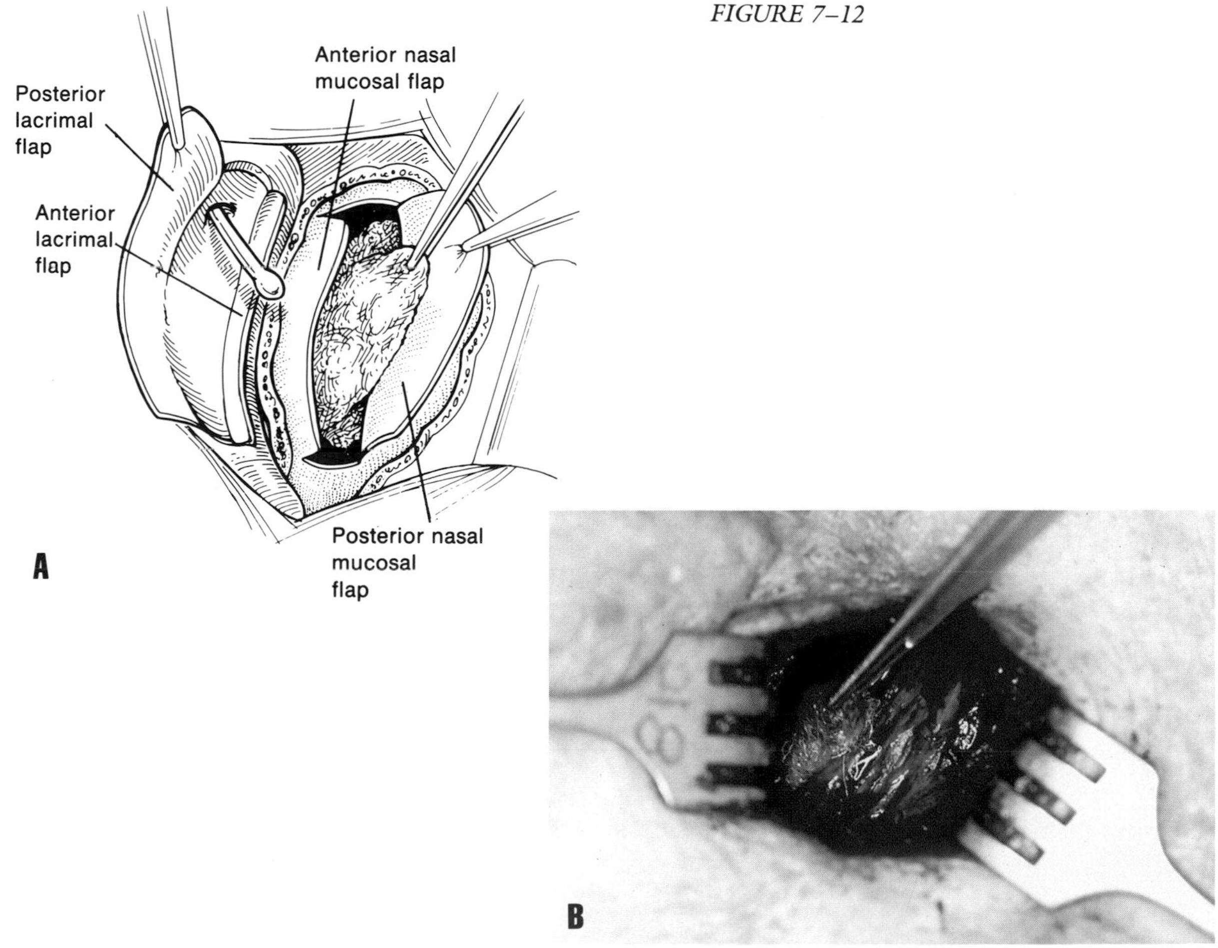

Anastomosis of Posterior Flaps

Figure 7–13A. The posterior flaps of the lacrimal sac and nasal mucosa are joined with two interrupted 4–0 Vicryl sutures on a semicircular needle. A short half-circle needle facilitates the passage of the suture in a tight, deep space. Union of the posterior flaps should overlap the posterior osteotomy edge.

Figure 7–13B. Lumen of the lacrimal sac (*arrow*) and middle meatus (*arrowhead*) should be inspected. Extreme care should be taken to avoid cheese-wiring of the flaps while passing the needle or tying the sutures. Occasionally, tying these preplaced sutures in a confined space can be difficult.

Figure 7–13C. One simple way of tying the sutures is the slipknot technique. Suture knots are tied external to the incision and slide into position without undue tension on the flaps. After passing the suture through the edges of the flaps, the suture is cut long. It does not matter which suture one starts with, as long as the proper sequence is followed while tying. The suture label *A* is looped over suture *B* as the first step. Suture *A* is looped under suture *B* and then over suture *A*. This creates the first loop in the knot. As one continues with the slipknot formation, a second loop identical with the first is created with the same sequence: *A* going over *B*, *A* under *B*, and then *A* over *A*. The final knot is tightened and should be firmly secured before sliding it down into the area of flap anastomosis. The sutures are then cut a few millimeters above the knot.

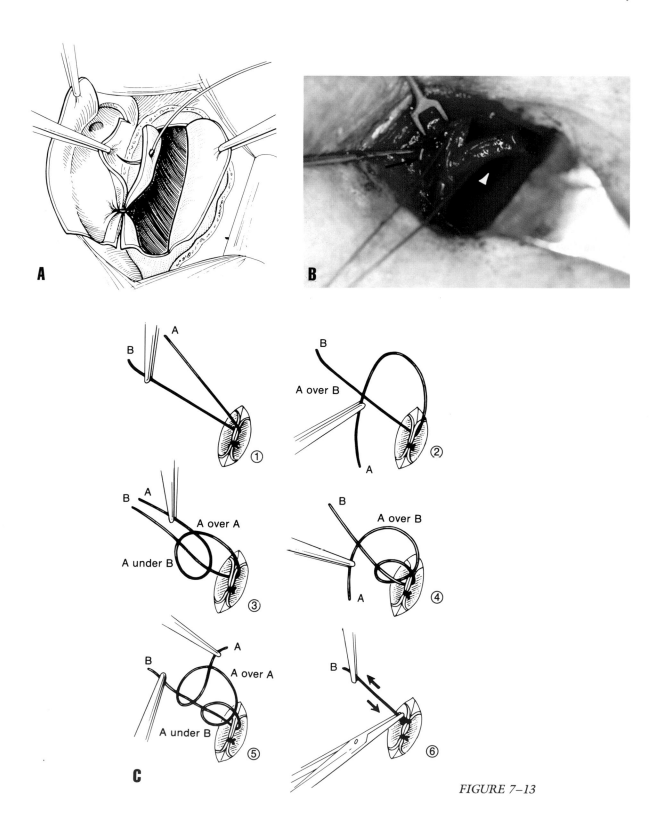

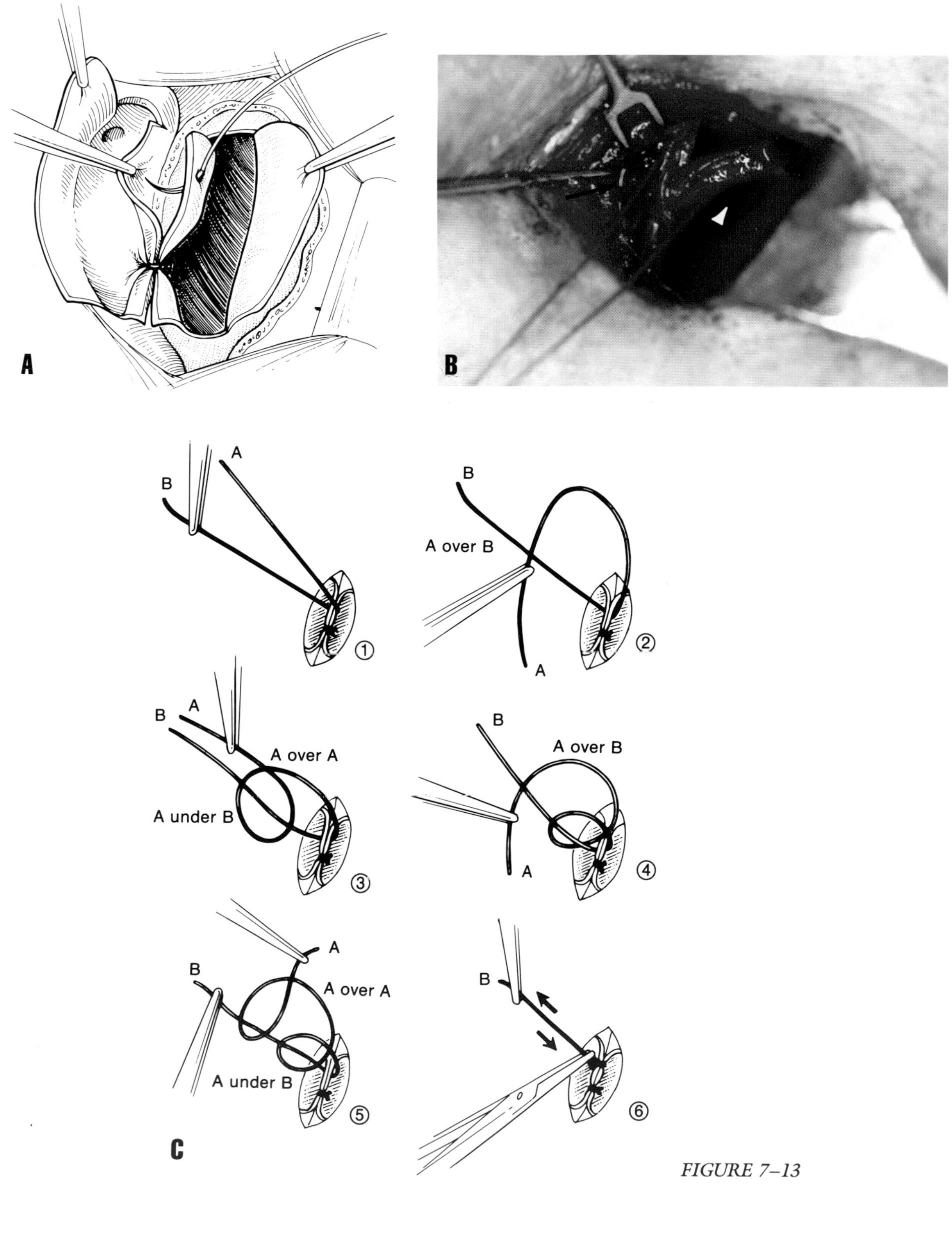
A
B
B
A
A over B
A
B
A
A over A
A under B
B
A over B
A
A
B
A over A
A under B
B
C
①
②
③
④
⑤
⑥

FIGURE 7–13

Silicone Stent Placement

After uniting the posterior flaps, both upper and lower puncta are dilated with a punctal dilator.

Figure 7–14. One end of a Crawford silicone tube is inserted into the upper canaliculus, through the newly created ostium, and into the middle meatus. The olive tip of the probe is guided out of the nasal cavity by a groove director. The probe is withdrawn from the external naris with the silicone tubing trailing. The procedure is then repeated through the lower canaliculus so that both ends of the tubing are delivered out of the nose.

Anastomosis of Anterior Flaps

Figure 7–15A. After placement of the silicone stent, the anterior lacrimal sac flap is united with the anterior nasal mucosal flap with two 4–0 Vicryl sutures.

Figure 7–15B. The silicone stent (*arrowhead*) can be seen under the flaps. The anterior flap should be tied with sufficient tension to prevent sagging of the flaps and to obstruct the internal ostium or scarring to the posterior flap anastomosis.

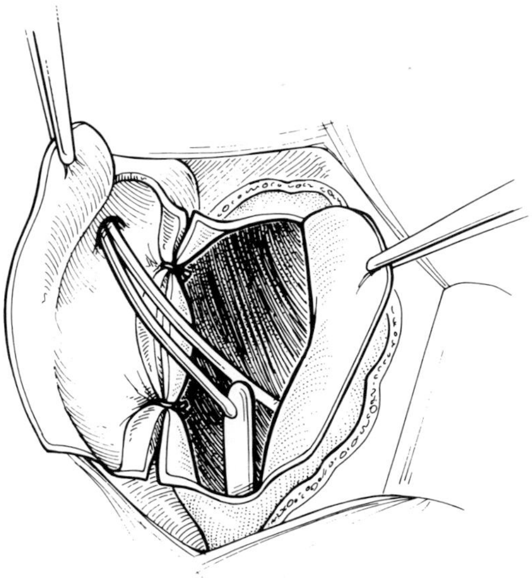

FIGURE 7–14

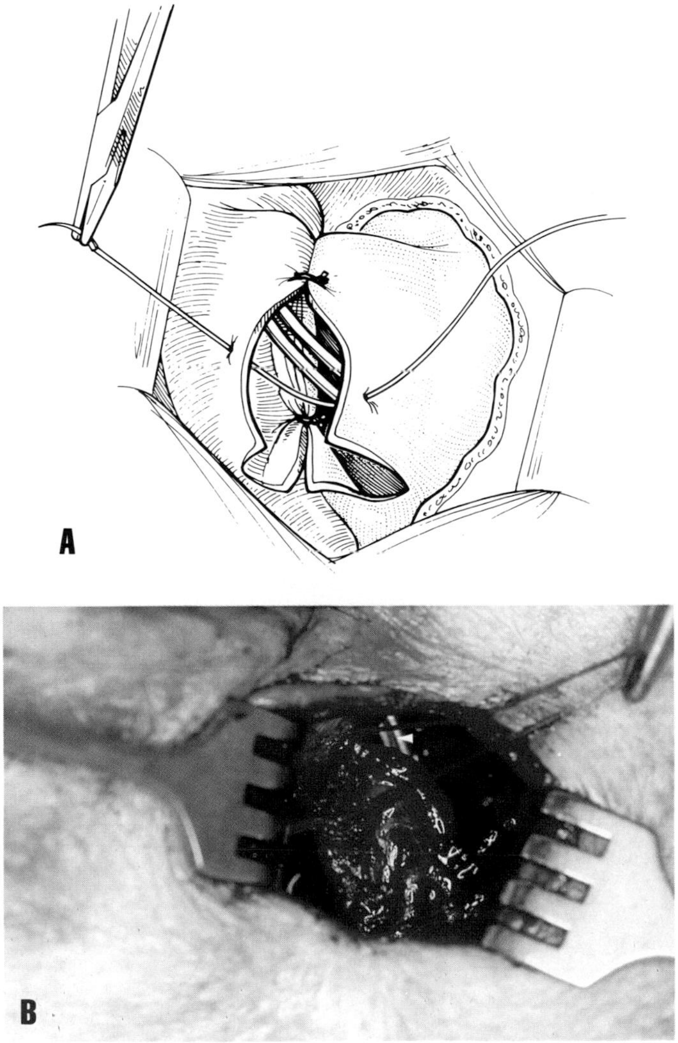

FIGURE 7–15

Skin Closure

Upon completion of the mucosal anastomosis and intubation with silicone stents, the cut edges of the periosteum are united with two 5–0 chromic sutures.

Figure 7–16. The orbicularis muscle layer is also reapproximated with 5–0 chromic sutures. The skin incision is closed with 6–0 nylon sutures in a vertical mattress fashion.

Tying of Silicone Stent

Figure 7–17. The tubing is tied tightly with four square knots under moderate tension over a metal probe placed across the external naris, while the portion of the tube at the medial canthal angle is held with a muscle hook. The ends of the silicone tube are cut close to the knots. The metal probe is removed, and the knots retract into the nostril and hang loosely in the middle meatus.

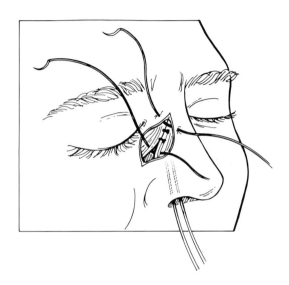

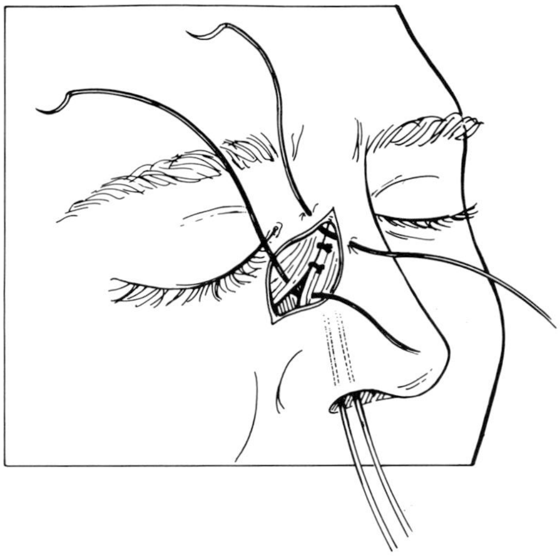

FIGURE 7–16

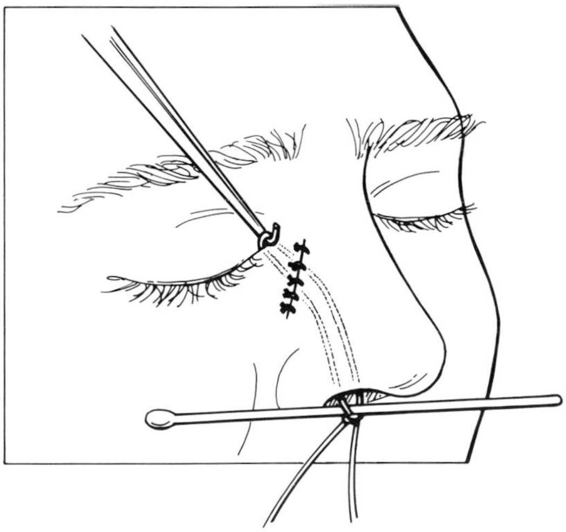

FIGURE 7–17

POSTOPERATIVE MANAGEMENT

Bacitracin ophthalmic ointment is placed on the incision site and Maxitrol (dexamethasone–neomycin–polymyxin B) eye drops are given three times a day for 1 week. In infected cases, bacitracin ophthalmic ointment and sulfacetamide (Sulamyd) 10% eyedrops are used. A 1-week course of oral antibiotic is also given.

The patient's activity is unrestricted, except for avoidance of nose blowing. A nasal decongestant spray is given twice daily for 1 week. Skin sutures are removed in 5 to 7 days, and the silicone stents are usually left in place for 3 to 6 months. The patient is instructed to wipe the eyelids in a unidirection toward the bridge of the nose, rather than outward toward the lateral canthus, minimizing the chance of catching the loop at the medial canthal region and pulling the stent out.

Chapter Eight

CONJUNCTIVODACRYO-CYSTORHINOSTOMY

David T. Tse

Conjunctivodacryocystorhinostomy (CDCR) is a lacrimal bypass procedure designed to circumvent stenosis or obstruction of the canalicular system by establishing a drainage conduit between the lacrimal lake and the nasal cavity. Common causes of canalicular obstruction include unsuccessful repair of a lacerated canaliculus, damage to the canaliculi from repeated probings, viral or chlamydia infections of the conjunctiva and lacrimal sac, chronic use of miotics or antiherpetic drugs, partial or total loss of the canalicular system secondary to tumor removal, congenital malformation of the lacrimal drainage system, inflammatory conditions such as sarcoidosis, iatrogenic thermal punctal closure, and idiopathy. Dacryocystorhinostomy (DCR) with Jones tube placement may also be indicated for failed DCR revisions in which the canaliculi are patent but nonfunctional.

PREOPERATIVE EVALUATION

Preoperative examination of the nasal cavity is imperative to rule out a deviated septum, enlarged middle turbinate, or any nasal abnormalities. A severely deviated nasal septum toward the operative side will invariably compromise proper placement and function of the Jones tube; hence, correction of this problem before CDCR surgery may be advisable. Preoperative recognition of an enlarged middle turbinate will alert the surgeon of a possible intraoperative need for partial turbinectomy to improve visualization and positioning of the tube.

Patients should be advised that the glass tubes will remain with them for the rest of their lives, and that direct trauma to the medial canthal region can cause breakage.

SURGICAL TECHNIQUE

A standard DCR is performed, as described in the previous chapter, up to the step of uniting the posterior flaps of the nasal mucosa and lacrimal sac. After anastomosis of the posterior flaps, the position of the middle turbinate is inspected. If the anteroinferior tip is situated above the plane of the posterior flaps and will likely affect the orientation of the Jones tube, it is then resected with a front-biting Takahashi forceps or angled scissors. Brisk bleeding will be encountered, but can be minimized by injecting lidocaine with epinephrine 15 to 20 minutes before resection. The use of a sheet of Surgicel (or Gelfoam soaked in thrombin) over the cut surface and packing with cocaine-moistened cottonoid will greatly enhance hemostasis.

The caruncle is infiltrated with a small amount of 2% lidocaine with 1:100,000 dilution of epinephrine on a 30-gauge needle. The needle then penetrates the conjunctiva medial to the caruncle and aimed toward the internal ostium in a 30° to 40° inferonasal direction. As the needle is advanced forward, anesthetic is infiltrated along this path.

Figure 8–1. Instead of excising the caruncle, as is frequently recommended, a horizontal snip incision is made on the caruncle with a Westcott scissors. Preservation of the caruncle permits it to serve as a collar for a snug fit of the canthal flange and prevents nasal migration of the tube.

Figure 8–2. A von Graefe knife is inserted through the incision on the caruncle and pushed along the needle track toward the posterior flap junction. The direction of the stab incision should be such that the tube will rest in a dependent drainage position once placed. Advancement of the knife blade through a dense fibrous tissue should be under firm digital control, as sudden "give" in tissue resistance may occur, thereby thrusting the knife forward. Once the tip of the knife is visualized within the internal ostium, the knife is moved up and down in small sawing movements to enlarge the track. Care should be taken not to inadvertently incise the lid margin with the sharp edges of the blade or to puncture the nasal septum with the knife tip.

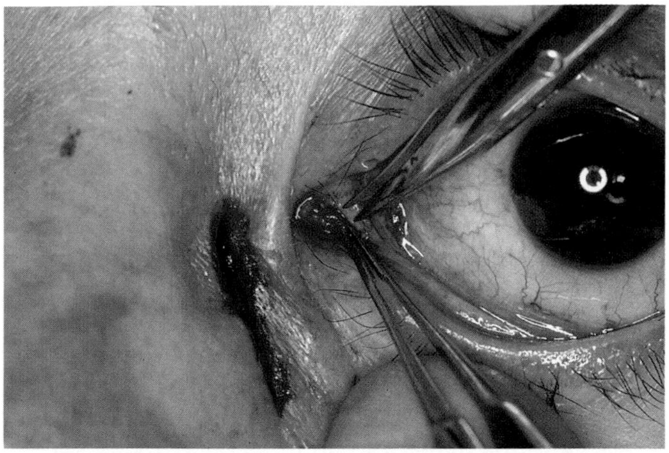

FIGURE 8–1

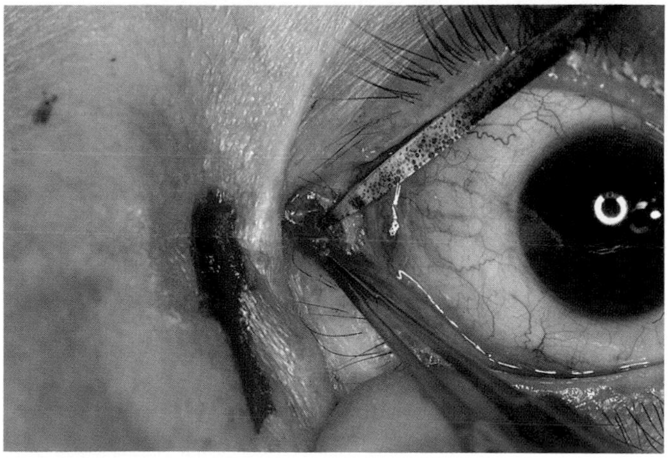

FIGURE 8–2

Figure 8–3. The von Graefe knife is withdrawn and a small-diameter Weiss gold dilator is introduced into the track to widen the aperture from the medial canthus to the nasal cavity. The use of a trephine to core out any tissue along the track to facilitate tube insertion is discouraged, since fibrous tissue is needed to envelop the tube and hold it into position. A Bowman probe is passed into the newly created tissue track, through the internal ostium until it makes contact with the nasal septum. A hemostat grasps the probe at the medial canthus, flush with the caruncle, and the length of the internal track is estimated. The distance from the probe end to the hemostat is measured, and a Jones Pyrex tube, 3 to 4 mm shorter than the recorded length, is selected from the tube kit. A 4-mm diameter flange is preferred, since it lessens the chance of inward tube migration; however, if it crowds the medial canthal region, it should be exchanged for a smaller-diameter flange.

Figure 8–4. A Bowman probe is passed into the lumen of the selected Jones tube; the probe is then inserted into the tissue tunnel until the tip is visualized in the osteotomy site. While using the Bowman probe as a guide, the Jones tube is pushed into the tunnel with the finger tip. One should not use excessive force to advance the tube into the ostium. If resistance is encountered, a larger-sized gold dilator should be used to progressively enlarge the aperture. Once the tube is embedded within the track, the flange should be partially hidden within the lacrimal recess at the medial canthus. Internally, the shaft of the tube should be resting over the posterior flap anastomosis, and its distal end at least 2 to 3 mm away from the nasal septum. If the tube abuts the nasal septum, or its distal end does not extend into the nasal cavity by about 2 mm, the tube should be removed and an appropriately sized tube reintroduced. Once satisfied with its placement, the position of the tube is again verified through a nasal speculum inspection with the aid of a headlight. One must be certain that the end of the tube is not in contact with the septum and that it is not hidden from view by the middle turbinate.

The anterior flaps are anastomosed with two 4–0 Vicryl sutures. The periosteal edges are also reapproximated with several 4–0 Vicryl sutures. The orbicularis muscle and skin are closed in separate layers. A 6–0 nylon suture is tied around the collar of the Pyrex tube, with both arms going beneath the orbicularis, exiting the skin, and tied in the medial canthal area. This is an elective step that ensures tube position and prevents accidental displacement in the perioperative period. The skin sutures are removed in 7 days. The suture anchoring the tube may be removed in 3 weeks.

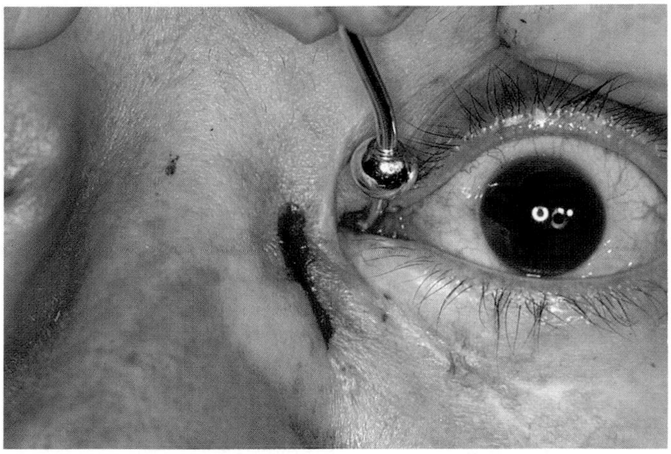

FIGURE 8–3

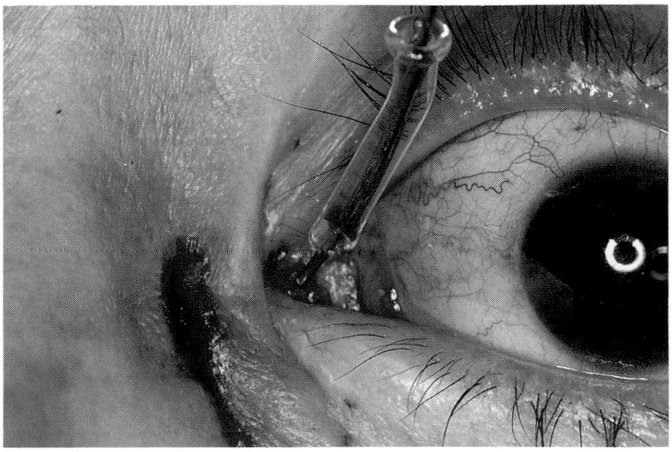

FIGURE 8–4

POSTOPERATIVE CARE

In addition to the routine postoperative care for a DCR procedure, Jones tubes require frequent cleaning and intermittent replacement. Four weeks after surgery, a nasal speculum examination is performed, without vasoconstricting the nasal mucosa. This assures a true topographic survey of the tube position relative to the nasal septum under normal conditions. The tube should be replaced if it is too long or too short. Similarly, the tube should be replaced if the flange is too large and is irritating the globe.

For the tube replacement or cleaning process, the medial canthal region is infiltrated with small amount of anesthetic: 4% cocaine nasal spray is used in the nose for anesthesia, and topical anesthetic drops are applied to the eye. The tube collar is grasped with a 0.3-mm forceps and pulled out of the CDCR ostium. Immediately, a dilator is inserted into the fistulous track as a temporary stent. The external surface of the tube is cleaned with soap and water. The inner lumen is cleaned by forcing a small wad of cotton through with a Bowman probe. After cleaning, the Jones tube is ready for reinsertion. The dilator is removed from the CDCR ostium. The clean Jones tube is slid onto the Bowman probe, and the probe is inserted into the ostium. The tube is returned to its well-healed fistulous track by gently pushing on the flange.

After the tube exchange, the patient is instructed to irrigate the Pyrex tube with sterile normal saline on a regular basis. The solution is instilled into the medial canthal region and the patient quickly sniffs in the fluid, flushing out the lumen. Ideally, the tube is removed, cleaned, inspected, and possibly exchanged once a year.

Chapter Nine

ENTROPION

Thaddeus S. Nowinski

Entropion, an inward turning of the eyelid margin and appendages, remains one of the most common eyelid malpositions seen in clinical practice. The involutional variety is the most frequently encountered, whereas those cases of cicatricial etiologies are the most difficult to treat. The true spastic and congenital types are less commonly seen.

It is important to distinguish between entropion and eyelash misdirection or aberrant growth. *Trichiasis* is a misdirection of normal lashes, whereas *distichiasis* represents an abnormal growth of lashes from the multipotential tarsal meibomian glands. Normal lashes may be mechanically misdirected by exaggerated folds of skin. *Epiblepharon*, a redundant horizontal pretarsal skin fold, epicanthal folds, or dermatochalasis may push lashes toward the globe.

PREOPERATIVE EVALUATION

The constant rubbing of the eyelashes and eyelid skin against the ocular surface results in abrasions of the cornea and conjunctiva. This often can progress to secondary stromal scarring, corneal thinning, and vascularization. Patients complain of a chronic foreign body sensation, redness, tearing, and discharge. Corneal ulceration and perforation may occur in extreme cases.

The approach to the evaluation and repair of entropion is intimately associated with knowledge of lower eyelid anatomy and function. The retractors of the lower eyelid are analogous to the levator aponeurosis and Mueller's muscle of the upper lid, and they greatly contribute to lower eyelid function and stability. An extension of the inferior rectus muscle, the capsulopalpebral head, travels forward in the inferior orbit, surrounds the inferior oblique muscle, and contributes to the formation of Lockwood's ligament. It then continues forward and superiorly, fuses with the orbital septum, and has multiple insertions, the strongest being to the inferior border of the tarsus (see Chapter 1). Attenuation or disinsertion of these attachments of the lower eyelid retractors renders instability of the tarsus and subsequent inward rotation of the lid margin. This is probably the most frequently encountered anatomic defect found in involutional entropion.

The lower eyelid retractors have fine extensions to the orbicularis and eyelid skin. A weakening of the extensions, along with loss of the attachments between the preseptal orbicularis muscle and the orbital septum, allows the preseptal orbicularis to override the pretarsal orbicularis. Spasms of the orbicularis may occur because of an acute inflammatory episode and result in a temporary entropion. However, almost all cases that were once termed *spastic* are now known to represent involutional entropion, with the associated lower eyelid anatomic pathology.

The lateral and medial canthal tendons rigidly anchor the lids to the orbital bony periosteum. Horizontal laxity of the lids results when stretching of these tendons, especially the lateral canthal tendon, allows displacement and loss of elasticity of the lower eyelid. These changes can be a factor in the functional abnormalities of both entropion and ectropion of the lower eyelid.

Eyelid Evaluation

The etiology of entropion may include multiple factors, including loss of the integrity of the lower eyelid retractors and the canthal tendons, secondary overriding of the preseptal orbicularis oculi muscle, and a decrease in orbital volume caused by trauma or relative enophthalmos secondary to aging changes. Cicatricial processes secondary to ocular or systemic disorders or trauma may produce shrinkage of the conjunctival fornices, symblepharon formation, and distortion and metaplasia of the lid margin and meibomian glands.

The lower eyelid retractors contribute to a 3- to 4-mm downward excursion of the lower eyelid on down gaze. Loss of this movement may indicate weakening or disinsertion of the lower eyelid retractors. Horizontal eyelid laxity, caused by canthal tendon laxity, can be quantitatively evaluated by noting the relative elasticity of the eyelid by pulling the lid downward and observing the movement of snapping back to its original position without allowing blinking. Another method of evaluation involves pulling the lid forward and noting the relative amount of dislocation away from the globe that is produced. Forceful squeezing of the eyelids by the patient may reproduce an intermittent entropion and permits observance of the overriding of the preseptal orbicularis on the tarsal eyelid.

Cicatricial components should be suspected if resistance to downward traction is encountered and if horizontal traction on the lid does not temporarily improve the entropion. Difficulty of lid eversion also may be present in these cases. The conjunctival fornices should be inspected for symblepharon and shallowing of the entire fornix, as well as conjunctival, lid margin, and meibomian gland abnormalities.

Procedural Choices

The techniques that have withstood the test of time have addressed the lower eyelid retractors as essential in the functional abnormality of entropion.

Full-thickness eyelid sutures remain a popular office or bedside procedure for involutional and spastic entropion. They indirectly tighten the lower eyelid retractors and transfer the eversion force to the anterior lamella (orbicularis and skin). This is accomplished by promoting an inflammatory cicatrix between the retractors and the orbicularis muscle and by anchoring the skin and orbicularis, preventing overriding of the preseptal orbicularis muscle. The use of full-thickness sutures is quick, easily performed, and gives immediate relief. However, its relatively high recurrence rate limits its usefulness for a definitive long-term correction.

Direct repair, including advancement and tightening of the lower eyelid retractors allows an anatomic correction of the defect in most patients. This repair is analogous to the aponeurotic repair of ptosis of the upper eyelid. Intraoperative adjustment and evaluation of lid contour and function yields more predictable results. Horizontal laxity is often present, and a lid-tightening procedure is indicated as an adjunct to eyelid retractors repair. For horizontal eyelid tightening, the lateral tarsal strip procedure is preferred (see Chapter 10). Medial canthal tightening, and excision of excess skin and orbicularis muscle, can also be utilized in selected cases.

Rotation of the eyelid margin can also be employed for involutional and mild-to-moderate cases of cicatricial entropion. A full-thickness horizontal incision disinserts all attachments of the lower eyelid at the level of the inferior border of the tarsus. This full-thickness defect is then repaired to transfer the eversion effect of the lower eyelid retractors to the anterior lamella of the remaining lid margin bridge flap. This is similar in concept to the full-thickness suture technique, but is done under direct visualization, and it promotes a much better-defined scar tissue barrier to shorten the retractors, evert the tarsal plate, and inhibit upward overriding of the preseptal orbicularis muscle.

A modification of this procedure is used in the upper lid for mild to moderate cicatricial entropion. In these cases, the upper eyelid tarsus is incised horizontally 4 to 5 mm above the lid margin. The posterior lamella is similarly sutured to the anterior lamella of the bridge flap to accomplish rotation of the upper eyelid margin.

SURGICAL TECHNIQUES

Full-Thickness Sutures

Topical tetracaine is applied, and 2% lidocaine with 1:100,000 epinephrine is injected subcutaneously and subconjunctivally. The lower eyelid is pulled away from the globe with forceps. One arm of a double-armed 4–0 chromic suture is passed in a perpendicular fashion through the eyelid, starting deep within the inferior fornix. The conjunctiva is entered well below the inferior border of the tarsus, and the retractors are engaged with the needle tip.

Figure 9–1. A sagittal view of suture passage through the lower eyelid. The skin and the preseptal orbicularis muscle are retracted downward with forceps, and the needle is then passed through the orbicularis and skin to exit about 2 to 3 mm below the lash line. The needle exit point can be placed higher or lower, depending on the amount of eversion effect desired.

The other arm of the suture is passed 3 mm from and parallel to the first arm. It is brought through all the layers of the lid in an identical fashion. The arms of the suture are tied to each other tightly to evert the eyelid.

Figure 9–2. Two or three additional sutures are placed in a similar fashion across the eyelid.

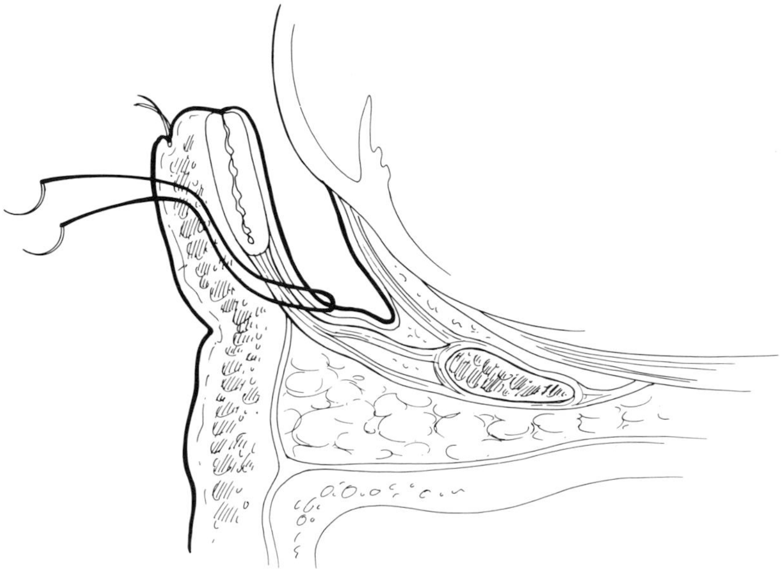

FIGURE 9–1

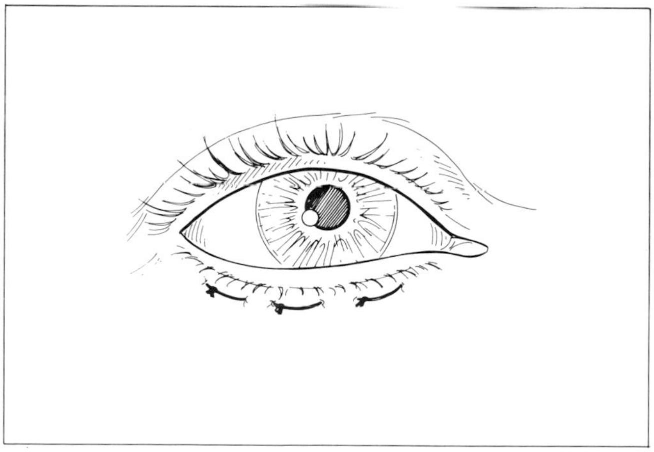

FIGURE 9–2

Retractors Approach

Subcutaneous infiltration is made with 2% lidocaine with epinephrine. A marking pen is used to mark a subciliary incision from just lateral to the lacrimal punctum to the lateral canthus. A 4–0 silk traction suture is placed at the central portion of the lower eyelid margin. The needle is passed horizontally in a lamellar fashion through the tarsal plate, and the suture is retracted superiorly. This places all the structures of the posterior lamella on tension, while allowing the anterior lamella of skin and orbicularis to be mobilized.

An incision is made through skin with a size 15 Bard–Parker blade. The skin and orbicularis inferior to the incision are grasped and tented anteriorly. The orbicularis muscle is then incised centrally with a Westcott scissors.

One blade of the scissors is passed bluntly laterally through the buttonhole, and the incision is extended with minimal dissection. This is also done medially, to expose the avascular postorbicular fascial plane.

Figure 9–3A, B. The orbital septum is placed on tension, and an incision is made below the fusion of the septum and the lid retractors with Westcott scissors. The septum is opened in both directions to expose the orbital fat pads.

The fat pads are the key anatomic landmarks to look for, since the retractors are located beneath them. Gentle pressure on the globe will facilitate forward herniation of the fat pads.

Figure 9–4A, B. The fat pads are retracted superiorly to fully expose the underlying white retractor band (grasped by forceps). The patient can be asked to look downward, and force-generating movement will also help identify the retractors.

The orbital fat pads are gently dissected from the anterior surface of the retractors. Inspection is made for dehiscence or disinsertion of the retractors.

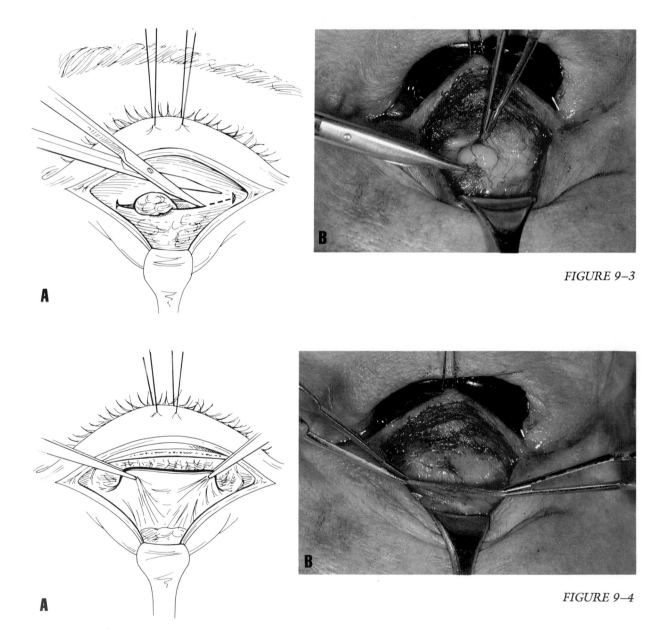

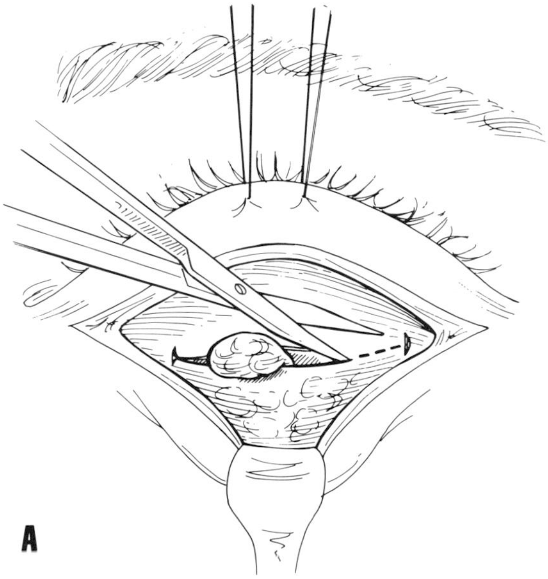

A

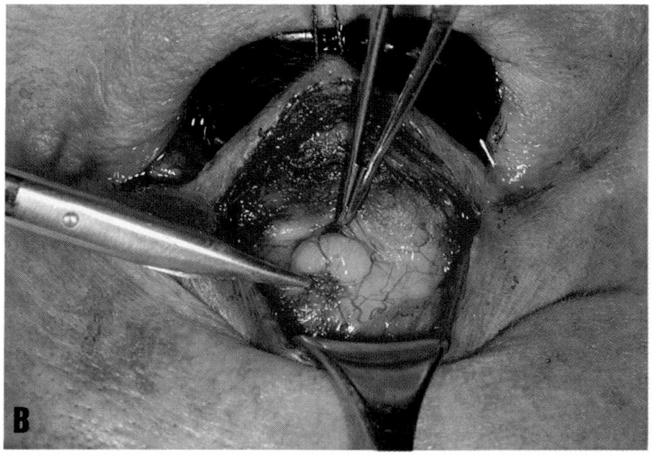

FIGURE 9–3

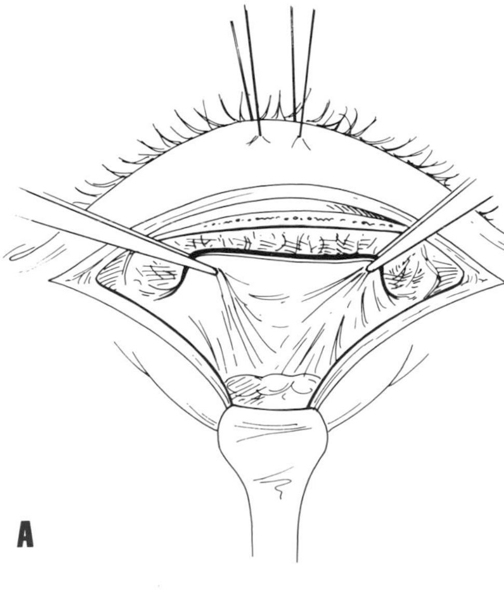

A

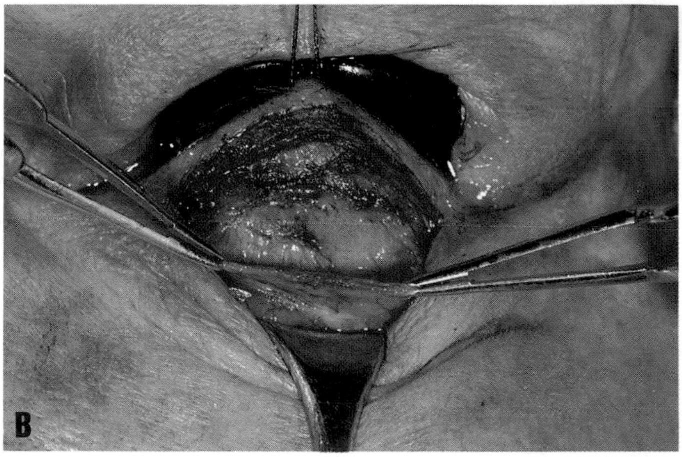

FIGURE 9–4

Figure 9–5. The disinserted edge of the retractors is then reattached onto the inferior margin of the tarsus with a 5–0 Vicryl suture.

Figure 9–6. A sagittal view of suture placement. The retractors should not be sutured to the anterior surface of the tarsal plate, as it may induce lid margin eversion. If the retractors were reunited with the tarsal plate properly, there should be a smooth downward movement of the lower eyelid on attempted down gaze.

Figure 9–7. Additional interrupted sutures are placed to complete the repair. Excess orbital fat can be removed if desired. If concomitant horizontal laxity is present, a lid-tightening procedure is performed. The lateral tarsal strip procedure is preferred.

A small amount of excess skin can be removed from the inferior edge of the incision. The lower lid incision is closed with a running 6–0 nylon suture. The lateral canthal extension can be closed with interrupted sutures if a tarsal strip has also been performed.

Marginal Rotation

A horizontal line is outlined with a marking pen on the lower lid, about 3 to 4 mm from the margin. The marking begins at about 1 to 2 mm lateral to the punctum and extends to the lateral canthal angle. Two percent lidocaine with epinephrine is injected subcutaneously across the entire lid. Two 4–0 silk traction sutures are placed through the lid margin and retracted superiorly.

Figure 9–8. A lid plate is placed in the lower fornix to separate the lid and the globe for protection. A size 15 Bard–Parker blade is used to create a full-thickness eyelid incision in the middle of the lid. The blade should be placed perpendicularly to the plane of the lid and parallel to the lid margin.

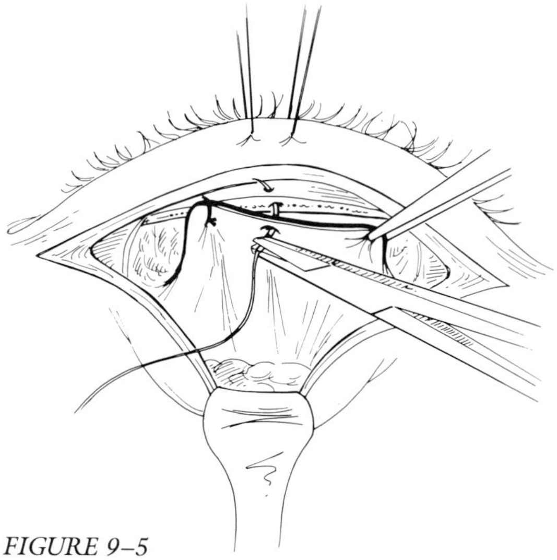

FIGURE 9–5

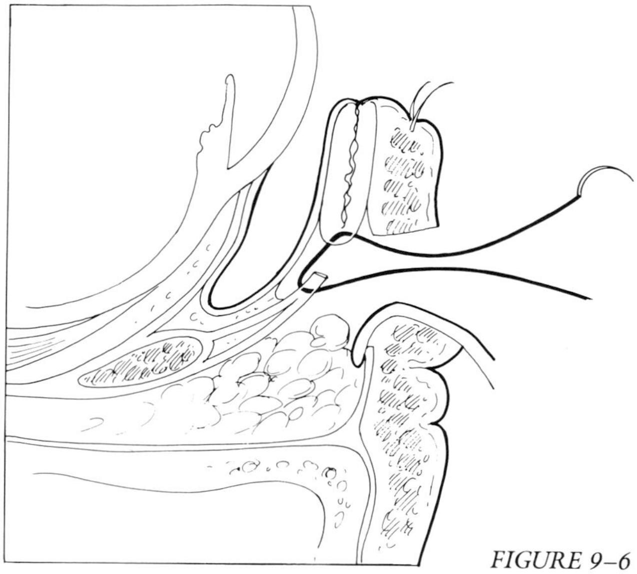

FIGURE 9–6

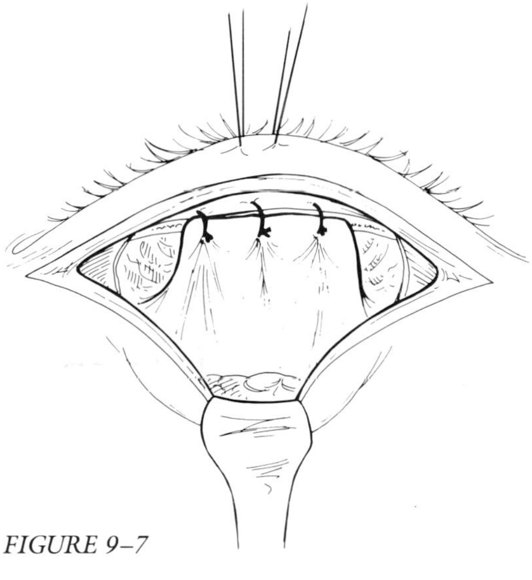

FIGURE 9–7

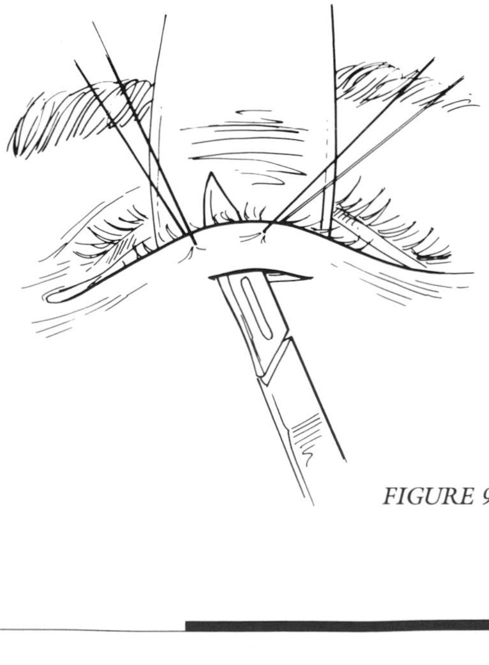

FIGURE 9–8

Figure 9–9. Straight scissors are used to extend the full-thickness incision laterally to the end of the lid, and medially to just lateral to the lacrimal punctum. For patients in whom the entropion is present only laterally, the incision is limited to the lateral two-thirds of the lid.

Figure 9–10. One arm of a double-armed 4–0 chromic suture is passed in a lamellar fashion through the tarsal stump on the inferior bridge. Two or three additional double-armed sutures are placed 3 to 4 mm apart. Each pair may be tagged with clamps to help avoid confusion. Each parallel pair of needle arms is then attached to the superior flap in a plane just anterior to the tarsus and posterior to the pretarsal orbicularis muscle.

Figure 9–11. The sutures are then passed through the orbicularis and skin 2-mm below the lash line. Before each pair is tied, the skin incision is closed with a 7–0 nylon suture in a running fashion. The double-armed sutures are each tied over a small cotton bolster, which serves as a fulcrum for eversion of the lid margin.

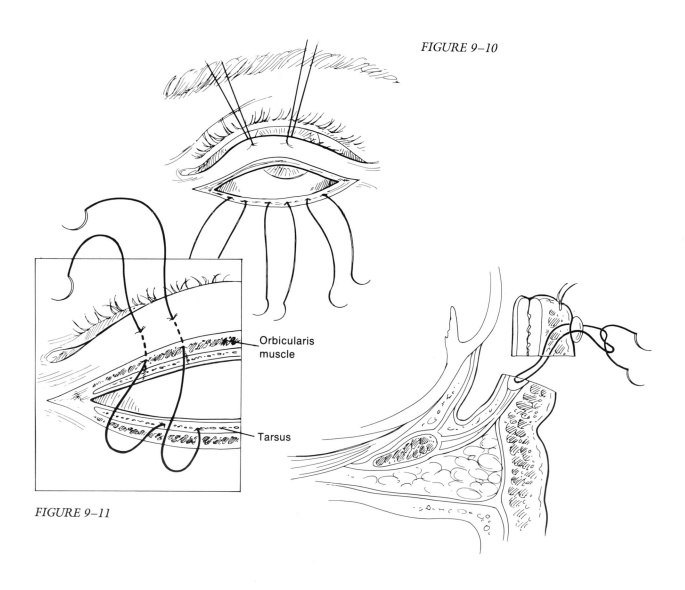

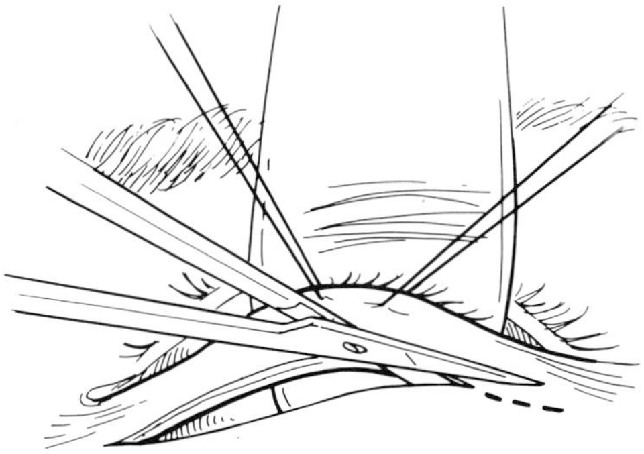

FIGURE 9–9

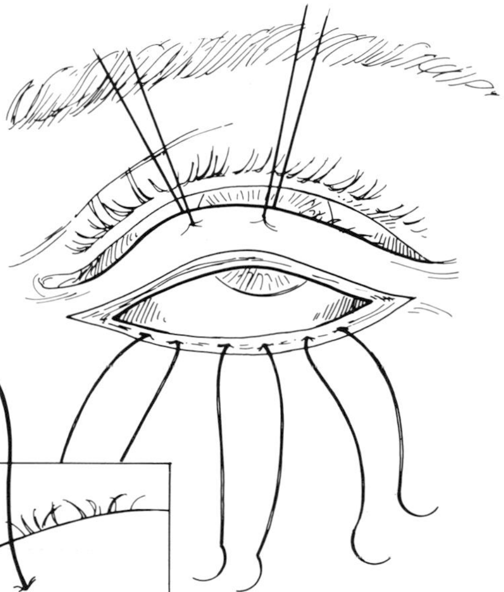

FIGURE 9–10

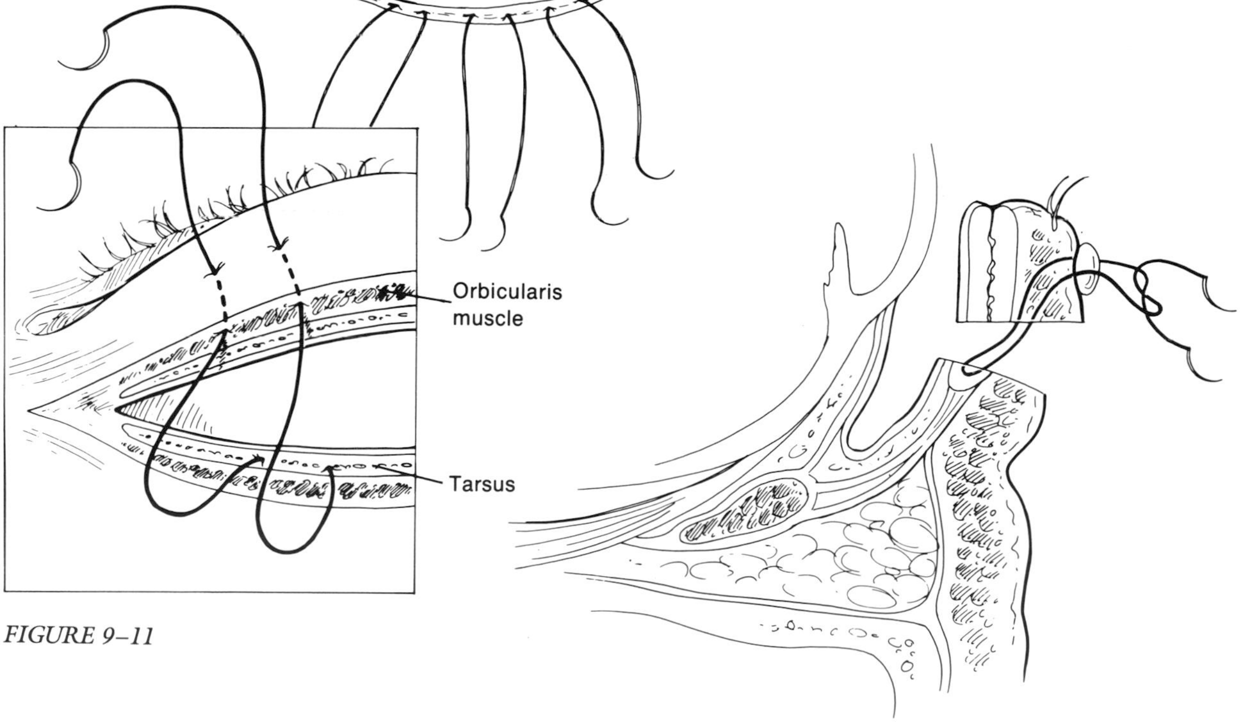

FIGURE 9–11

POSTOPERATIVE CARE

Antibiotic–steroid ointment is applied, a light dressing is placed overnight and is removed the next day. Ice packs may be used for 2 days, and ointment is continued four times daily for 1 week. Nylon sutures are removed at 1 week.

AVOIDANCE AND MANAGEMENT OF COMPLICATIONS

A small overcorrection at the time of the procedure is desired in those techniques for entropion repair that use full-thickness sutures or marginal rotation. However, ectropion with punctal eversion may result if the sutures are placed through the anterior lamella too close to the lid margin. One or more sutures can be removed at 1 week and massage of the lid will help remedy any overcorrection. For those patients in whom the entropion mainly exists temporally, the full-thickness sutures need be placed only in the lateral two-thirds of the eyelid. Ectropion may also result in those procedures that advance the retractor band under direct visualization, if the retractors are reapproximated to the anterior tarsal surface, rather than to the inferior border of the tarsus. Local anesthesia is preferable, since lid height, contour, and movement of the lid can be evaluated and adjusted intraoperatively to decrease this possibility.

Overzealous shortening or advancement of the retractors will exaggerate their effect, leading to eyelid retraction and scleral show. Close monitoring of the lid's relative position to the globe during the procedure will minimize this complication. Excessive removal of lower eyelid skin may also exaggerate this effect, and should be avoided.

Failure to recognize horizontal laxity of the lids will exaggerate the effect of the lower lid retractors and the instability of the lateral canthal tendon. Lower lid retraction and ectropion are both common if a lid-tightening procedure is not performed simultaneously when needed at the time of surgical repair. The lateral tarsal strip procedure usually corrects horizontal laxity and maintains the almond-shaped canthal angle, while avoiding phimosis and lid notching.

Eyelid margin necrosis may occur with the marginal rotation procedure if the marginal arcade is violated. The full-thickness incision in lower lids should be placed at or below the inferior border of the tarsus and, in the upper lid, should be placed through the tarsus above the marginal arcade; at least 4 mm from the lid margins, to avoid vascular compromise. Fistula formation may occur in lid-splitting procedures and should be excised and repaired.

Chapter Ten

ECTROPION

David T. Tse

Ectropion is a condition commonly encountered in clinical practice. The pathogenesis of ectropion varies. Frueh and Schoengarth (1982), in an excellent paper, succinctly summarized in a systematic manner the evaluation and treatment of the six elements of pathology that may be present in an ectropic eyelid. These factors include horizontal lid laxity, medial canthal tendon laxity, punctal malposition, vertical tightness of the skin, orbicularis paresis secondary to seventh nerve palsy, and lower eyelid retractors disinsertion.

The presence of each factor is determined by clinical examination. One or more of these components may be present in an ectropic eyelid. Proper recognition of the underlying anatomic defect will enable the surgeon to select the appropriate surgical procedure for correction. There are many procedures described for the treatment of each of these eyelid malpositions. In this chapter, one technique will be recommended for each of the conditions.

HORIZONTAL LID LAXITY

Horizontal lid laxity is most likely a result of stretching of the lateral and medial canthal tendons, rather than actual elongation of the tarsal plate. This produces a redundancy in the lid tissues, causing the lid margin to fall away from the globe. Horizontal lid laxity can be corrected surgically by several procedures. One popular method is full-thickness excision of a wedge of eyelid tissue and closing the defect primarily. One disadvantage of this method of horizontal lid shortening is that it often leads to lateral canthal deformities, such as blunting of the lateral canthal angle. Additionally, a block resection technique often exaggerates the laxity of the medial and lateral canthal tendon and may produce a horizontally narrowed palpebral fissure. More importantly, surgical correction is not aimed at the underlying defect, namely, stretching of the lateral canthal tendon.

In correcting this element of lid malposition, the *lateral tarsal strip* procedure advocated by Anderson (1979) is preferred. In this technique, the eyelid is shortened at the lateral canthal end of the lid. The advantages of this technique are that (1) surgery is directed at correcting the anatomic defect, (2) there are no marginal lid sutures, (3) the danger of lid notching or misdirected lashes irritating the cornea is avoided, (4) canthal malposition and lid shortening may be corrected simultaneously, (5) the procedure can be performed quickly, and (6) the almond-shaped canthal angle is preserved.

The procedure is also useful in correcting eyelid laxity and canthal malposition in an anophthalmic socket. This technique provides immediate lid strength, allowing it to support weight, as is needed when there is an ocular prosthesis.

Procedure: Lateral Tarsal Strip

Lidocaine 2% with 1:100,000 epinephrine is injected into the lateral canthal region with a 30-gauge needle. A small amount of anesthetic is also delivered to the periosteum of the lateral orbital rim and the temporal inferior fornix.

Figure 10–1. Surgeon's view from the head of the operating table. The procedure is being performed on the left lower eyelid. A lateral canthotomy is made with a Stevens scissors until the lateral orbital rim is exposed.

Figure 10–2. The tip of the Freer periosteal elevator is inside the bony rim. The periosteum is exposed. One should avoid cutting into the periosteum, as it will serve as an anchoring structure for the lid later on.

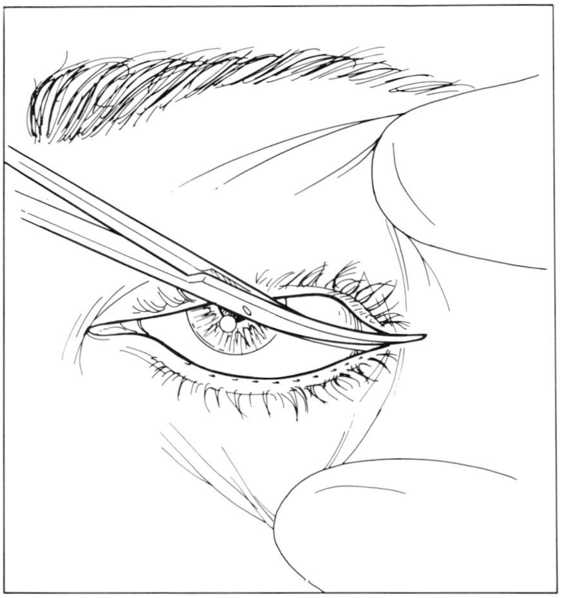

FIGURE 10–1

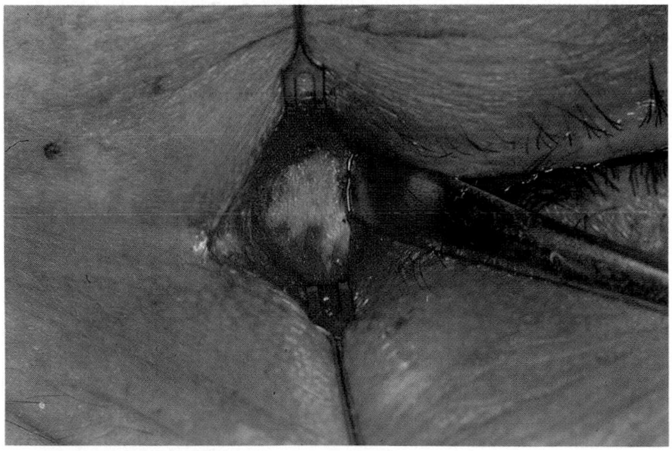

FIGURE 10–2

Figure 10–3A, B. An inferior cantholysis is performed by incising the attachment of the inferior crus of the lateral canthal tendon from the lateral orbital rim. Once the inferior crus of the lateral canthal tendon is severed, the entire eyelid becomes mobile. Occasionally, the temporal pocket of the preaponeurotic fat pad may prolapse through this incision. The prolapsing fat pad can be cauterized with a bipolar cautery.

Figure 10–4A, B. With a straight scissors, the eyelid is separated horizontally at the gray line into anterior and posterior lamellae. Incision should be made in the gray line, without cutting into the tarsal plate. At times, the gray line may be indistinct owing to erythema from chronic irritation. One way to identify this landmark is to gently pinch on the lid margin with a nontoothed forceps to look for secretions from the meibomian gland openings. The gray line is located immediately anterior to the secretions. The length of incision along the gray line depends on the amount of lid shortening needed.

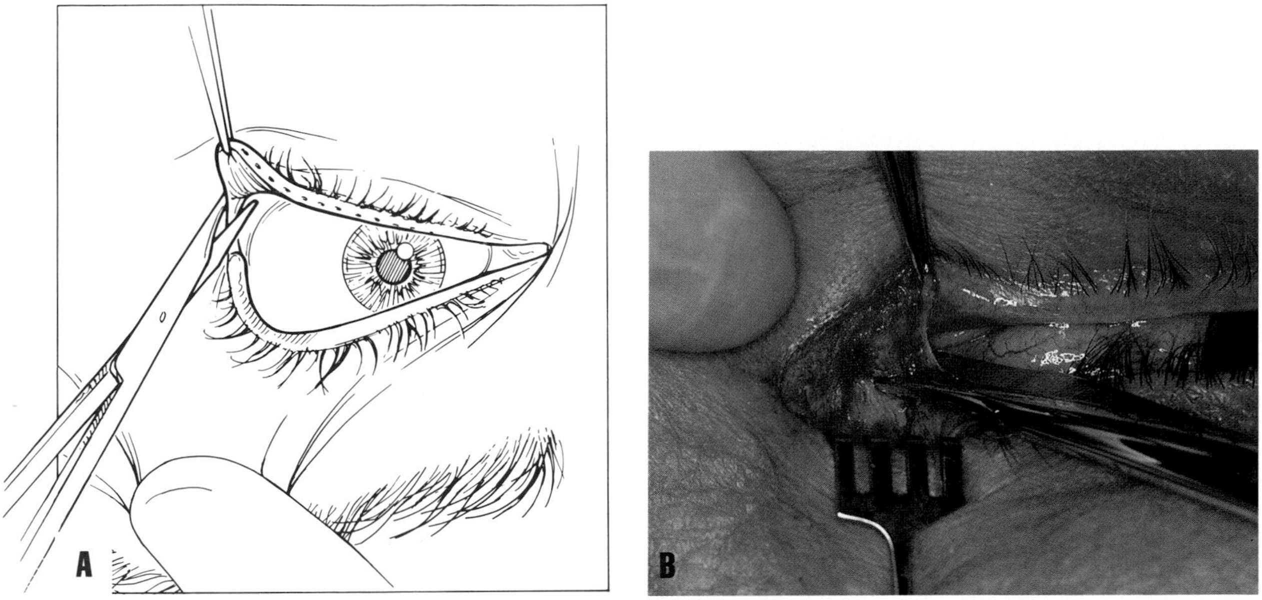

FIGURE 10–3

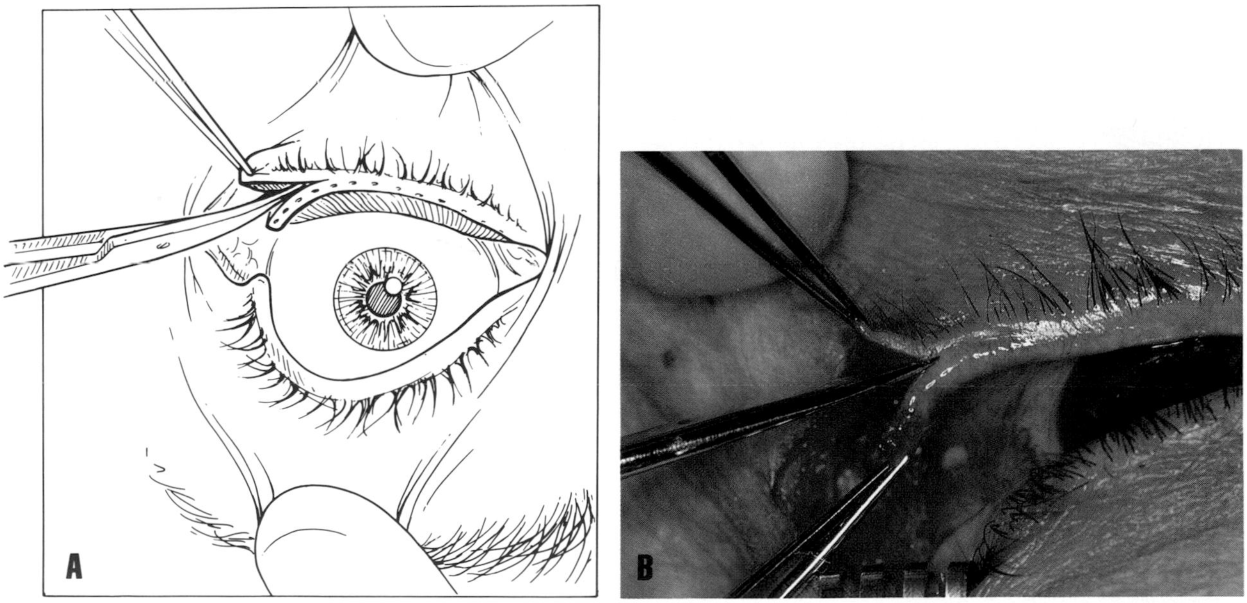

FIGURE 10–4

Figure 10–5A, B. A horizontal incision, equal in length to the amount of lid splitting, is made with a scissors at the inferior margin of the tarsal plate. This maneuver severs the conjunctiva and lower eyelid retractors from the tarsal plate, thereby creating a 4- to 4.5-mm wide strip of tarsus.

Figure 10–6A, B. The mucosal lining at the superior margin of the tarsal plate is then trimmed off with a straight scissors. One should avoid excising any tarsal substance. While the tarsal plate is stabilized by a tissue forceps over a metal plate, a size 15 Bard–Parker blade is used to scrape the palpebral conjunctiva off the tarsus. The tarsus must be denuded of conjunctiva to avoid epithelial inclusion cyst formation in the area of the new lateral canthus.

The tarsal plate is grasped with a tissue forceps and pulled with sufficient tension in a lateral direction to place the lower punctum slightly lateral to the upper punctum.

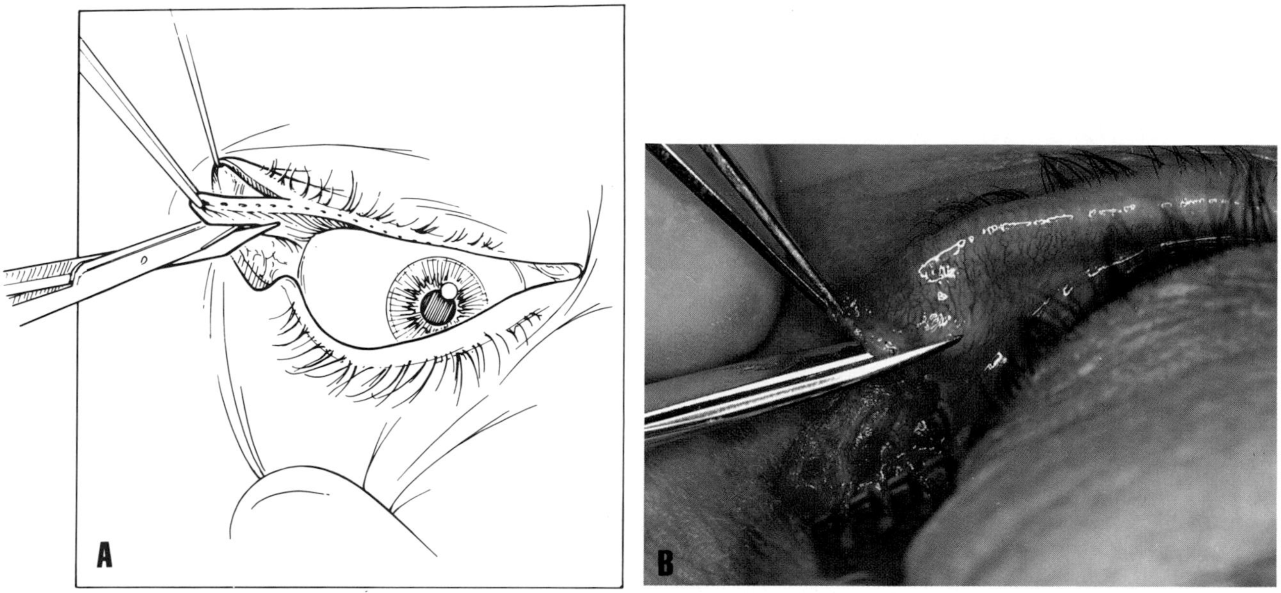

FIGURE 10–5

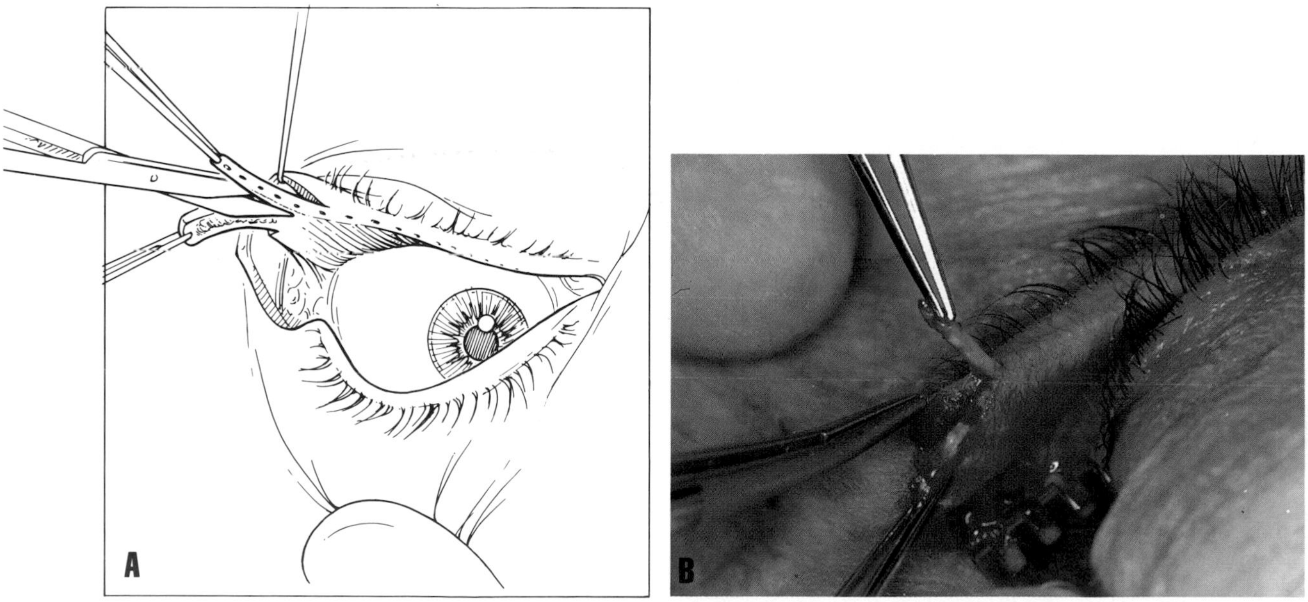

FIGURE 10–6

Figure 10–7. The amount of redundant lid tissue is determined by draping the tarsal plate over the lateral orbital rim. The excessive tissue is excised with a scalpel blade. A strip of tarsus, free of any epithelial lining, is thus fashioned.

Figure 10–8. The tarsal strip is sutured to the periosteum on the inner aspect of the lateral orbital wall with a 4–0 polygalactin 910 suture (Vicryl) on a small half-circle spatula needle. The needle is first passed full-thickness through the superior pole of the tarsal strip. A firm bite, at least 1.5 to 2 mm from the tarsal edge should be taken; this avoids the potential problem of suture "cheese-wiring" through the tarsal substance.

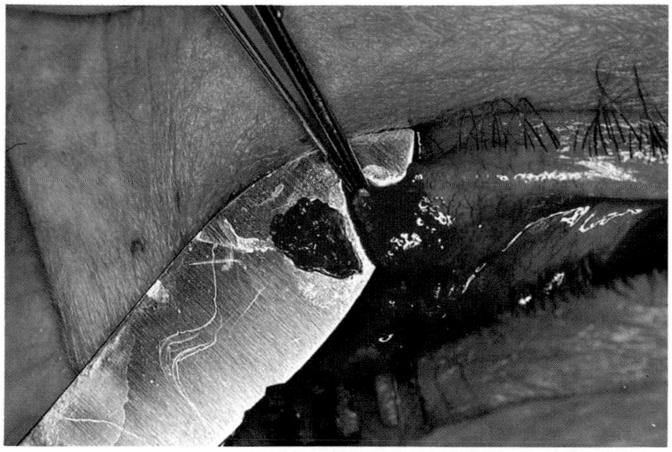

FIGURE 10–7

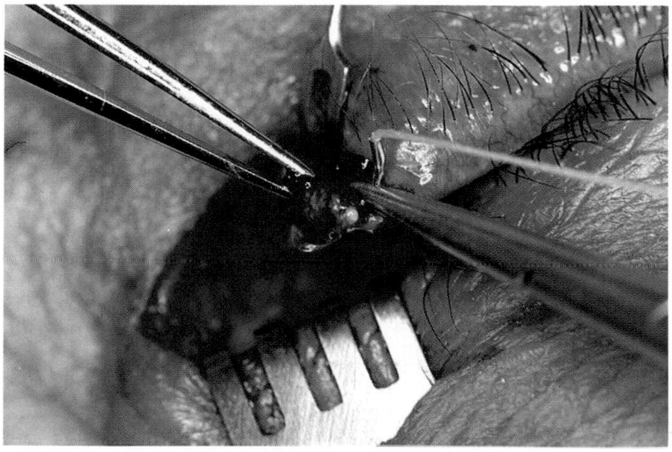

FIGURE 10–8

Figure 10–9A, B. The needle then engages the periosteum immediately inside the lateral orbital wall and exits at the anterior surface of the rim to prevent anterior displacement of the canthus. Another suture is passed through the inferior pole of the tarsal strip and engages the periosteum in the same fashion. When correcting lid laxity and canthal malposition in an anophthalmic socket, an additional suture may be placed to augment lid support of the prosthesis. Larger needles are difficult to maneuver at the tight lateral orbital rim region, and needles with a smaller curvature may bend or break on attempted passage through the periosteum. A slight overcorrection in both tightness and elevation at the lateral canthus should be achieved at surgery to allow for slight stretching of tissue in the early postoperative period.

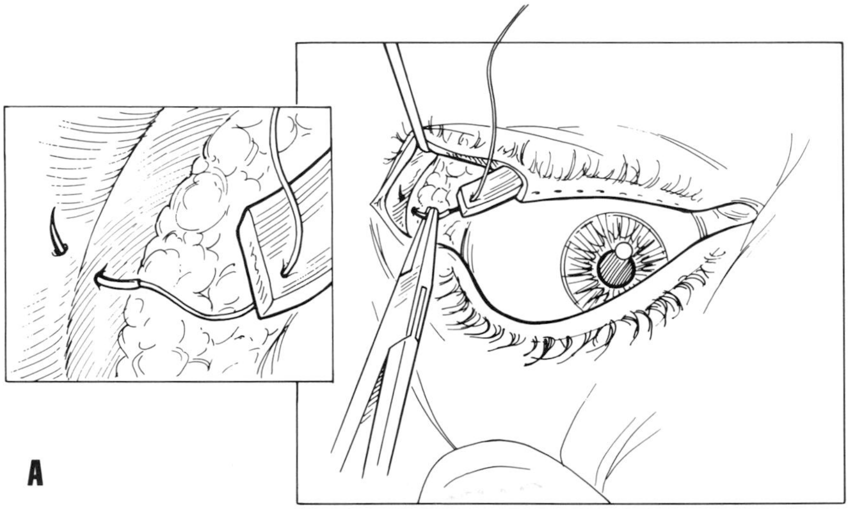

A

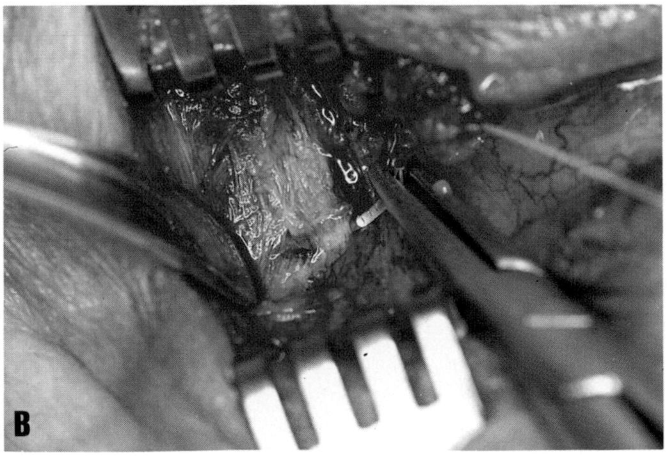

B

FIGURE 10–9

Figure 10–10. After securing the tarsal strip to the orbital rim, a wedge of anterior lamella, including the eyelash follicles, is excised.

Figure 10–11. The lateral canthotomy incision is closed with 6–0 nylon sutures in an interrupted fashion. The skin sutures are removed in 1 week.

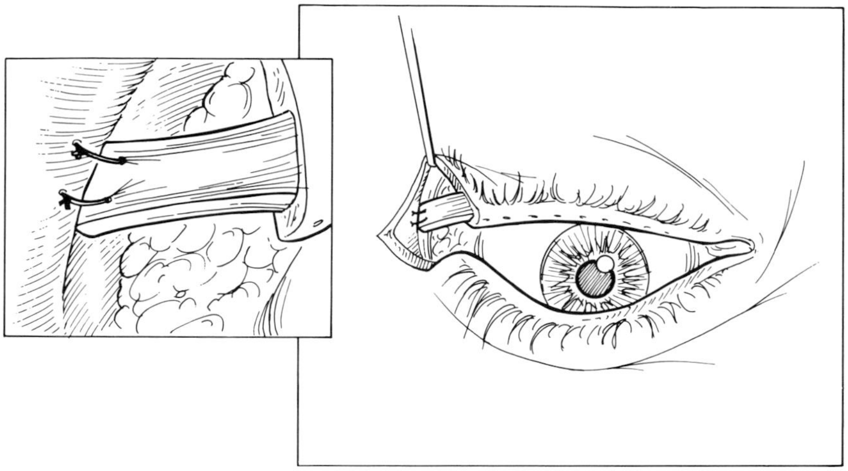

FIGURE 10–10

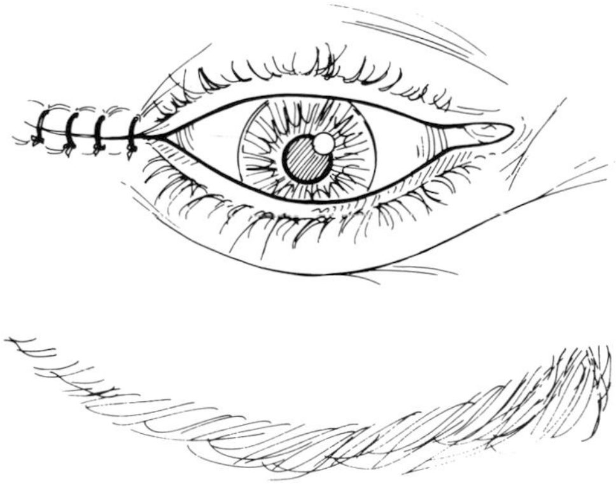

FIGURE 10–11

MEDIAL CANTHAL TENDON LAXITY

Medial canthal tendon laxity is detected by observing the lateral displacement of the lower punctum with lateral traction on the nasal eyelid. When the lower punctum is no longer aligned vertically with the upper punctum and can be displaced to the nasal limbus when the eye is in primary position, the medial canthal tendon should be repaired. It is unusual to find medial canthal tendon laxity alone, without concomitant lateral canthal laxity. The medial canthal laxity should be corrected first, before proceeding with the horizontal-shortening procedure. The aim of medial canthal tendon plication is to restore the anatomic position of the inferior punctum, so that it is in apposition with the globe and tear lake. The technique involves the exposure of the tendon, anchoring the lid nasally and posteriorly, and protecting the inferior canaliculus.

Procedure: Medial Canthal Tendon Plication

A curved, vertical incision is made over the medial canthal tendon and continued inferiorly to the medial lid margin, about 3 mm below the punctum.

A Bowman probe is placed in the lower canaliculus to identify and protect the structure throughout the operation. Blunt dissection is carried through the orbicularis muscle fibers with a Freer periosteal elevator to expose the medial canthal tendon and the nasal-most end of the tarsus beneath the punctum.

A double-armed 4–0 Polydek suture on an ME-2 half-circle needle is used.

Figure 10–12. The suture passes through the nasal-most end of the tarsal plate, tunnels beneath the orbicularis muscle, and exits at the superior margin of the medial canthal tendon insertion. The other arm of the suture is passed parallel to the first in the same fashion. While passing the needle through the orbicularis, it is important to always keep the needle anterior to the Bowman probe. Passing the needle behind the Bowman probe will incarcerate the canaliculus and compromise lacrimal drainage when the sutures are tied. Care should also be taken to avoid injuring the canaliculus. The two arms of the sutures are tied with sufficient tension to bring the lower punctum to a point just slightly lateral to the superior punctum. Do not tie too tightly, because this will bunch up the inferior canaliculus and displace the punctum away from the tear lake.

The skin incision is closed with interrupted 7–0 nylon sutures. Horizontal laxity is then reassessed. If needed, a lateral tarsal strip procedure can be performed.

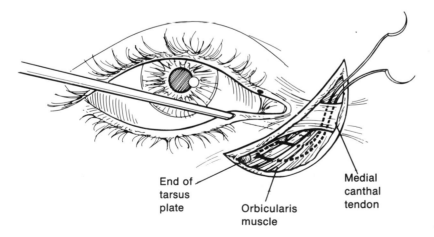

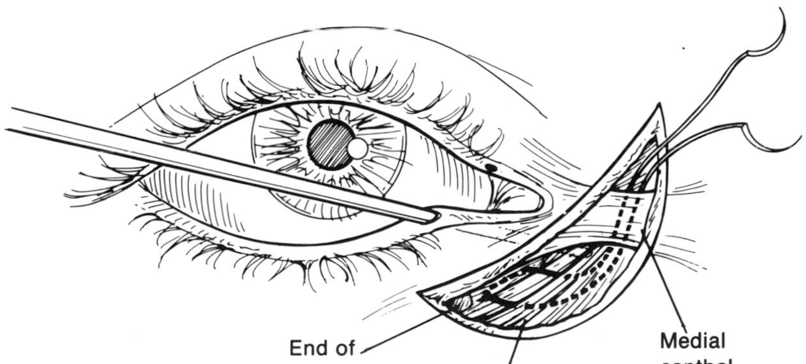
End of
tarsus
plate
Orbicularis
muscle
Medial
canthal
tendon

FIGURE 10–12

PUNCTAL MALPOSITION

The inferior punctum is normally in apposition with the globe and in vertical alignment with the superior punctum. Occasionally, punctal eversion without horizontal eyelid laxity or anterior lamellae cicatrix can be seen. The exact cause of this condition is unclear, but dehiscence or disinsertion of the lower eyelid retractors along the medial lid may be contributory.

If punctal eversion is severe and the patient is symptomatic, surgical correction will be necessary so that the punctum may return to its normal anatomic position and serve as a conduit for tears. A common approach is excision of tarsus, conjunctiva, and eyelid retractors as a horizontal, fusiform wedge at the lower margin of the tarsal plate. The conjunctiva is closed with three or four 7–0 absorbable sutures. However, inadequate punctal inversion and recurrent punctal ectropion are frequent drawbacks of a simple ellipse closure. Failure to unite the lower eyelid retractors to the tarsal plate and lack of a cicatrix to maintain the punctum in an inverted position are factors contributing to the lack of precise and lasting correction of the condition. A modification of the simple closure technique is preferred, which emphasizes the union of the lower eyelid retractors, not just the conjunctiva, to the tarsal plate, and the formation of a cicatrix to help keep the punctum in its normal anatomic alignment. This technique can be combined with a horizontal-shortening procedure of the eyelid, if laxity of the lower lid accompanies the punctal eversion; if not, it can be performed alone.

Procedure: Medial Spindle

A small amount of anesthetic is infiltrated under the skin about 10 mm below the punctum as well as along the medial forniceal conjunctiva.

Figure 10–13A. Surgeon's view from the head of the operating table. The medial eyelid is severed, a Bowman probe is inserted into the inferior canaliculus, and a diamond-shaped fusiform wedge of conjunctiva and lower lid retractors are excised inferior to the lower margin of the tarsal plate. The conjunctiva and underlying retractors are removed with the vertical height being about 4 to 6 mm and the horizontal dimension approximately 6 to 8 mm. The vertical height of the fusiform excision depends on the amount of punctal ectropion. Its greatest vertical dimension should lie beneath the punctum. The inferior edge of this diamond-shaped incision points toward the inferior fornix and exposes the superior margin of the lower lid retractors. One should avoid cutting into the horizontal preseptal orbicularis muscle fibers.

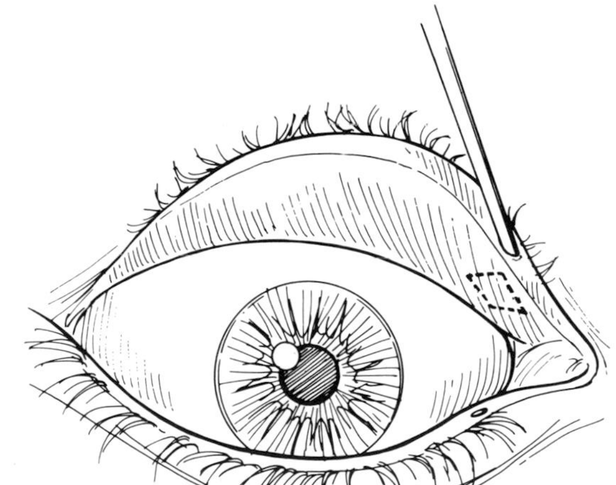

FIGURE 10–13

Figure 10–13B. The defect is closed with a double-armed 5–0 chromic suture in a horizontal mattress fashion. The suture is initially passed through the retractors at the lower edge of the incision in a backhanded pass.

Figure 10–13C. The needle passes through the upper edge of the ellipse, uniting the tarsal plate and conjunctiva on the upper edge. After passing both arms of the suture, the suture is pulled superiorly, joining the edge of the retractors to the inferior tarsal border.

Figure 10–13D. With forceps grasping the conjunctival edge of the lower border of the incision, the suture is passed full-thickness through the eyelid. The needle should be brought through the skin 12 to 15 mm inferior to the lid margin. The other arm of the suture is passed in the same fashion. The sutures are tied on the skin surface. The suture tension should be adjusted as needed to invert the punctum to the proper position. Care should be taken not to tie too tightly as to overcorrect the medial eyelid margin and produce entropion. It may be helpful to have the patient sit up while tying the sutures. The suture is left in place until it is absorbed.

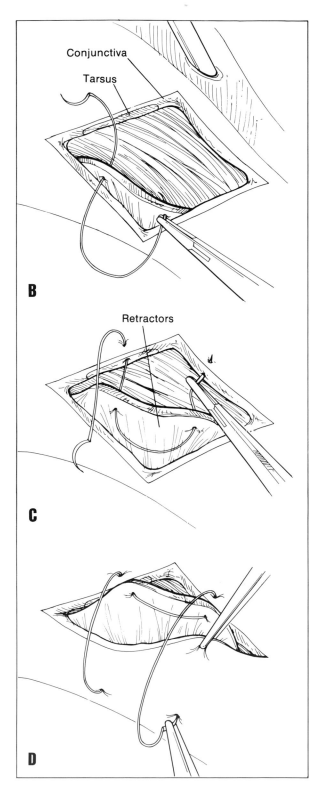

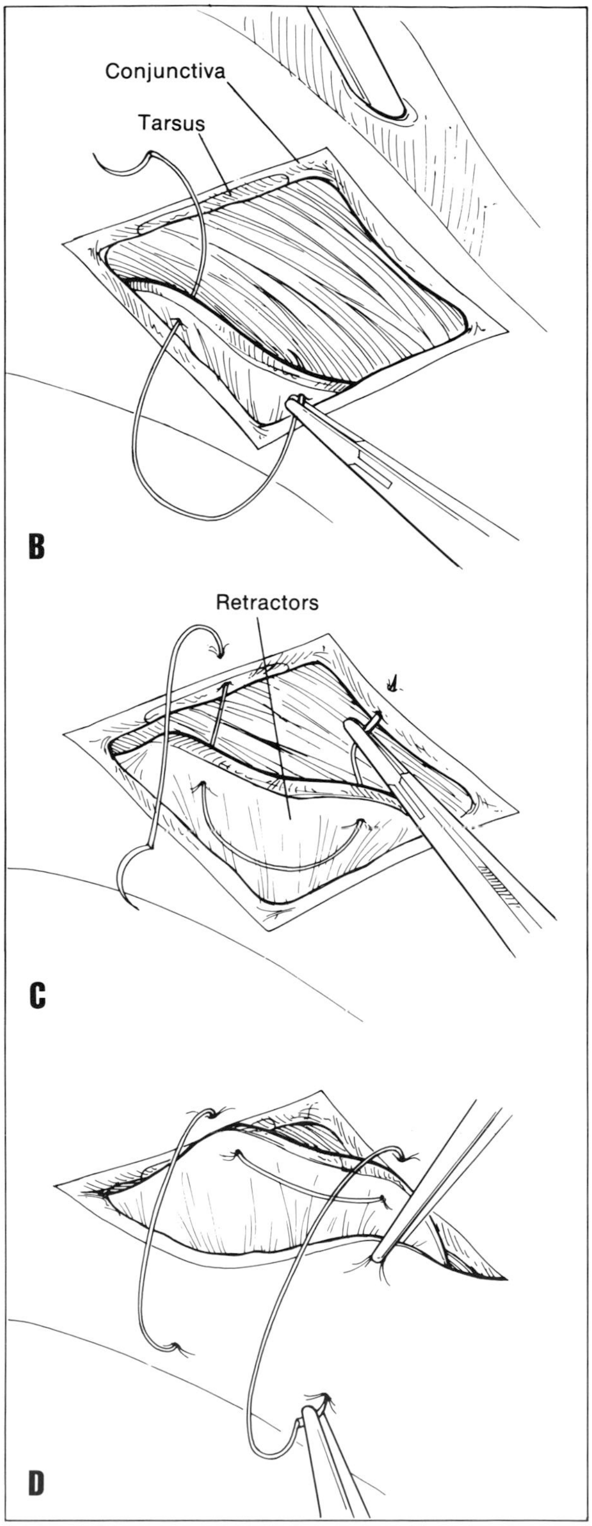

FIGURE 10–13 (Continued)

Figure 10–14. The looping passage of the suture induces a vector force that pulls the tarsal plate downward and rotates the punctum posteriorly.

Figure 10–15. The passage of the suture through full-thickness of the lower eyelid produces enough inflammatory reaction to create a cicatrix, augmenting the inversion effect and helps to keep the punctum in position after absorption of the suture.

This procedure corrects mild and moderate degrees of punctal ectropion. In patients with concomitant horizontal lid laxity, a lateral tarsal strip procedure may also be required.

VERTICAL TIGHTNESS OF THE SKIN

Cicatricial ectropion is caused by abnormal vertical shortening of the anterior lamella, which pulls the lid away from the globe. Conditions that cause excessive scarring or shrinkage in the skin or subcutaneous tissue (e.g., trauma, skin disease, burns) can lead to ectropion. If lid retraction is due to one vertical line of scar tissue, a Z-plasty can be performed. However, if vertical tightness of the skin is diffuse, a skin graft is indicated.

Procedure: Z-Plasty

Z-plasty is a procedure designed to release a line of tension and to transpose the contractile forces in an appropriate direction. Z-plasty works on the principle of transfer of tissue to reduce pull in one direction at the expense of a line perpendicular to it. It is better than V- to Y-plasty for vertical contracture of the skin near the lid margin.

The Z is formed by triangular flaps in which all sides of the triangle are equal. The flaps are usually made at 60° angles. The angle can vary between 30° and 90°. A 60° angle is the optimum angle that will permit transposition of the flaps, and it yields the maximum increase in length. In general, with an angle of 30°, there is an increase in length equal to 25% of the central line; with an angle of 45°, there is a 50% increase in length; however, with an angle of 60°, the increase in length rises to 75%. The vertical limb of the Z is always placed parallel to the direction of the scar tension line.

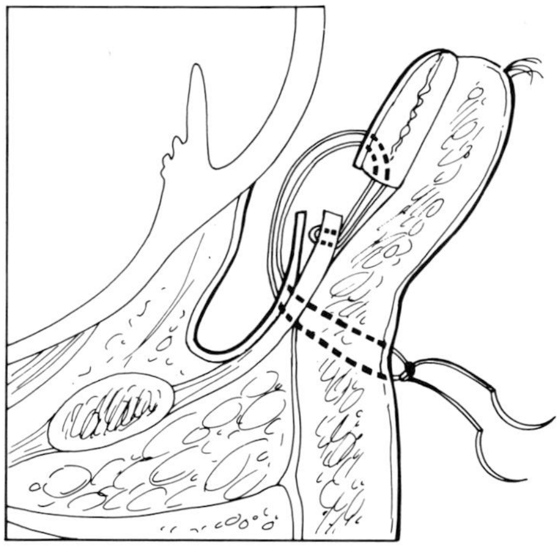

FIGURE 10–14

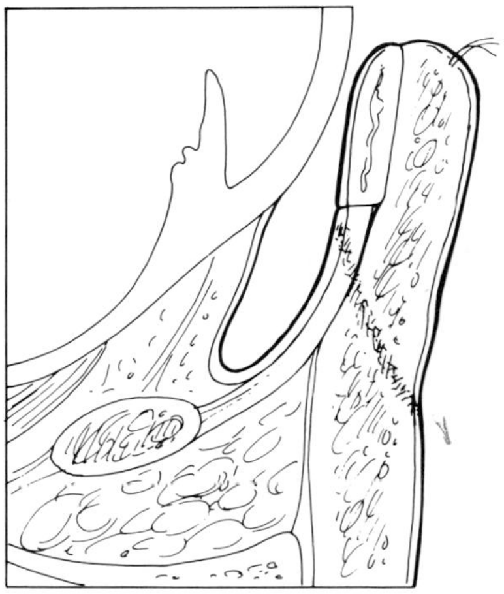

FIGURE 10–15

Figure 10–16. With a marking pen, a vertical line is drawn directly over the scar band, beginning about 1 mm from the cilia and extending the length of the scar. A line is drawn 60° from the superior and inferior ends of the vertical line, each measuring the same length as the vertical line. After local infiltration with anesthetic, a 4–0 black silk traction suture is passed through the gray line at the apex of the vertical cicatrix. The eyelid is placed on slight tension by anchoring the suture to the surgical drape superiorly.

Incision over the preplaced marking is made with a size 15 Bard–Parker blade. Subcutaneous scar bands are severed with a Westcott scissors until the eyelid can be easily stretched.

Figure 10–17. The resultant skin flaps are undermined widely and transposed into proper position without undue tension on adjacent skin. Only skin hooks should be used to manipulate and transpose the skin flaps, to avoid tissue damage. Care should be taken not to macerate the tip of the flap. The cutaneous edges of the flaps are approximated using interrupted 6–0 nylon sutures.

Figure 10–18. The entire eyelid is placed on slight tension by taping the marginal traction sutures above the brow for 1 week. Skin sutures are removed in 7 days.

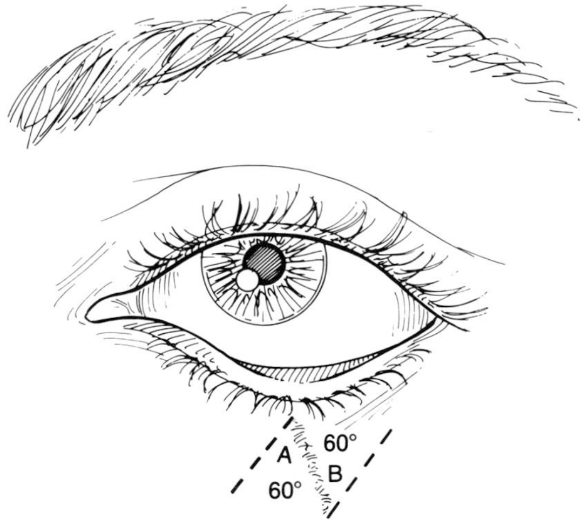

FIGURE 10–16

FIGURE 10–17

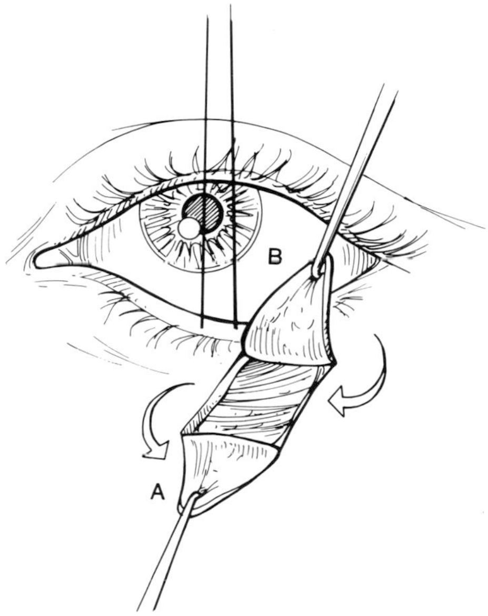

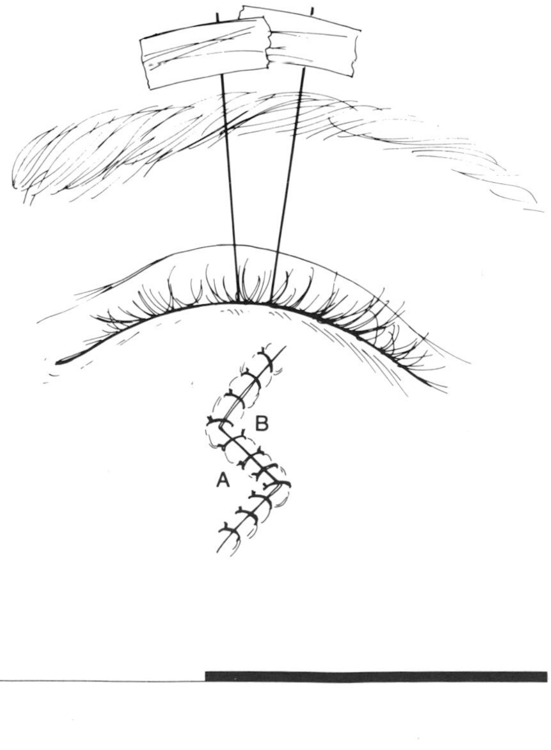

FIGURE 10–18

Procedure: Full-Thickness Skin Graft

Two percent lidocaine, with 1:100,000 epinephrine, is injected subcutaneously over the involved eyelid. Two 4–0 silk marginal traction sutures, placed temporally and medially to the limbus, are anchored to the surgical drape superiorly with a hemostat.

Figure 10–19. A horizontal incision 3 to 4 mm below the lash margin is made with a scalpel. Bands of vertical scar tissue are incised with a scissors or blade.

Figure 10–20. The incision should be carried down to whatever depth is necessary until all scar bands have been released and the eyelid returns to its normal position. This maneuver is absolutely essential. Thorough hemostasis should be obtained before placement of the graft. Hematoma formation under the graft may prevent graft survival.

Figure 10–21. A template of the defect is fashioned from a Telfa pad. The Telfa template, matching the defect, is transferred over the graft donor site (here the retroauricular skin) and outlined with a marking pen. The donor skin graft should be slightly larger than the recipient defect to allow for contour differences and graft shrinkage. The ideal source of donor skin for an upper lid defect is the upper eyelid skin fold from the contralateral lid; for the lower lid, they are acquired from the retroauricular (first choice) or supraclavicular (second choice) regions. When harvesting skin from the retroauricular area, equal amount of skin should be removed from either side of the retroauricular crease to facilitate closure (see Figure 10–21). The donor skin should not be hair-bearing.

The skin edges on the posterior surface of the ear and the mastoid area are undermined and advanced. Closure is accomplished by using 5–0 Vicryl material as tension-bearing subcutaneous sutures. Skin edges are closed with multiple interrupted 6–0 nylon sutures. Sterile gauze cut to the shape of the retroauricular crease is placed over the incision and a light dressing is applied. The skin sutures are removed in 7 days.

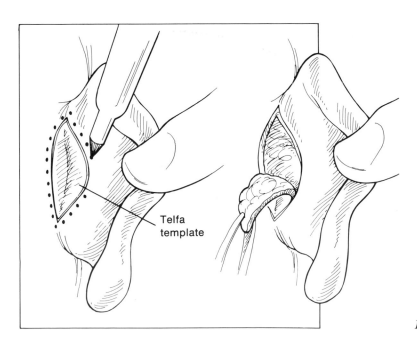

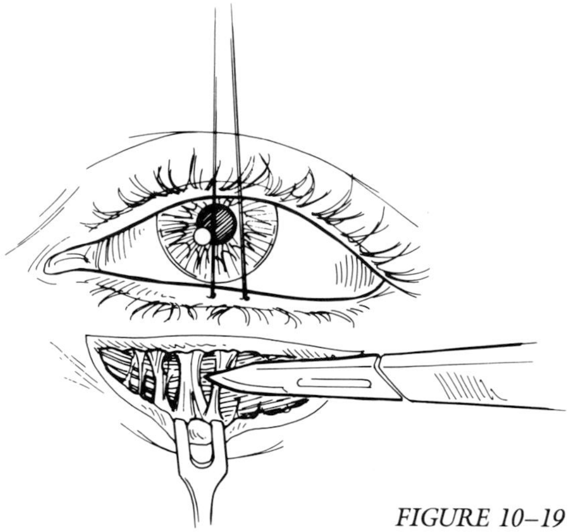

FIGURE 10–19

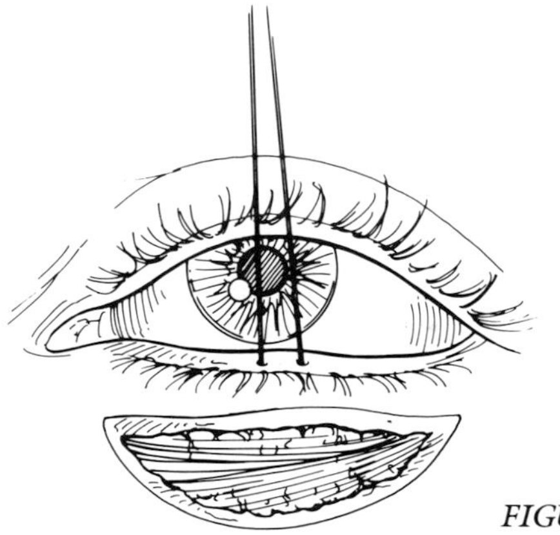

FIGURE 10–20

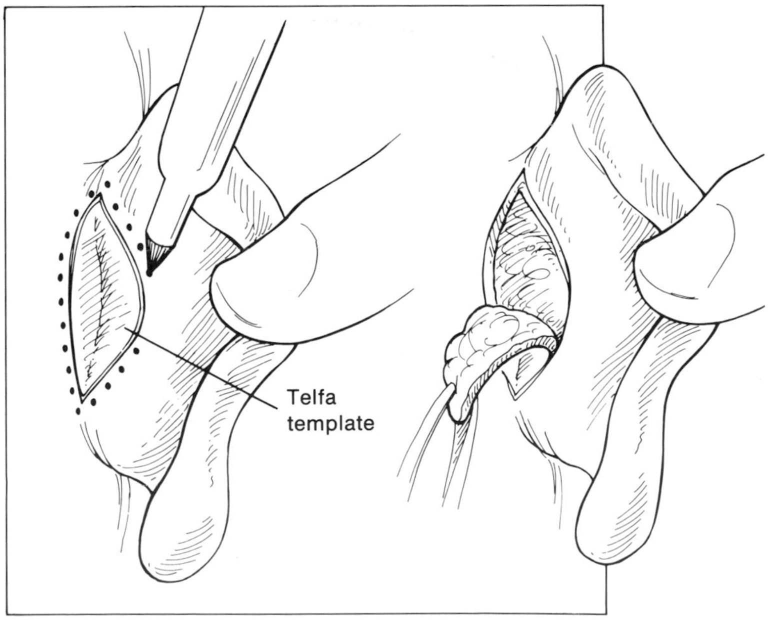

FIGURE 10–21

Figure 10–22. The ellipse of donor skin is placed on the finger of the surgeon and the subcutaneous tissue is trimmed with a Stevens scissors applied against the finger. Removal of the subcutaneous tissue is complete when the dermal follicles are visible. Stab incisions may be placed on the graft to facilitate the egress of serosanguinous fluid from under the graft.

Figure 10–23. The donor skin graft is then placed over the recipient bed, and the edges are trimmed to conform to the shape of the defect. The graft is sutured in position with multiple, interrupted 6–0 silk sutures. The ends of the sutures are left long and later tied over a sponge bolster on top of the graft.

Figure 10–24. A sterile sponge, cut into the shape of a cylinder, is enveloped with a Telfa dressing (without the cotton). This sponge stent is then firmly tied over the graft with the long ends of the preplaced 6–0 silk sutures. The transmarginal traction sutures are taped to the forehead to place the recipient bed on stretch and to minimize graft contracture. A light pressure dressing is applied over the sponge. The sponge, Telfa dressing, and sutures are removed in 1 week.

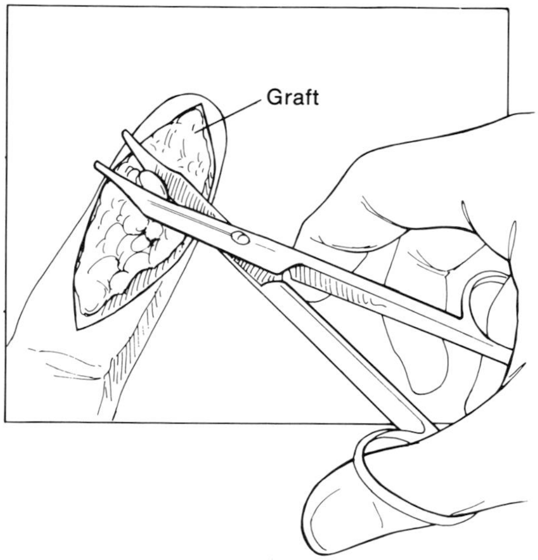

FIGURE 10–22

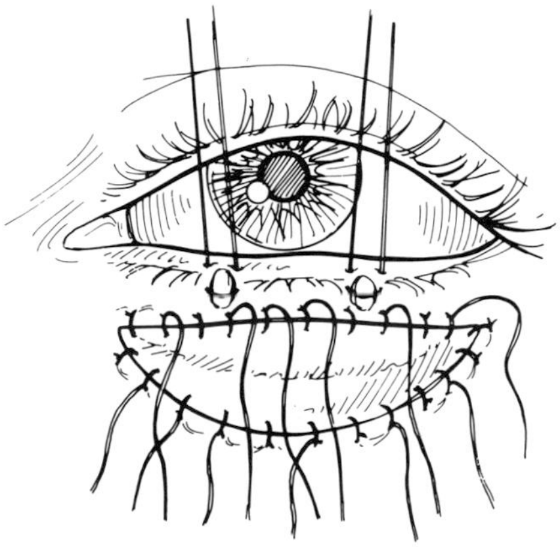

FIGURE 10–23

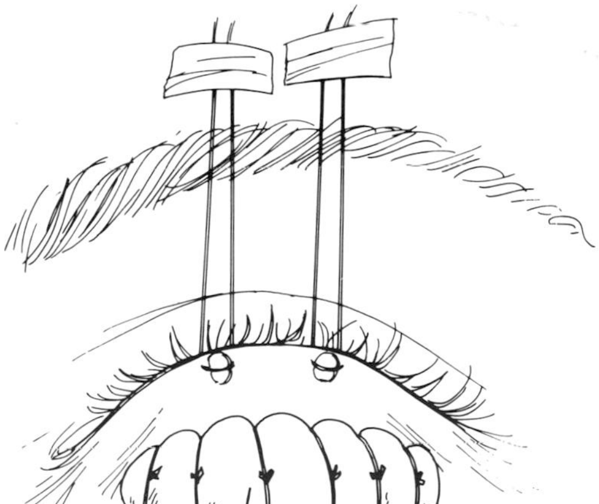

FIGURE 10–24

ORBICULARIS PARESIS SECONDARY TO SEVENTH NERVE PALSY

The lateral tarsal strip procedure is recommended, since it provides an immediate support to the paretic lower eyelid. In some cases, palpebral spring or lid-loading with a gold weight helps to augment lid closure and minimizes exposure (see Chapters 18 and 19).

LOWER EYELID RETRACTORS DISINSERTION

The lower eyelid retractors are referred to both the capsulopalpebral fascia and the Mueller's muscle. The capsulopalpebral fascia originates as the capsulopalpebral head with delicate attachments to the inferior rectus muscle and tendon. The capsulopalpebral head divides into two portions as it extends around and fuses with the sheath of the inferior oblique muscle. Anterior to the inferior oblique muscle, the two portions of the capsulopalpebral head rejoin to form the Lockwood's ligament. The fascial tissue anterior to the Lockwood's ligament is termed the capsulopalpebral fascia. A large portion of the capsulopalpebral fascia proceeds anteriorly to insert on the inferior fornix and to form the Tenon's capsule on the globe. The rest of the capsulopalpebral fascia then proceeds upward to insert onto the inferior margin of the tarsal plate (see Chapter 1 for further review of lower eyelid anatomy).

Disinsertion of the retractors of the lower eyelid may manifest either as ectropion or entropion. Differential vector forces between the anterior and posterior lamella often determine whether ectropion or entropion will result. Lower eyelid retractors disinsertion in the absence of horizontal laxity or anterior lamella shortage is the most difficult element of an ectropic eyelid to recognize clinically. In patients with lower eyelid retractors disinsertion or dehiscence, there are four clinical clues one can look for. These clinical clues are similar to those found in an entropic eyelid: (1) Deeper inferior fornix (because the capsulopalpebral fascia sends attachments to the inferior fornix, when the retractors are disinserted, it pulls the inferior fornix inward, thereby deepening the inferior fornix). (2) A higher resting lower lid position (because the retractors are no longer attached to the inferior margin of the tarsal plate, when the involved eyelid is pulled out of its ectropic position, it often has a higher resting position of the lid margin). (3) Diminished lower eyelid excursion on down gaze (owing to absence of attachment of the retractors to the tarsal plate). (4) A horizontal infratarsal red band and the edge of the disinserted retractors can be seen. This red band is thought to be the orbicularis muscle fibers showing through the area of retractors disinsertion. However, this sign has not been too useful because the inferior fornix is often injected as the result of chronic lid eversion.

Occasionally, tarsal ectropion, a striking and unusual form of ectropion may be seen. In these patients, the lid is completely everted, with the tarsal plate turned essentially upside down. The palpebral conjunctiva is turned outward and the lower border of the tarsus is flipped upward to the level of inferior limbal margin. Putterman corrected this condition by reattaching the disinserted Mueller's muscle and capsulopalpebral fascia to the inferior tarsus by an anterior approach. Wesley (1982) described an internal approach in which a wedge of redundant conjunctiva was excised and the retractors reattached to the inferior tarsal edge. An alternative treatment method, analogous to the medial spindle technique in correcting punctal ectropion is described in the following section. For this procedure, a transconjunctival approach is used, but without excision of any forniceal conjunctiva. The looping passage of the fornix sutures through full-thickness eyelid and the formation of an inflammatory cicatrix, produce a vector force that helps to effect and maintain an inward rotation of the lid margin. The key to success in this method is to unite the lower eyelid retractors, not just the conjunctiva, to the tarsal plate, as the retractors are responsible for the inversion effect.

Procedure: Suture Inversion Technique

The lower lid is anesthetized with lidocaine 2% with 1:100,000 epinephrine. Anesthetic is also injected under the conjunctiva along the infratarsal border. A 4–0 silk suture is placed through the central lid margin for traction. An infratarsal conjunctival snip incision is made with a Westcott scissors until the postorbicular fascial plane is identified. The horizontal preseptal orbicularis muscle fibers can be seen through this opening. Medial and lateral infratarsal incisions are made across the length of the eyelid. Sharp dissection within this plane is carried toward the inferior orbital rim until the orbital fat pads are identified. The orbital fat pads are retracted anteriorly with a Desmarres retractor. Once the orbital fat is retracted, the disinserted anterior edge of the retractors can usually be seen several millimeters below the conjunctival incision.

To identify the lower eyelid retractors with certainty, the disinserted edge of the retractors is grasped with a tissue forceps and the patient is asked to look downward. One should feel a downward pull if the retractors are grasped by the forceps.

Figure 10–25A, B. The disinserted edge of the lower eyelid retractors is then reattached onto the inferior border of the tarsal plate by using three sets of double-armed 5–0 chromic sutures. These sutures should be evenly spaced along the length of the lid. One arm of the suture is initially passed horizontally through the retractors at the lower edge of the incision.

Figure 10–26A, B. While a tissue forceps is everting the infratarsal edge, the needle is passed through the tarsus in a backhanded fashion. The second arm is passed about 5 to 6 mm from the first in the same manner. After passing both arms of the suture, the suture is pulled superiorly, joining the edge of the retractors to the inferior tarsal border.

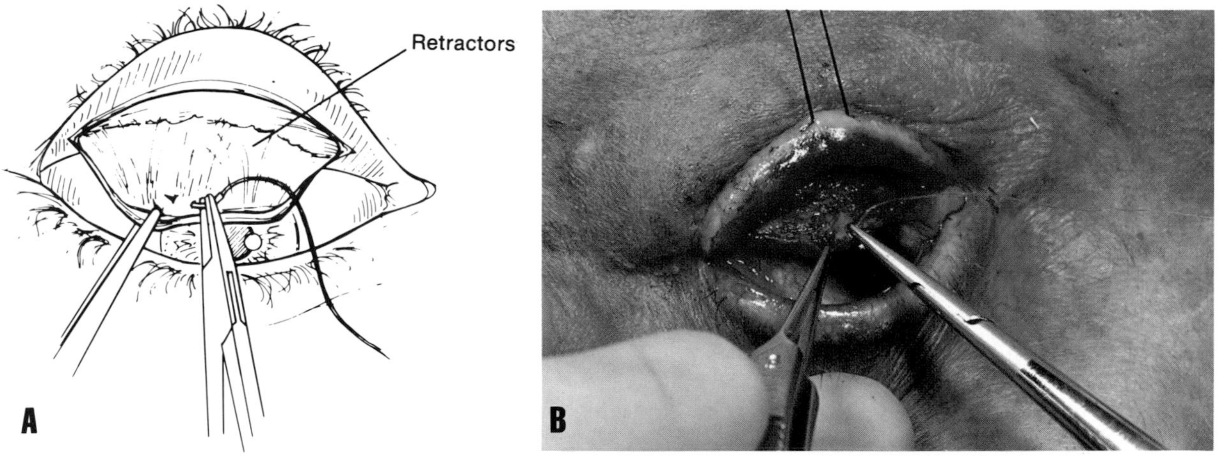

FIGURE 10–25

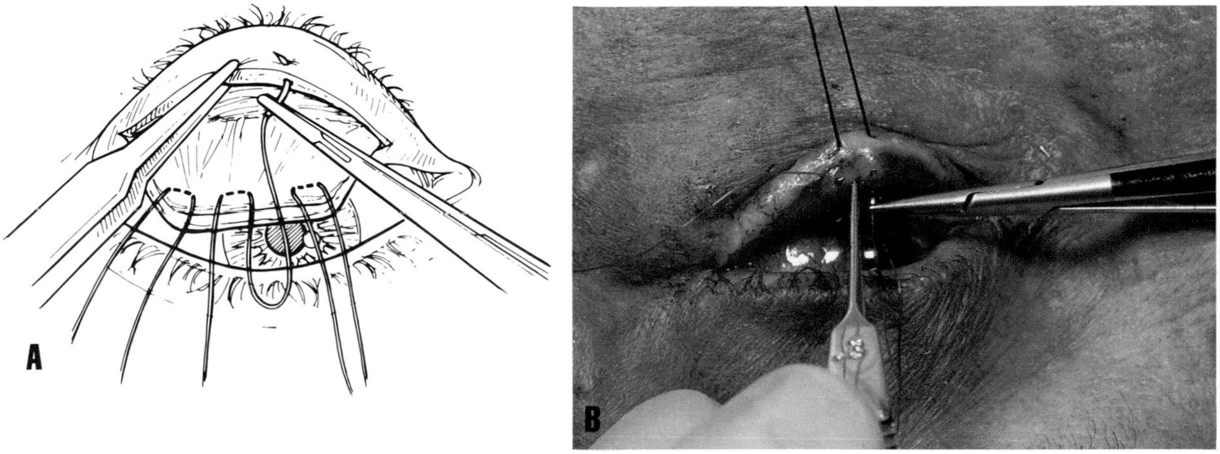

FIGURE 10–26

Figure 10–27A, B. With forceps grasping the conjunctival edge of the incision, the needle is passed deep into the inferior fornix, through the full-thickness of the eyelid, to emerge from the skin surface about 12 to 15 mm inferior to the lid margin.

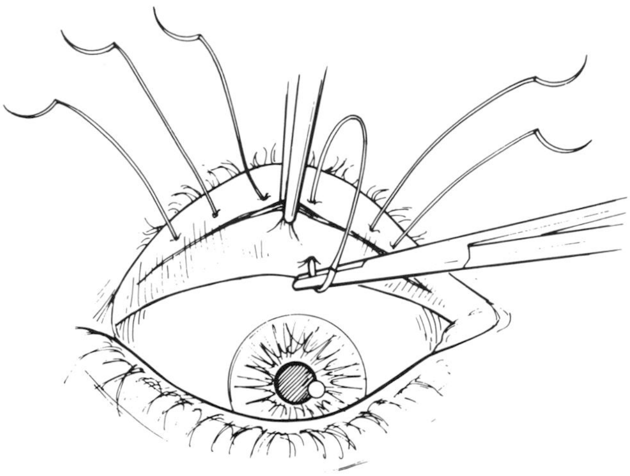

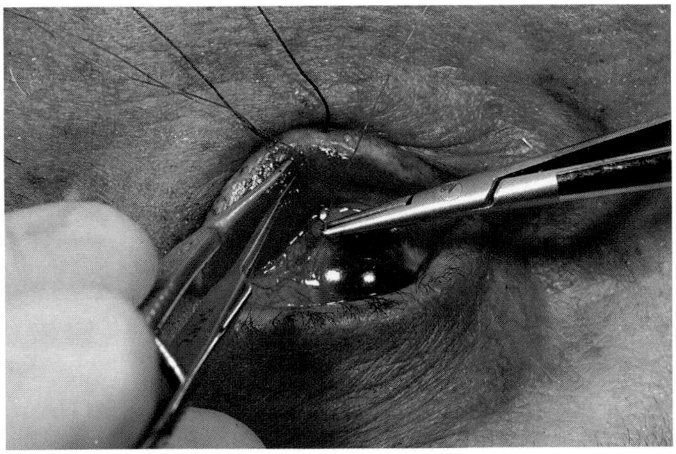

FIGURE 10–27

Figure 10–28. The other arm of the suture is passed in the same fashion. The other two sets of suture are passed 4 to 5 mm apart, in an identical manner to form three sets of evenly spaced sutures across the lid.

Figure 10–29. The three sets of sutures are then tied on the skin surface, without the use of bolsters. Upon tying of the sutures, there will be an immediate inversion of the lid margin. The sutures should not be tied so tightly that they overinvert the lid margin and produce entropion. To verify the proper reattachment of the retractors to the tarsal plate, the patient is asked to look downward, and one should see a smooth downward excursion of the lower lid.

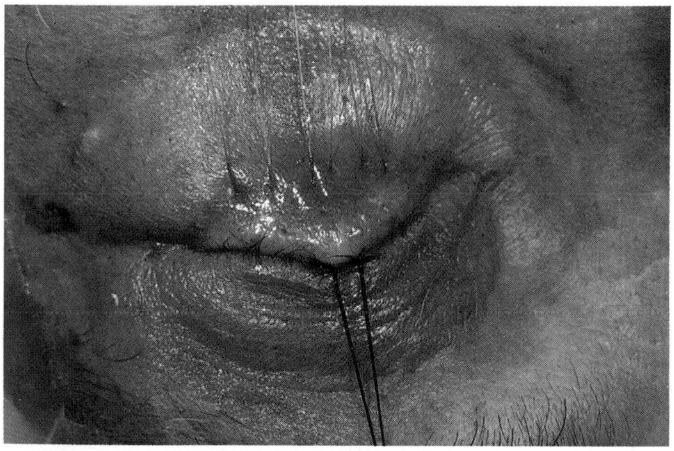

FIGURE 10–28

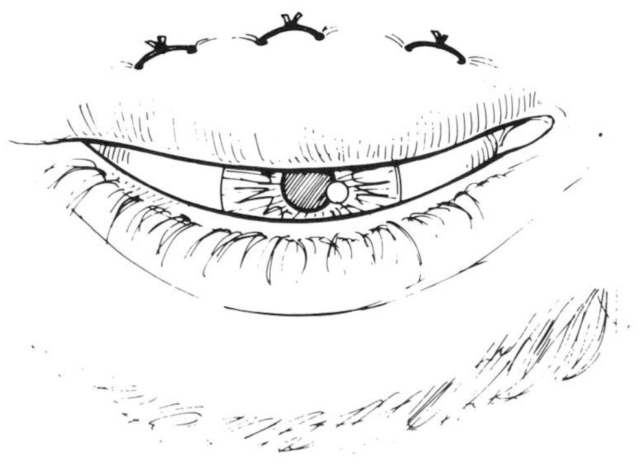

FIGURE 10–29

Figure 10–30. Sagittal view of the eyelid showing the path of the sutures. The looping passage of the sutures induces a vector force that pulls the tarsal plate downward and rotates the lid margin posteriorly. This inversion vector force counteracts any outward pulling effect imparted by the anterior lamella. The subsequent formation of an inflammatory cicatrix induced by the absorbable sutures helps to maintain the eyelid in an upright posture. If concomitant horizontal lid laxity is present, a lateral tarsal strip procedure can be performed. Bacitracin ophthalmic ointment is applied on the suture knots and in the inferior fornix. The chromic sutures usually are absorbed within 10 to 14 days.

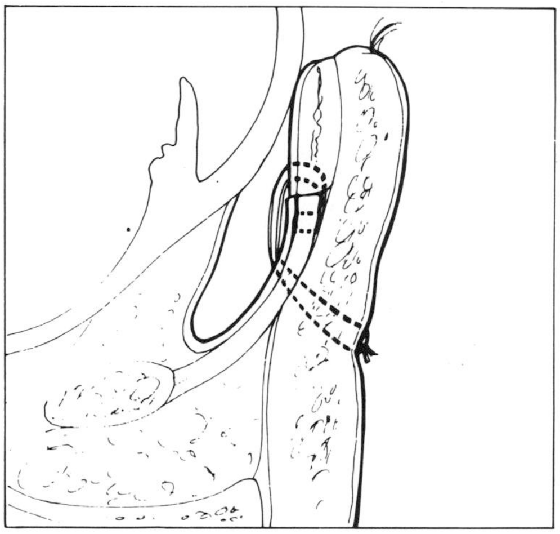

FIGURE 10–30

Chapter Eleven

CRYOTHERAPY

Thaddeus S. Nowinski

Clinical research evaluating cryotherapy of benign and malignant eyelid tumors produced an unexpected side effect—the loss of eyelashes in the treated area. Follow-up studies confirmed its usefulness, and cryotherapy became a standard of treatment for aberrant eyelashes.

Trichiasis is a misdirection or inturning of previously normally placed eyelashes, allowing abrasions of the globe. *Congenital distichiasis* represents a local or diffuse growth of an extra row of lashes from the multipotential tarsal meibomian glands. Metaplasia of previously normal meibomian glands may occur as an acquired condition secondary to trauma or chronic inflammation.

MASQUERADE

Aberrant lashes should be distinguished from eyelid malpositions that result in secondary inturning of normal lashes. Skin folds seen in severe dermatochalasis, epiblepharon, and in epicanthus varieties mechanically push normally positioned lashes toward the globe. *Entropion* is an inturning of the entire lid margin and lashes. Although involutional entropion is usually easily diagnosed, cicatricial entropion secondary to trauma or conjunctival shrinkage disorders may be difficult to distinguish from trichiasis or distichiasis. The presence of symblepharon and metaplasia of the lid margin and meibomian glands with acquired distichiasis blurs its distinction from cicatricial entropion, and multiple therapeutic approaches may be necessary.

INDICATIONS FOR TREATMENT

The patient with trichiasis or distichiasis often seeks treatment because of ocular discomfort, redness, and foreign body sensation owing to corneal and conjunctival abrasions. Chronic irritation of the cornea may lead to localized thinning or vascularization, with risk of subsequent ulceration or perforation.

MECHANISM OF CRYODESTRUCTION

A double freeze–thaw method with thermocouple monitoring of tissue temperature to −20°C has been most effective in the treatment of aberrant lashes. Two cycles of rapid freezing, followed by a slow thaw, induce destruction of the thermally sensitive lash follicles, while allowing recovery of the relatively resistant conjunctiva, tarsus, skin, and lacrimal outflow apparatus. Multiple factors contribute to the effect, including intracellular ice crystal formation and recrystallization, disruption of intracellular membranes and cell walls, intracellular pH changes, vascular thrombosis, and a posttreatment inflammatory response.

SURGICAL ANATOMY

The normal eyelashes arise in the anterior lamella of the eyelid and consist of a few irregular rows exiting the skin anterior to the intermarginal sulcus. The normal follicles lie in the pretarsal space near the marginal arterial arcade. The meibomian sebaceous glands are located in the fibrous tarsus and their orifices are located in the posterior lamella (i.e., posterior to the intermarginal sulcus) (see Chapter 1). Lack of differentiation of these glands during development may be accompanied by association of the glands with lash follicles.

ALTERNATIVE THERAPIES

Frequent mechanical epilation and the use of topical lubricants is preferred by some patients. The use of contact lenses is of limited value to protect the cornea. Electrolysis can be used to destroy isolated small numbers of lashes. Placement of the needle is difficult and results in a relatively high recurrence rate. Localized lid scarring can also be produced. Argon laser ablation at the slit lamp can also be used for individual lashes, but this has similar limitations.

Microscopic surgical excision of individual follicles is tedious and difficult. Lid splitting combined with cryotherapy may be useful in certain cases of congenital distichiasis. Surgical excision of a localized full-thickness section of eyelid can be utilized for small to moderate areas of lashes. Marginal rotation procedures can direct the entire lid margin away from the globe (see Chapter 9). A combination of surgical treatment, oral therapy, and cryotherapy may be indicated in conjunctival shrinkage disorders.

OTHER USES OF CRYOTHERAPY

Cryotherapy has been employed with variable success for benign and malignant tumors of the eyelid and ocular adnexa. It has proved very effective in the treatment of epithelial and pigmented malignancies of the conjunctiva. Cryotherapy combined with surgical excision has become an acceptable alternative to exenteration in selected patients, in an attempt to preserve a useful eye. This is especially true in the monocular or otherwise ophthalmically compromised patient, or in those who refuse or cannot undergo more extensive treatment.

The addition of cryotherapy to simple excision of conjunctival intraepithelial dysplastic lesions and squamous cell carcinoma has decreased the recurrence rate and improved the long-term prognosis. This combination has become the treatment of choice in cases without intraocular and intraorbital invasion and allows the treatment of large areas with relatively minimal destruction of normal tissue. It also can be used in selected patients who have localized scleral invasion of epithelial malignancies.

Malignant melanomas of the conjunctiva usually begin as radial intraepithelial proliferations of atypical melanocytes, followed by an invasive nodular progression. Radical surgical exenteration has been the treatment of choice, but does not prevent metastatic disease. Although radical surgery is still considered necessary for lesions with a deep invasive component, cryotherapy combined with localized excision of nodules has become an important alternative treatment.

Melanocytes are selectively sensitive to freezing. Cryotherapy is optimal for flat, noninvasive intraepithelial disease before nodule growth is present. Freezing large areas of acquired melanosis is preferable to huge conjunctival excisions with resultant symblepharon formation and globe limitations. Surgical excision of localized nodular disease combined with cryotherapy to the underlying excision bed and to the surrounding areas of flat pigmentation allows sloughing of the treated epithelium, while sparing the substantia propria, which acts as a framework for reepithelialization. Extensive areas of flat pigmentation can be treated serially in the office. Although some migration of adjacent pigmented cells may occur in treated areas, the overall number of cells is greatly reduced and prognosis is dramatically improved. Posttreatment biopsies, especially in pigmented areas, will distinguish between tumor recurrence and melanin accumulation in macrophages. Recurrences can be managed by repeat cryotherapy or more radical surgery.

PROCEDURE

Topical anesthesia is applied, and 2% lidocaine with epinephrine is infiltrated subcutaneously in the lid. Epinephrine facilitates rapid freezing and slow thawing by vasoconstriction. A hand-held cryoapplication unit is used, and the tissue temperature is monitored by a thermocouple probe.

Figure 11–1. A thermocouple 23-gauge probe is placed in the pretarsal space, at the base of the lash follicles. The tip of the cryoprobe is placed adjacent to the tip of conjunctival surface of the lid margin in a position perpendicular to the lid and, thus, parallel to the hair shaft. The globe can be protected with a scleral shell if desired.

Figure 11–2. Pulling the pistol grip then begins the freezing process. An iceball will develop closest to the tip and spread outward slowly. The lid can easily be pulled away from the globe once the iceball formation begins. The tissue will become white and hard near 0°C; it is difficult to predict tissue temperature clinically. Freezing should continue until monitoring through the thermocouple indicates a temperature of −20°C at the tissue plane of the follicles. This should occur in less than 1 minute, the more rapid the better.

The tissue is then allowed to thaw spontaneously. Freezing treatment is again applied to −20°C, followed by a slow thawing. The aberrant lashes are then epilated with a forceps.

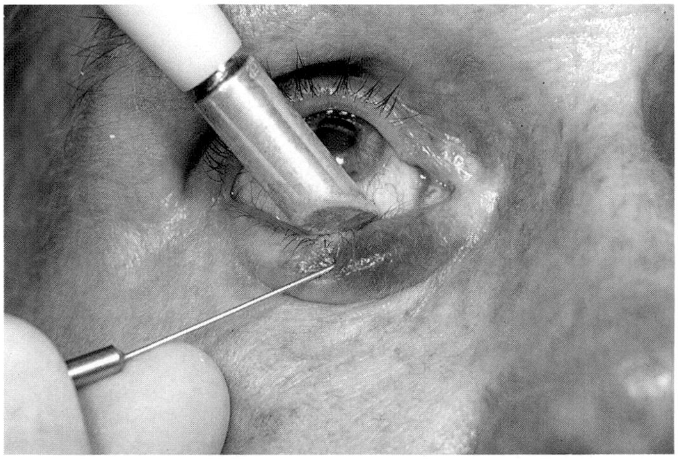

FIGURE 11–1

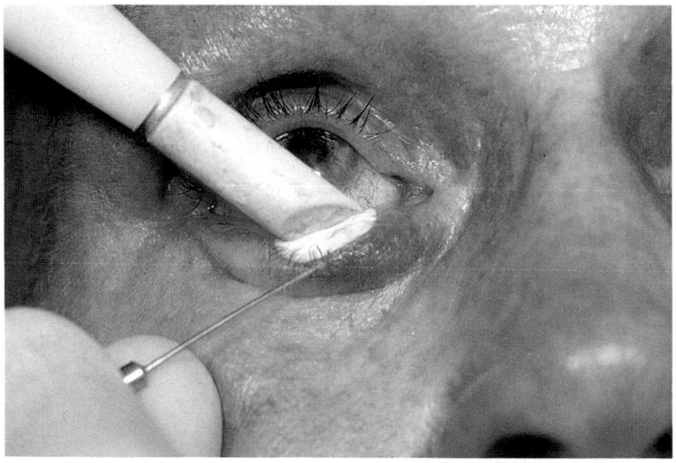

FIGURE 11–2

POSTOPERATIVE MANAGEMENT

Compresses may be helpful for comfort. Topical antibiotic–steroid ointment combination is useful four times daily for 1 week. Analgesics are given for moderate pain. Aberrant cilia may be pulled immediately or after a few days. Conjunctival discharge and lid edema are common and most marked at 48 to 72 hours after treatment.

RESULTS AND AVOIDANCE OF COMPLICATIONS

Ablation of aberrant lashes in otherwise normal eyelids by cryotherapy is successful in approximately 90% of treated lids. The treatment is nonselective and destroys surrounding normal lash follicles. Proper cryoprobe placement, thermocouple monitoring, a double freeze-thaw cycle to −20°C, and patient selection helps minimize complications. The use of a nitrous oxide-cooled cryoprobe permits more accurate placement and control and increased safety, than does a liquid nitrogen spray-delivery system.

Melanocytes are sensitive to cryotherapy to −20°C. Skin depigmentation can often occur, and discussion and proper patient selection is imperative. Many treated eyelids show thinning and transient erythema. Chronic erythema, lid notching, misdirection of previously normal lashes, activation of herpes zoster, and lid necrosis may occur and require further appropriate treatment.

Edema of the lids is common, and moderate or severe edema is not unusual during the first few days after treatment. This often extends to the cheek and surrounding areas of the face. Localized cellulitis may be simulated by this edema, but true infection is an uncommon complication. Inadvertent freezing of the globe must be avoided during lid treatment. Severe corneal or intraocular damage may occur. Patients with previous lid surgery or reconstruction, borderline tear film, neuropathic lids, or compromised vasculature have a significantly higher complication rate.

MUCOUS MEMBRANE PEMPHIGOID

Patients with aberrant lashes caused by conjunctival shrinkage disorders remain difficult to treat. These irregularly placed lashes are difficult to eradicate, and the cycle of inflammation and cicatricial changes may be exacerbated by cryotherapy or surgery. These patients should be as stable as possible before treatment. Sulfones or systemic steroids may be useful in selected cases. Initial freezing to −10°C may be prudent in severe or active immune-related conjunctival shrinkage disorders. Recurrences or poor results are common, and cryotherapy alone may not be sufficient in these difficult cases. It may be necessary to combine cryotherapy with reconstructive procedures in selected cases.

Chapter Twelve

BLEPHAROPTOSIS

John B. Holds
Richard L. Anderson

ACQUIRED PTOSIS

PREOPERATIVE EVALUATION

The vast majority of cases of acquired ptosis are aponeurogenic. Nonetheless, the causes of acquired ptosis are diverse, and it is helpful in evaluation and treatment to classify acquired ptosis into the following: aponeurogenic, from involutional or other disinsertional changes in the aponeurosis; myogenic, associated with decreased levator muscle function, as seen in myasthenia gravis or congenital progressive external ophthalmoplegia (CPEO); neurogenic, as seen in third-nerve palsy or Horner's syndrome; mechanical, associated with eyelid masses or scarring of the eyelid lamellae. Traumatic ptosis may be considered as a separate category, although it actually is a subcategory of each of the foregoing categories.

In the patient workup and evaluation, one must begin with a careful history, with attention to duration and progression of ptosis, daily variation in the severity of ptosis, and any history of dry eye complaints. Examination should focus on determining the severity of ptosis, levator function, lid crease height, and coexisting eye problems, such as lower eyelid retraction, overhanging skin on the upper lid, or contralateral upper eyelid retraction, creating a pseudoptosis on the side in question. Clinical features of a patient with acquired aponeurosis disinsertion consist of good levator function, higher than normal eyelid crease, and a ptotic eyelid that assumes a lower position on down gaze. If a history consistent with myasthenia gravis is suspected, tests for fatigability as well as an edrophonium (Tensilon) test should be performed. The examiner should be cognizant of the frequency of bilateral ptosis that is more apparent on one side. Because of the equal innervation to both levator muscles, correcting only one upper lid may result in worsening the appearance of ptosis on the opposite side. This phenomenon follows Hering's law and is especially frequent in aponeurogenic ptosis.

INDICATIONS FOR SURGERY

Adult ptosis is typically sympatomatic, whether the complaints relate to visual obstruction or a tired, inattentive appearance. A patient may also complain of forehead fatigue caused by constant brow elevation in an effort to help lift a ptotic eyelid. If repair is being performed for functional indications, it is vital to document the severity of ptosis with diagrams, facial photographs, and perimetry, showing the superior visual field constriction produced by the ptosis. It is also helpful to have photographs and notes available for reference at the time of surgery. A ptosis repair may be performed in most patients at any time. After trauma, it is prudent to wait 6 months before ptosis repair, as function may improve during that time. In myasthenia gravis, or any medical or neurologic condition that may remit with therapy, it is wise to delay surgery until the condition is stable and optimally controlled.

MAKING PROCEDURAL CHOICES

With few exceptions, acquired ptosis can be treated by an aponeurotic resection or repair. An external aponeurotic approach directly treats the most common cause for acquired ptosis, aponeurotic rarefaction or disinsertion. Aponeurotic surgery is also the preferred approach in myogenic or neurogenic ptosis with adequate levator function. Frontalis suspension procedures (see section on congenital ptosis) may be required in severe neurogenic, myogenic, or traumatic ptosis with the loss of levator function. In acquired unilateral ptosis with poor levator function, it is unnecessary to extirpate the contralateral levator and then suspend both lids. It is much easier for an adult without longstanding visual suppression to learn to use brow function to help elevate a ptotic eyelid. When performing sling procedures or aponeurotic surgery on individuals with ptosis associated with weak eyelid closure (CPEO, myasthenia gravis) one must avoid overcorrection and exposure keratopathy.

SURGICAL PROCEDURE

The eyelid crease is marked, with a marking pen, to correspond with the natural skin crease of the opposite upper lid. Anesthesia is obtained by subcutaneous infiltration along the preplaced skin marking with 1.0 to 2.0 ml of 2% lidocaine with 1:100,000 epinephrine. It is important not to inject too deeply into the eyelid, thereby anesthetizing Mueller's muscle which can influence intraoperative lid height adjustments. Topical tetracaine is instilled onto the cornea.

Figure 12–1. After subcutaneous infiltration, a 4–0 double-armed silk traction suture is placed at the central upper lid margin and secured to the surgical drape below with a hemostat. The suture is placed through the gray line at the lid margin to avoid the marginal arcade, thereby preventing unnecessary bleeding. When secured inferiorly, this traction suture puts all eyelid structures posterior to the orbicularis muscle on tension, while allowing the anterior lamella to be mobilized. The skin is incised along the previously marked lid crease with a scalpel.

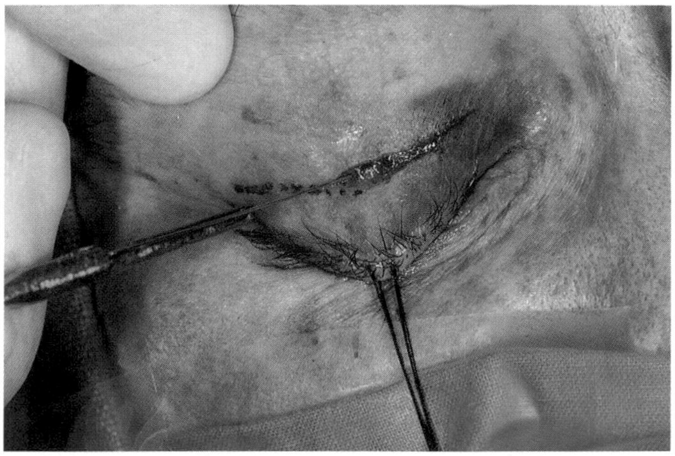

FIGURE 12–1

Figure 12–2. The orbicularis is tented anteriorly with a toothed forceps, and its full-thickness is incised centrally with a Westcott scissors oriented perpendicularly.

Figure 12–3. It is a key maneuver in this technique to make a full-thickness incision through the orbicularis muscle, as this avoids unnecessary bleeding from multiple cuts into the muscle, and permits identification of the avascular posterior orbicular fascial plane (*needle*).

Figure 12–4. One blade of a scissors is then passed bluntly into the avascular plane and the incision is completed medially and laterally. The superior edge of the incision is retracted upward with a skin hook, and the disinserted edge of the levator aponeurosis can oftentimes be identified through the translucent postorbicular fascia. The postorbicular fascia is recognized as a delicate layer overlying the aponeurosis. In this fascial plane, vertically oriented peripheral nerve fibers can sometimes be seen. Further dissection is required to expose the levator aponeurosis.

While retracting the superior edge of the incision with a double-pronged skin hook, gentle pressure is applied on the globe. With retrograde orbital pressure, the preaponeurotic fat pad bulges forward to tent up the orbital septum.

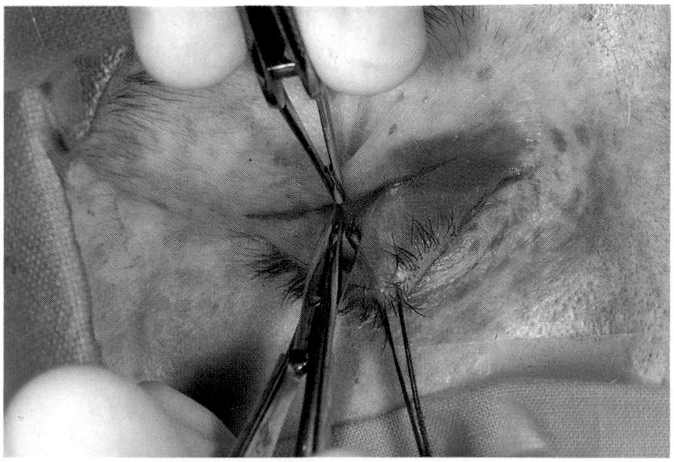

FIGURE 12–2

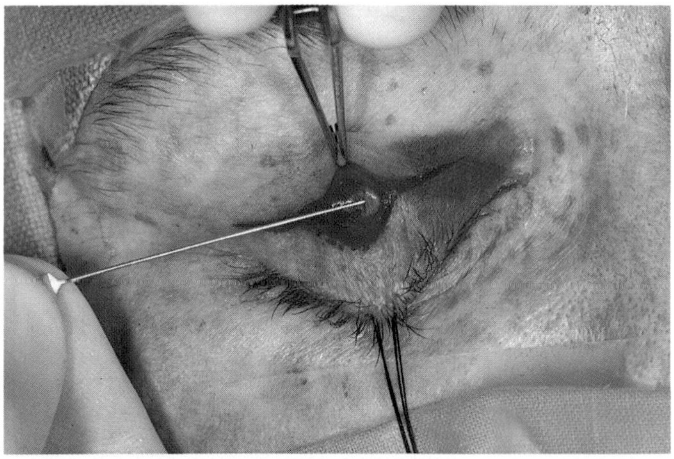

FIGURE 12–3

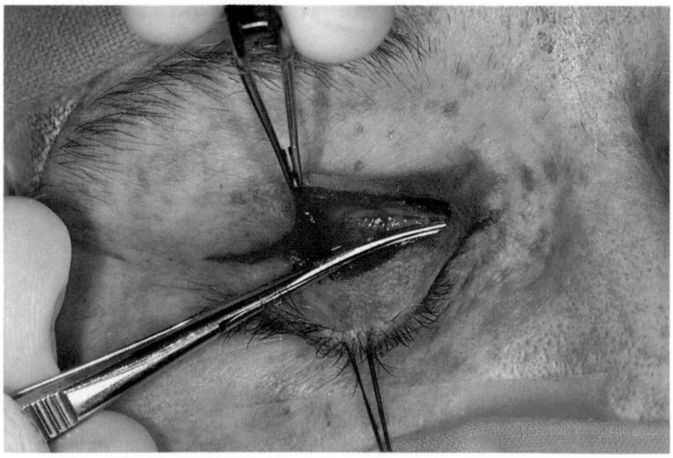

FIGURE 12–4

Figure 12–5. A horizontal incision is made with a Westcott scissors to buttonhole the orbital septum above its fusion with the aponeurosis. The incision should be directed superiorly to avoid transecting Mueller's muscle or the conjunctiva. This allows the preaponeurotic fat to herniate through the buttonhole. The entire orbital septum is then opened by placing one blade of the scissors behind the orbital septum and extending the incision medially and laterally.

The foregoing maneuvers are important to identify the preaponeurotic fat pad and to avoid making iatrogenic defects in the aponeurosis.

Figure 12–6. The skin and orbicularis muscle are retracted with a forceps. The preaponeurotic fat pad (indicated by the *top needle*) is the key anatomic landmark in this surgery, since the levator aponeurosis is located immediately beneath this structure (*lower needle*). Mueller's muscle lies immediately under the levator aponeurosis. In cases of repeated operation, trauma, or in eyelids infiltrated by tumor, such as neurofibroma, the preaponeurotic fat pad may be the only identifiable structure.

Figure 12–7. The preaponeurotic fat pad is retracted superiorly with a Desmarres retractor, and fine attachments to the underlying levator aponeurosis are lysed with a Westcott scissors.

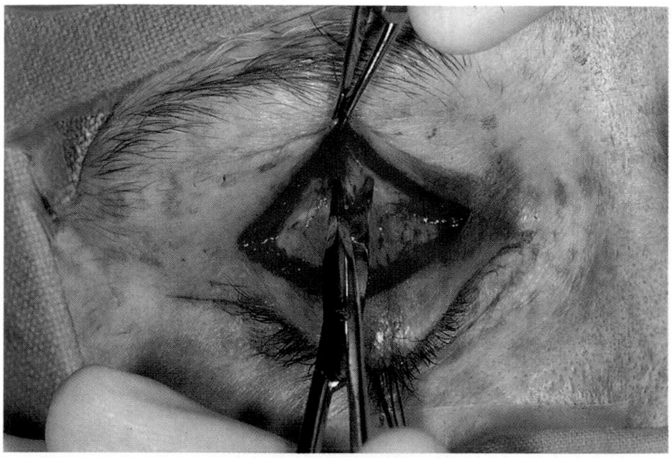

FIGURE 12–5

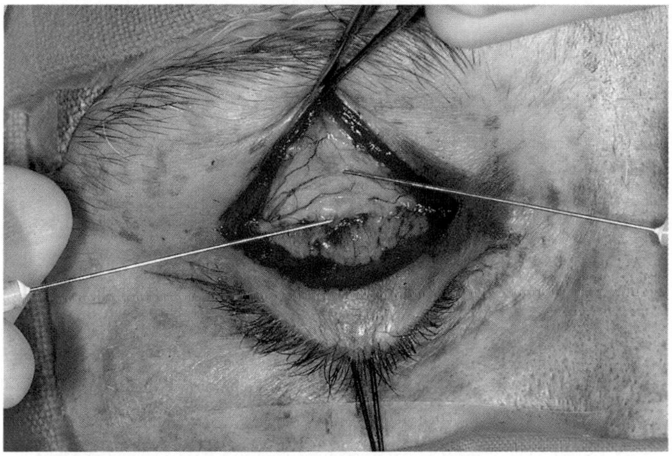

FIGURE 12–6

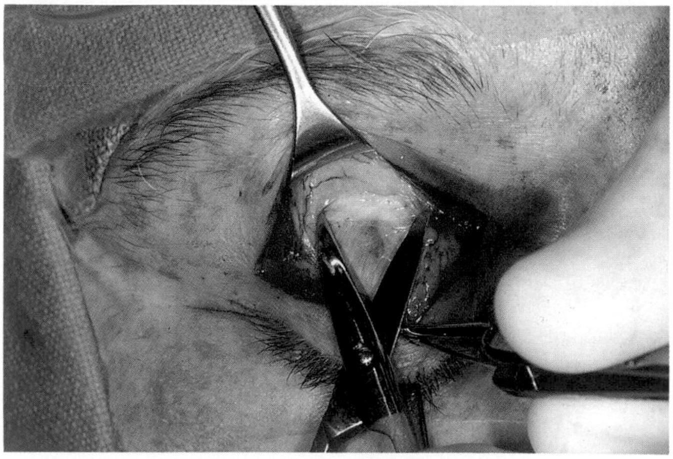

FIGURE 12–7

Figure 12–8. The disinserted edge of the levator aponeurosis is grasped with forceps. When the patient is asked to look superiorly, the surgeon can feel the force generated against the forceps, confirming the structure to be the aponeurosis. The Whitnall's ligament can be seen at the superior limit of the aponeurosis (*needle tip*). Frequently, the disinserted edge of the aponeurosis can be recognized.

Figure 12–9. A strip of pretarsal orbicularis muscle, at the superior margin of the tarsus, is excised by bluntly undermining with a Westcott scissors, thus baring the anterior surface of the tarsal plate. In ptosis cases in which the levator aponeurosis is intact, the appropriate amount of aponeurosis is resected with Westcott scissors. In patients in whom a rarefaction or dehiscence of the aponeurosis is present, it is important to excise the rarefied area to create a free healthy muscle edge for anchoring onto the tarsal plate.

If the aponeurosis has been disinserted, the disinserted edge is grasped with a forceps and sutured to the anterior surface of the tarsal plate. If there has been no obvious disinsertion, the aponeurosis is then detached from the upper border of the tarsal plate. The peripheral vascular arcade in Mueller's muscle helps to identify this structure. If bleeding occurs in this plane, one should pick up the tissue with the bipolar tip before cauterizing, thereby preventing thermal injury to the underlying cornea.

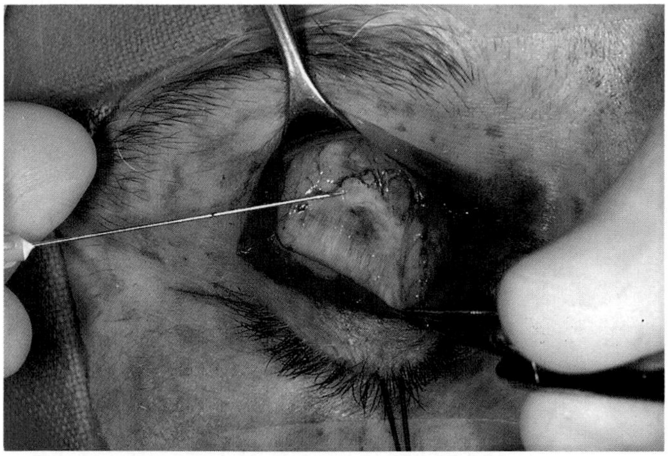

FIGURE 12–8

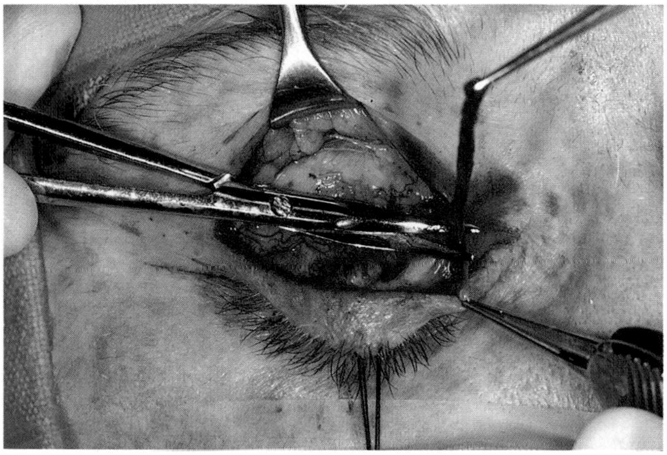

FIGURE 12–9

Figure 12–10. Once the full expanse of the aponeurosis has been separated from the tarsal plate and the appropriate amount of aponeurosis resected, it is then reattached onto the upper midportion of the tarsal plate with a 5–0 polygalactan 910 (Vicryl) suture on a spatula needle. A spatula needle facilitates a partial-thickness tarsal pass; the lid may be everted to confirm that full-thickness passes have not occurred. Full-thickness tarsal sutures should be avoided to prevent buckling of the tarsal plate and corneal abrasion. The first suture is placed just medial to the pupil, which is the highest point of the normal eyelid. The aponeurosis should be advanced and firmly fixed to the tarsus with a temporary tie first. "Tucking" of the aponeurosis does not result in a permanent correction, as no raw surfaces are opposed. The aponeurosis should be resected in all cases, except a complete disinsertion, to create a healthy, strong edge to suture to the tarsus. If the aponeurosis is advanced too low on the tarsal plate, eversion of the eyelid margin may occur.

Figure 12–11. After the central suture is adequately placed, three or four medial and lateral sutures are placed to adjust eyelid contour and height.

Figure 12–12. The lid height should be overcorrected about 1 to 1.5 mm at surgery to compensate for anesthetic paralysis of the orbicularis and to counteract slight postoperative fall.

When local anesthesia is used, the lid height and contour should be evaluated while the patient sits upright on the operating table. Eyelash position and lid crease should be evaluated at the same time. Once the lid height and contour are judged to be satisfactory, additional sutures are used to firmly secure the aponeurosis to the tarsal plate. The eyelid is then everted to look for any exposed sutures on the tarsoconjunctival surface.

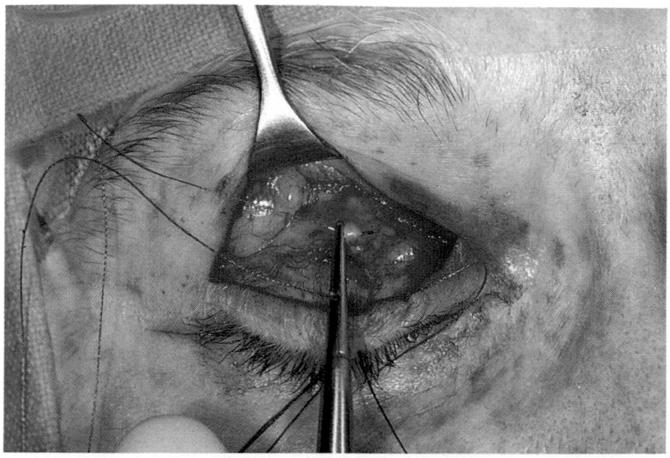

FIGURE 12–10

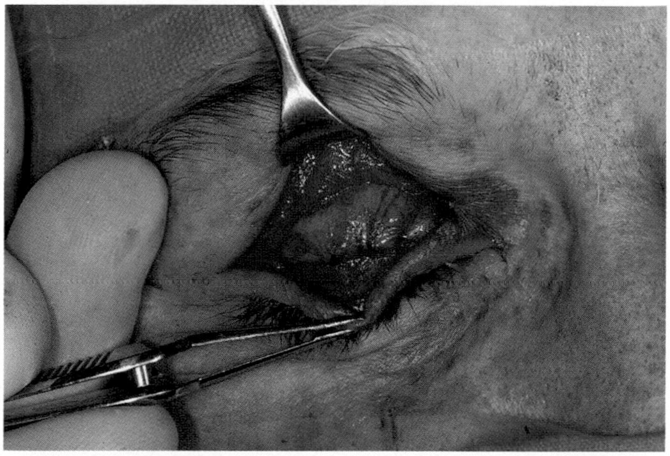

FIGURE 12–11

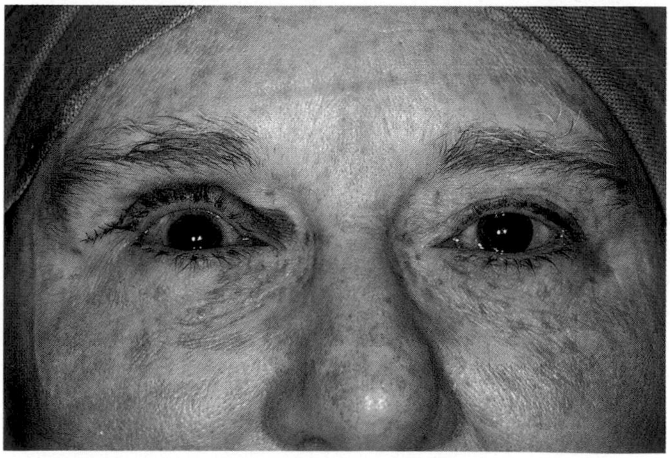

FIGURE 12–12

Figure 12–13. Frequently, excess skin and orbicularis are marked and excised from above the original incision site. This is almost invariably necessary and enhances the skin fold. However, one must be conservative on skin removal unless a blepharoplasty is to be performed on the contralateral eyelid as well.

The skin incision is closed with a running 7–0 nylon suture or 6–0 plain gut interrupted sutures. An antibiotic ointment is placed onto the incision. An ice pack is applied to reduce swelling.

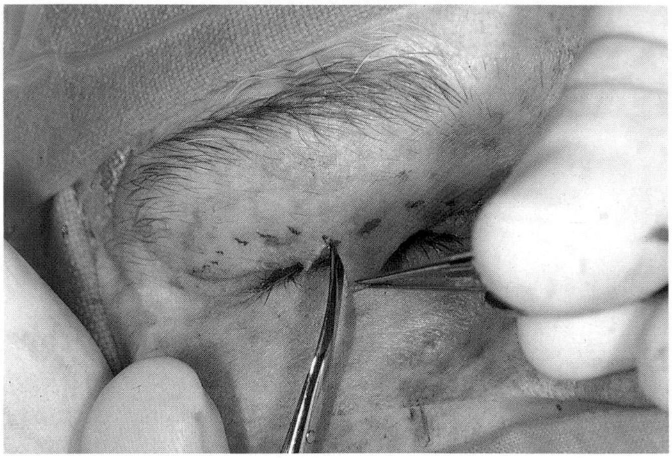

FIGURE 12–13

POSTOPERATIVE CARE

The patient is given a mild analgesic and instructed to apply an icebag on the operated eyelid intermittently for a few days. Patients should not take any aspirin-containing products. They are instructed to contact the physician should they experience severe orbital pain that may signal the development of an orbital hemorrhage. A lubricating ophthalmic ointment is applied onto the cornea, since most patients experience a mild degree of lagophthalmos in the perioperative period. Patients are seen the first postoperative day to check for hematoma or exposure keratopathy; they are again seen 1 week later for suture removal.

During the first 3 weeks after surgery, if over or undercorrection is apparent that is unrelated to eyelid edema, an adjustment may be performed. The eyelid crease incision is opened and eyelid height adjusted by advancing or recessing the levator aponeurosis.

CONGENITAL PTOSIS

PREOPERATIVE EVALUATION

The proper workup of a child with ptosis should begin with a careful history. It is important to establish the severity of ptosis at birth, of birth trauma or other injuries, and of progression. It is useful to inquire about the presence of a head turn, head tilt, or noticeable strabismus.

The examination of young children is frequently limited because of their short attention span, which may necessitate a rapid assessment. The vision must be assessed as well as ocular motility. Other eyelid abnormalities or decreased superior rectus function should be documented. The most important measurements relating to ptosis repair are the levator function (measured with the brow immobilized) and the amount of ptosis. The height of the lid creases is also essential to note preoperatively. It is useful to have an infant suck on a bottle or have a child chew gum to determine whether a jaw-winking ptosis is present, as the parents may be unaware of this. An explanation of this phenomenon is far better received preoperatively than if the jaw-winking is noted postoperatively. The vast majority of cases presenting in the pediatric age range will typically be the congenital variety, owing to an idiopathic developmental dystrophy of the levator muscle. Additionally, in "unilateral" congenital ptosis, the levator function is often diminished in the contralateral normal-appearing eye. One should bear in mind that the pediatric patient may present with acquired ptosis. Aponeurogenic ptosis on a congenital basis, neurogenic ptosis from third-nerve injury or a Horner's syndrome, mechanical ptosis secondary to an upper eyelid hamartoma, CPEO, or even a myogenic ptosis associated with myasthenia gravis may present in the pediatric-aged group. Appropriate treatment requires recognition of the etiologic basis of the ptosis.

It may be useful to use a grading scheme described by Beard (1979). Congenital ptosis with a lid droop of 2 mm or less is considered mild, 3 mm moderate, and 4 mm or more severe. Likewise, levator function of 8 mm or more may be considered good, 5 to 7 mm fair, and 4 mm or less poor. These arbitrary measures are useful in deciding on the appropriate surgical approach.

INDICATIONS FOR SURGERY

As children 8 years of age and younger are at risk for occlusion amblyopia, ptosis that is causing visual obstruction should be repaired as soon as possible. In addition, the surgeon should consider early correction of a ptosis that is causing an abnormal head posture or other functional problems. In congenital ptosis that is not causing visual impairment or other functional problems, it is wise to wait until the child is at least 3 years of age before repair. This allows the levator function to be measured on several different occasions, and yet completes the surgical repair before the child begins school.

The parents must be counseled concerning the chance of an under- or overcorrection and the possibility of the child needing additional surgery. It is also essential to discuss the expected postoperative appearance, as the lid will be low in up gaze and retracted in down gaze if there is diminished levator function and unilateral surgery is performed.

MAKING PROCEDURAL CHOICES

Although numerous approaches have been described in congenital ptosis, almost all ptosis cases can be managed with one of two procedures: (1) the aponeurotic approach and its modifications and (2) frontalis suspension procedures. The techniques of Fasanella-Servat or levator muscle resection provide no additional advantages in ptosis repair, and there are some significant disadvantages to these procedures. In mild or moderate congenital ptosis, with good or fair levator function, the ptosis may be corrected with an aponeurotic resection procedure (Table 12–1). In patients with poor levator function, it is usually not possible to achieve an ideal lid height with a unilateral levator procedure of any sort, although considerable improvement may be obtained with a maximal aponeurotic resection (Whitnall's sling) procedure. In this procedure, the Whitnall's ligament is sutured onto the tarsal plate. In unilateral ptosis with very poor function (<2 mm function), only a bilateral fascia sling, with extirpation of the levator muscle on the normal side, will produce adequate lid height and symmetry. As parents are often opposed to surgery on the normal eye, considerable improvement may be obtained and further surgery deferred or avoided if a maximal aponeurotic resection (Whitnall's sling) procedure with a superior tarsectomy is performed first. The authors have used a superior tarsectomy of 5 mm of tarsus to augment the elevation achieved by the Whitnall's sling procedure, expanding its application to some cases of congenital ptosis with poor levator function.

Congenital ptosis cases with good levator function respond to aponeurotic surgery in a fashion similar to adult ptosis. Patients with congenital aponeurotic defects and normal levator function will not demonstrate lid lag on down gaze, unlike the more typical patients with dystrophic levator muscles and diminished levator function. In patients with good levator function, a 3- to 4-mm resection of the levator apo-

TABLE 12–1
Procedure Selection for Congenital Ptosis

LEVATOR FUNCTION	SURGICAL PROCEDURE
Good (>8 mm)	Levator aponeurosis resection (3–4 mm aponeurosis resection per millimeter ptosis)
Fair (5–7 mm)	Levator aponeurosis resection or Whitnall's sling (5–6 mm aponeurosis resection per millimeter ptosis)
Poor (3–4 mm)	Maximal aponeurosis resection (Whitnall's sling with or without superior tarsectomy), Supramid sling, fascia lata sling
No function (<3 mm)	Supramid sling for infants (temporizing); bilateral fascia lata sling with extirpation of opposite levator muscle after age 3

neurosis for each millimeter of ptosis will usually provide the proper elevation. Under general anesthesia, the lid should be opened to approximately midpupil heights with only mild resistance to traction. Patients with fair levator function will require an aponeurosis resection of 5 to 6 mm or more for each millimeter of ptosis to obtain an adequate correction. Poor function cases will generally require a Whitnall's sling procedure, with or without a superior tarsectomy. A 5-mm superior tarsectomy will usually provide an additional 1 to 1.5 mm of elevation in these children. Alternatively, one may use the formula proposed by Tse to determine the amount of aponeurosis advancement in congenital ptosis: Amount of aponeurosis advancement (mm) = [Difference in levator function (mm) + Difference in eyelid fissure (mm)] + 3 (mm). (This formula is appropriate only for unilateral congenital ptosis cases.)

In children with poor function ptosis that is either severe or has not responded adequately to maximal aponeurotic surgery, bilateral frontalis suspension surgery will be required. As the patient is habituated to the ptosis, there is little drive to maintain a normal lid fissure in an eye with severe congenital ptosis. Unilateral frontalis suspension procedures are generally unsuccessful in achieving equivalent lid heights. The levator muscle must be cut or extirpated on the nonptotic side at the time of bilateral frontalis suspension if equal lid heights are to be achieved. In patients younger than 3 years of age, the iliotibial tract in the leg is not fully developed, precluding the use of autogenous fascia lata to suspend the lid. In this age group, we prefer to perform a frontalis sling, with an alloplastic material, Supramid, and defer a more permanent correction until an age at which an adequate piece of fascia lata can be harvested.

SURGICAL PROCEDURES

Maximal Aponeurotic Resection (Whitnall's Sling)

The steps leading up to the attachment of the Whitnall's ligament to the tarsal plate are identical with the steps illustrated earlier for levator aponeurosis advancement in acquired ptosis. Instead of advancing a predetermined amount of aponeurosis, the Whitnall's ligament is sutured onto the upper border of the tarsus with several interrupted 5–0 Vicryl sutures. Lid height adjustment is limited, since the Whitnall's ligament is a relatively fixed and nonmobile structure. Lid contour adjustment can be accomplished by varying the level of attachment on the tarsal surface. If inadequate lid elevation is obtained, a 5-mm superior tarsectomy is performed, and Whitnall's ligament is sutured to the cut edge of the tarsus. Skin closure is the same.

Pentagonal Supramid Sling

Five incision marks are placed on the lid, brow, and forehead to form a pentagonal configuration. The two lid incisions are placed approximately 2 mm above the lid margin. The medial incision is 1 to 2 mm medial to the medial limbus; the lateral incision 1 to 2 mm lateral to the lateral limbus. The brow incisions correspond to the medial and lateral canthi. The forehead incision is located midway between the two brow incisions and 1 cm above the brow line. Eyelid incisions are made with a lid plate in place to protect the globe. Forehead and brow stab incisions are similarly made with a size 15 blade. A hemostat or large needle-holder is used to pass the 4–0 Supramid suture with a swaged-on needle. A Wright needle may be used for passage of other suspensory materials.

The needle is first passed deep to the frontalis muscle through the forehead incision and exits the lateral brow incision. The needle reenters the lateral brow incision, passed deep to the orbicularis plane and exits from the lateral lid incision. The needle is then inserted into the lateral lid incision, passing superficial to the tarsus and exiting the medial lid incision. To complete the pentagonal configuration, the needle is passed in a retrograde fashion. The needle reenters the nasal lid incision, passing under the orbicularis toward the nasal brow incision. Passage of the suture is completed when the needle is brought out through the forehead incision. The ends are tied to elevate the lid above the superior pupillary margin. The ends of the suture are cut, and the knot buried deep in the forehead tissue. The skin incision is closed with 6–0 plain gut suture to avoid the need for suture removal. An antibiotic ointment is applied onto the incision sites.

Harvesting an Autogenous Fascia Lata Sling

The leg is prepared and draped from the knee to the anterosuperior iliac crest. An incision is marked 2 cm superior and slightly anterior to the lateral condylar process of the femur, where a distinct iliotibial tract can be palpated. A vertical incision is made extending up the leg for 2.5 to 3.0 cm. The incision is carried down through skin and fat to expose the white, glistening fascia. Once the dissection plane is identified, a long (12″) Metzenbaum scissors is used to bluntly dissect the overlying subcutaneous fat off the anterior surface of the fascia. Subcutaneous dissection is extended superiorly along the thigh for 12 to 15 cm. The wound is retracted, and two parallel incisions, 12-mm apart are made along the direction of the fascial fibers. Through these incisions, the fascia is bluntly separated from the underlying muscle for several centimeters with the Metzenbaum scissors. The fascial incisions are then bluntly extended superiorly for several centimeters with the Metzenbaum scissors, splitting the horizontally oriented fascial fibers. It is easier to make these two fascial incisions with a Metzenbaum scissors than with the stripper, as the cutting edge of the stripper is often quite dull, causing shredding of the fascia. Alternatively, a U-shaped stripper can be used to make these two fascial incisions. At the proximal end of the fascia, a vertical incision across the fascial fibers is made to connect the two parallel incisions. This strip, measuring 1 to 1.2 cm, is threaded into the tip of a Crawford fascia stripper. The end of the strip is grasped with a hemostat, and the stripper is firmly, but gently, pushed upward. When the stripper is fully up the leg, with 15 to 20 cm showing on the scale, the distal end of the fascia is transected by the cutting mechanism of the stripper. The stripper, along with a strip of fascia are withdrawn from the wound. Any subcutaneous fat adherent to the fascia is excised with a Westcott scissors. This broad strip of harvested fascia is then divided longitudinally into strips, each 2 mm wide. The subcutaneous layer is reapproximated with 4–0 chromic sutures and the skin is closed with 5–0 nylon sutures. An elastic bandage is applied to the thigh for 2 days. The strips are now ready for brow suspension.

Brow Suspension With Fascia Lata (Crawford, Modified)

The upper eyelid crease and several millimeters of redundant skin above the crease are outlined with a marking pen. The skin and orbicularis are excised to expose the orbital septum. All bleeding points are cauterized with a wet-field cautery.

A lid plate is placed under the upper eyelid, and three stab incisions are made about 2 mm above the lid margin. The medial incision is 2 mm medial to the medial limbus; the lateral incision is 2 mm lateral to the lateral limbus. The central incision is slightly medial to the pupil. The depth of the incision is down to the epitarsal surface. Two stab incisions are made above the brow ½ cm medial and lateral to vertical lines drawn from the medial and lateral lid incisions. A third incision is made midway between the brow incisions and 1 cm superior to the brow line. The brow incisions are made to the periosteum of the frontal bone. Bleeding from the incisions can be stopped by pressure. It is unnecessary to apply cautery.

With the lid plate in place, an empty Wright needle is inserted into the medial brow incision to the depth of the periosteum. It is passed across the orbital rim, directed inferiorly and posteriorly to penetrate behind the orbital septum and then superficially along the anterior lamella, to emerge through the medial lid incision.

Figure 12–14. The fascia is threaded through the eye of the needle.

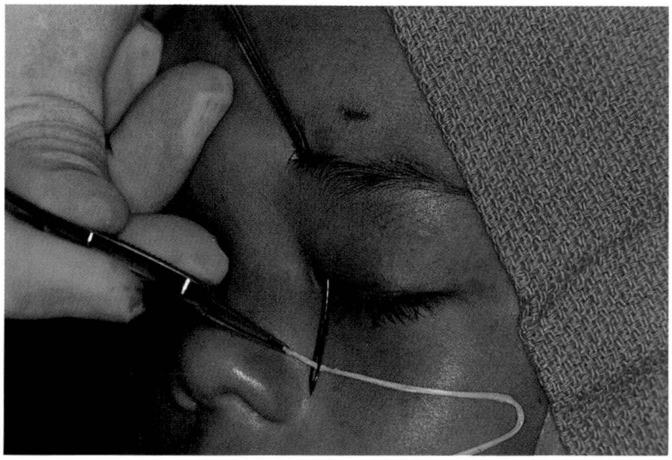

FIGURE 12–14

Figure 12–15. The needle is withdrawn, pulling the fascia through the lid incision and out of the brow incision. Care should be taken not to pull any cilia into the tract. The empty Wright needle is inserted into the middle lid incision, coursing horizontally along the epitarsal surface to exit the medial lid incision. The end of the fascial strand is threaded through the needle and drawn out through the central lid incision.

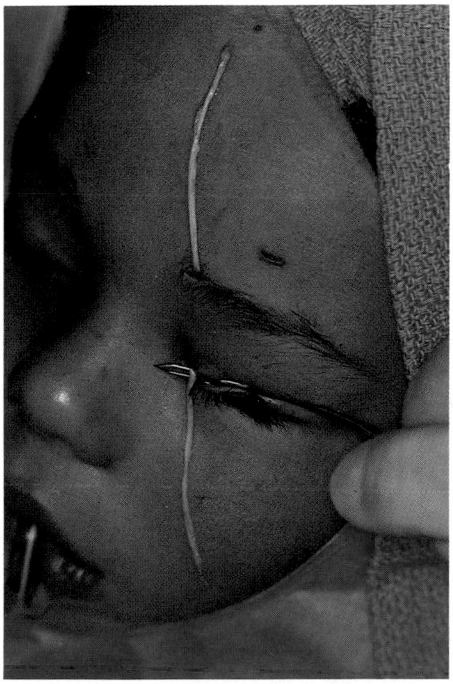

FIGURE 12–15

Figure 12–16. To complete the triangular configuration placement of the fascia in the lid, the Wright needle is reinserted into medial brow incision, traversing downward in the same fashion to emerge from the central lid incision. The fascia is withdrawn upward through the brow incision, uniting the two ends of the fascia.

After similar placement of another fascial strip to form the lateral triangle, the ends of the fascia are ready for tying at the brow incisions. If the suspension procedure is performed for bilateral ptosis, two fascial strips are placed in the identical manner for the fellow eye. Before tying the strips, a 6–0 polypropylene suture is used to secure the fascial strips to the epitarsal surface at each of the four points where the ascending fascia crosses the upper border of the tarsus. Care must be taken to avoid passing these sutures full-thickness and to cut the ends of the suture short. The eyelid crease incision is closed with a 6–0 plain gut suture.

Figure 12–17. The medial strip of fascia is tied first. A 5–0 polygalactin 910 (Vicryl) suture is laid between the two ends of the fascial strip, which are then pulled up and tied with sufficient tension to elevate the lid margin to 1 or 2 mm below the upper limbus with the eye in primary position. One square knot in the fascia is reinforced with the 5–0 Vicryl suture to prevent slippage. The knots are buried under the brow incision. The lateral strip is tied and reinforced in the same fashion.

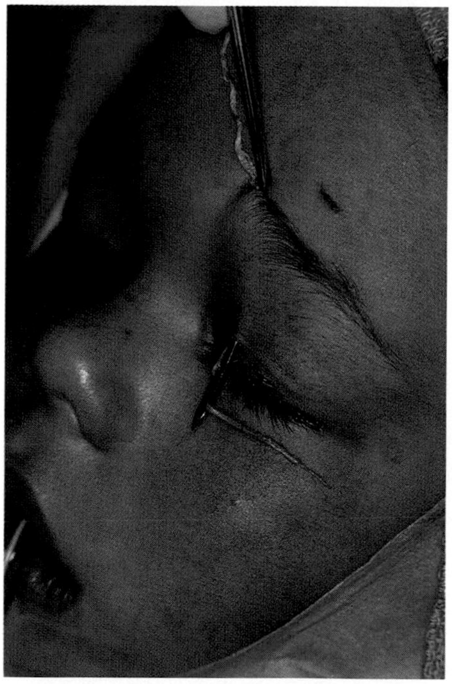

FIGURE 12–16

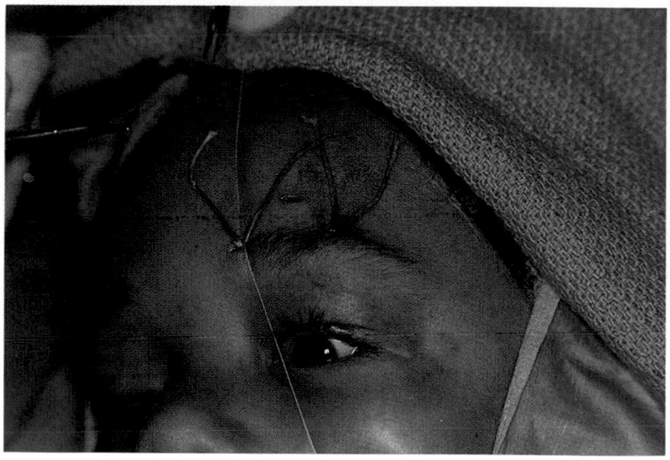

FIGURE 12–17

Figure 12–18. The long central end of each strip projecting from the brow is retrieved through the forehead incision using the Wright needle. By using traction and relaxation on each strip separately, the eyelid contour can be adjusted. The ends of the fascia are tied and the knots buried under the incision.

Figure 12–19. Once eyelid height and symmetry are assured, the stab skin incisions are closed with 6–0 plain gut sutures. Two 4–0 black silk traction sutures are placed in the lower lid and anchored to the forehead with adhesive tape. Antibiotic ointment is applied onto the cornea and to the incision sites.

The Frost sutures are removed the following day. The nylon sutures on the leg are removed in a week, and the wound is reinforced with a Steri-strip bandage.

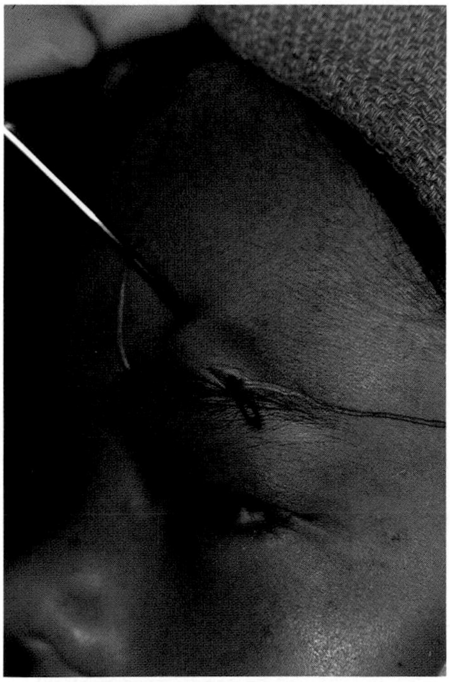

FIGURE 12–18

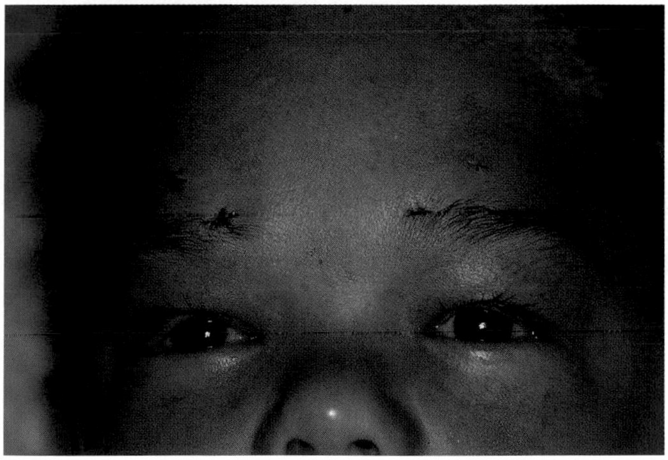

FIGURE 12–19

POSTOPERATIVE CARE

Initially it is recommended that ointment be instilled at least four times daily. The patient is seen the day after surgery and, if doing well, in 1 week. Usually, the ointment can be tapered to at bedtime only after 1 week, and artificial tear drops every 2 to 4 hours during the day. In many patients, it is possible to discontinue all lubricants after 1 month, although occasional patients will require lubricants indefinitely.

COMPLICATIONS

With aponeurotic resection for congenital ptosis, permanent overcorrection is uncommon. A slight overcorrection is desirable in the early postoperative period, and overcorrections of 2 mm or less will generally fall over time to a near-ideal lid height. Greater amounts of overcorrection may require massage or adjustment by recessing the aponeurosis.

In cases of undercorrection, it is best to wait to assess the final lid height until the swelling has resolved, as it is generally impossible to perform an adjustment under local anesthesia in a child. It is important to carefully note how much aponeurosis was initially resected. If the entire aponeurosis was initially resected to the level of Whitnall's ligament, additional lid elevation through a repeat anterior approach may not be feasible. In this situation, consideration may be given to extirpating the opposite normal levator muscle and performing a bilateral frontalis sling procedure. If only a partial aponeurotic resection was originally performed, it is possible to resect additional aponeurosis in a second procedure or perform a superior tarsectomy in addition.

Following frontalis suspension surgery, if marked lid asymmetry is noted the first postoperative day that is not related to swelling, consideration should be given to immediately reoperating and adjusting the fascia sling. Because of this possibility, one should always save any leftover fascia in a sterile specimen jar overnight so that the leg incision would not have to be reopened. For late undercorrections, repeating the fascia sling is generally the best approach.

Chapter Thirteen

UPPER EYELID BLEPHAROPLASTY

Russell S. Gonnering

PREOPERATIVE EVALUATION

The Periorbital Relaxation Syndrome

The majority of patients who present to the ophthalmologist for correction of "fullness" of the upper eyelids do so because of a constellation of abnormalities, best termed *the periorbital relaxation syndrome.* These patients will, to a greater or lesser degree, exhibit anatomic disturbances of all the supporting structures of the orbital unit and are best viewed as part of a continuum. Manifestations of this syndrome in the upper lid include dermatochalasis (lax eyelid skin and underlying orbicularis muscle), herniation of orbital fat, true ptosis, inferior displacement of eyebrow fat with or without eyebrow ptosis, and hypermobile lacrimal glands (Table 13–1). In the lower eyelid, manifestations include dermatochalasis, herniation of orbital fat, canthal laxity, and entropion or ectropion.

The preoperative evaluation must recognize the level of participation of each of these components of this syndrome in each individual patient so effective surgery can be planned. It is most helpful to sequentially tape structures into normal anatomic position to unmask the extent of involvement of other structures.

Associated Ophthalmic Abnormalities

It is obvious to the ophthalmic surgeon that all patients who present for eyelid surgery need a complete ophthalmic examination. Planned alterations in eyelid anatomy may have significant implications for

TABLE 13–1
Clinical Manifestations of the Generalized Periorbital Relaxation Syndrome

Upper Eyelid	Lower Eyelid
Brow ptosis	Dermatochalasis (skin and orbicularis muscle)
Inferior displacement of brow fat pad	Herniation of orbital fat
Dermatochalasis (skin and orbicularis muscle)	Laxity of canthal tendons
Herniation of orbital fat	Entropion or ectropion
Aponeurogenic ptosis	
Hypermobile lacrimal glands	

ophthalmic function. For patients in whom upper eyelid blepharoplasty is contemplated, particular attention needs to be focused on assessment of tear quality and quantity, presence or absence of a protective Bell's response, and possible underlying corneal lesions in which increased exposure may have import. Alterations in lid position and function may affect contact lens fitting after surgery.

Associated Conditions

The cause of the periorbital relaxation syndrome is multifactorial. In many instances, it is associated with solar elastosis, or the loss of elastic fibers in the dermis secondary to cumulative exposure to sun and weather. Such patients are also at risk for development of actinic keratoses and basal cell carcinoma.

Thyroid-associated orbitopathy commonly causes marked herniation of orbital fat, with concomitant relaxation of supporting structural elements of the orbital unit. In addition, such patients exhibit increased orbital vascularity, which may technically complicate the surgery.

The relatively rare condition of true blepharochalasis can be recognized by periodic, often unilateral, episodes of inflammatory edema of the eyelids without other cause. The repeated mechanical swelling causes a condition that mimics isolated acceleration of the normal-aging process of the orbital unit.

Periorbital edema can result from generalized edema caused by metabolic, cardiac, or hematologic abnormalities. It is also seen in a localized idiopathic form, and it can be confused with the fullness or orbital fat herniation. Rare causes of periorbital edema include the Melkersson–Rosenthal and Ascher syndromes, both with associated edema of the lips, buccal mucosa, or other parts of the face.

SURGICAL INDICATIONS

Objective Indications

A somewhat arbitrary distinction can be made between "reconstructive" blepharoplasty and "aesthetic" blepharoplasty. The reality is that most patients seeking relief of objective symptoms are also very concerned with achieving an optimum aesthetic result.

Perhaps the most persistent and easily quantified objective indication for upper eyelid blepharoplasty is a peripheral visual field defect. Many patients will volunteer that they can see much better when they manually elevate the upper eyelid. Visual field testing, with and without eyelid taping, will objectively document the presence of the peripheral field defect, as well as the expected improvement with surgery. Preoperative photography, taken in full-face and lateral or three-quarter views, can further document the existence of objective abnormality. Most insurance companies now demand such objective evidence for certification of the reconstructive nature of the proposed surgery.

Other objective indications include eyelash ptosis, with corneal irritation from contact of the lashes with the cornea. Pain from hypermobile lacrimal glands is also described by patients and is relieved with repair.

Subjective Indications

In the preoperative evaluation of the upper eyelid blepharoplasty, it is absolutely essential to identify the patient's expectations of surgery and to balance these against realistic surgical goals. A blepharoplasty will not improve brow ptosis, nor is it a substitute for a facial rhytidectomy. It may be helpful to give the patient a hand mirror and ask them to point out their expectations of surgery. All patients undergoing upper eyelid blepharoplasty need to be given a detailed informed consent form that includes the planned surgical procedure, its goals, anticipated benefits, and possible risks.

SURGICAL ANATOMY

The relatively thin, uniform skin of the upper eyelid merges with thicker skin at the nose, eyebrow, and lateral orbital rim. Ideally, the skin excision in upper eyelid blepharoplasty should be confined to this area of thin skin. In distinction to other areas of the face, there is no subcutaneous fat in the eyelid, with tight adhesion between lid skin and the underlying thin anterior investing fascia or the orbicularis muscle. This adhesion effectively joins the skin and orbicularis as a single unit.

The upper eyelid crease and overhanging fold divide the eyelid into a tarsal and orbital portion. Below this crease, pretarsal orbicularis muscle is tightly adherent to, in turn, the postorbicular fascia, levator aponeurosis, and tarsus. Superior traction on the skin in this region will be directly transmitted to the underlying layers.

Above the lid crease, preseptal and orbital portions of the orbicularis are also adherent to the underlying postorbicular fascia. However, the adherence to the underlying orbital septum is tenuous, and superior traction on skin in this area will elevate the skin, muscle, and fascia away from the orbital septum.

Formation of the lid crease is classically ascribed to skin attachments of the levator aponeurosis extending through the orbicularis muscle to terminate in the dermis. An alternative theory explains the formation of the lid crease as a union of the postorbicular fascia with the levator aponeurosis.

Perhaps the most clinically useful landmark in upper eyelid surgery is the orbital septum. This nonelastic connective tissue membrane arises from the arcus marginalis at the orbital rim and extends inferiorly to terminate and insert upon the levator aponeurosis. The exact point of attachment is variable, with inferior termination largely responsible for formation of the Oriental upper eyelid. Beneath the septum is the orbit proper, with variable amounts of orbital fat, divided into a preaponeurotic portion and a medial portion, split by the tendon of the superior oblique muscle and associated fascia. No true "lateral" fat compartment is present, although the preaponeurotic portion may extend laterally over the anterior aspect of the lacrimal gland.

Anterior to the septum is the postorbicular fascia, in which run the terminal fibers of the facial nerve. This layer may also contain considerable fat, contiguous with the eyebrow fat pad. The presence of such "preseptal" fat, especially laterally, is probably responsible for the elusive lateral fat compartment of the upper eyelid. This fat, unlike the easily prolapsed orbital fat, is contained within fibrous septa.

The levator aponeurosis fans out from the muscular portion of the levator, and inserts in a broad attachment along the anterior surface of the tarsus, with possible extensions to the skin, as described by Whitnall. The lateral expansion, or horn, splits the orbital and palpebral portions of the lacrimal gland to join the lateral retinaculum and insertion on Whitnall's lateral orbital tubercle. The course of the medial expansion is less delineated, but function attachments to the medial canthal tendon exist.

The orbital portion of the lacrimal gland occupies the lacrimal gland fossa and is held in place by "ligaments," or capsular connections within the orbital connective tissue network, particularly at its posterior extent.

An important precept that follows from a knowledge of upper eyelid anatomy is that alterations of anatomy will produce alterations in form and function. Indeed, that is the purpose of upper eyelid blepharoplasty. Most patients want a more youthful appearance. Although some Oriental patients may desire an Occidental appearance postoperatively, to create such an appearance when it is not desired will have disastrous consequences.

To this end, it is most important to plan the surgical incision to coincide with the desired eyelid crease, as the closure of this incision will locally unite the orbicularis muscle, postorbicular fascia, and levator aponeurosis. Superior traction on this unit produced by levator contraction will create the lid crease and associated lid fold. Most women desire this crease to be high. Most men would be very unhappy with such a "feminine" lid. The crease in the Oriental patient may be only a few millimeters from the cilia.

SURGICAL PROCEDURE

General Preparation of Patient

In most patients, upper eyelid blepharoplasty should be done under local anesthesia with intravenous relaxation. Provisions for monitoring vital functions, optimally to include pulse oximetry, must be made. Medications with anticoagulant properties, particularly aspirin, should be discontinued at least 7 days before surgery. If this is medically impossible, the intraoperative use of topical hemostatic agents, such as thrombin, should be anticipated.

Following intravenous relaxation and application of topical ophthalmic anesthetic, the patient is prepared in a sterile fashion for lid surgery. Care is exercised in the draping of the patient, to avoid artificial tension of the eyelid from the drape.

Although some surgeons successfully inject local anesthetic before skin margin and preparation, the distortion produced by the injection may make accurate skin margin impossible.

Surgical Technique

With superior traction on the skin at the brow, the redundant skin and orbicularis muscle is effaced. The site of incision and proposed upper eyelid crease is marked, extending from the lacrimal punctum to the lateral palpebral commissure. In the male patient, the crease should be marked approximately 7.5 to 8.0 mm from the lid margin at its highest extent in midlid. The crease in female patients is higher, approximately 9.0–9.5 mm from the lid margin. In both male and female patients, the medial and lateral extremes of the lid crease are approximately 1.0 to 1.5 mm lower than its central height. From the lateral termination of the lid crease incision marking, an extension is drawn at about a 20° angle, terminating at the outside border of the lateral orbital rim.

Figure 13–1. At several points along the lid crease incision, the redundant skin and underlying orbicularis is grasped with a smooth forceps. The forceps is closed at various levels until the amount of skin pinched eliminates excessive eyelid skin and minimally everts the lashes. The points are marked with the marking pen and are then connected to create an ellipsoid segment to be excised.

Figure 13–2. The contralateral upper eyelid is marked in a similar manner, and the amount of skin outlined is compared. A measurement is made from the upper lid margin to the lid crease line, making sure that both sides are symmetric. The exact form of the segment will be dictated by the amount and location of redundancy. To avoid standing cones or "dog-ears," terminal angles of excised tissue should approximate 30° to 40°. If this angle is too small to accommodate the redundancy, Burrows' triangles or *M*-plasties should be employed. Incisions should be confined to eyelid skin and not extend onto the nasal root or beyond the orbital rim. Final trimming of these can be left until closure, to ensure exact fit.

Infiltration anesthesia is then injected subcutaneously into the segment to be incised. I use a 1:1 mixture of 2% lidocaine with 0.75% bupivacaine with 150 units of hyaluronidase, with 1 to 2 ml injected in each eyelid.

Figure 13–3. After waiting 5 to 7 minutes, skin incision over the preplaced marking is made with a scalpel blade. The segment of skin and orbicularis muscle is excised with a Stevens scissors. Hemostasis is obtained with a wet-field cautery.

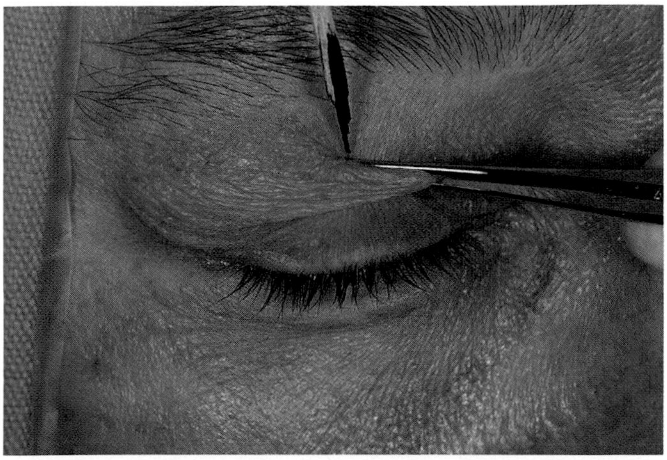

FIGURE 13–1

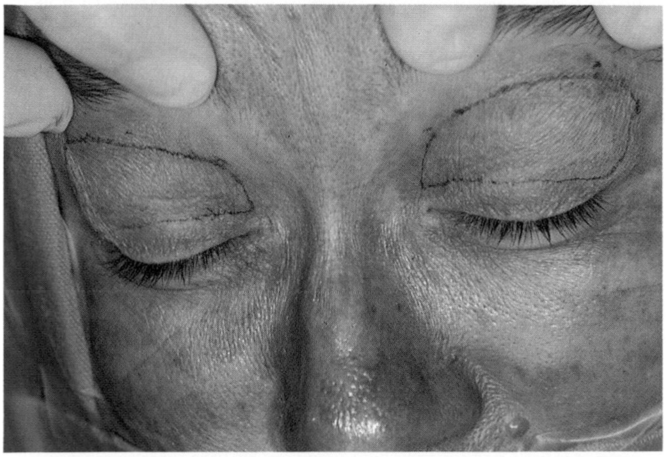

FIGURE 13–2

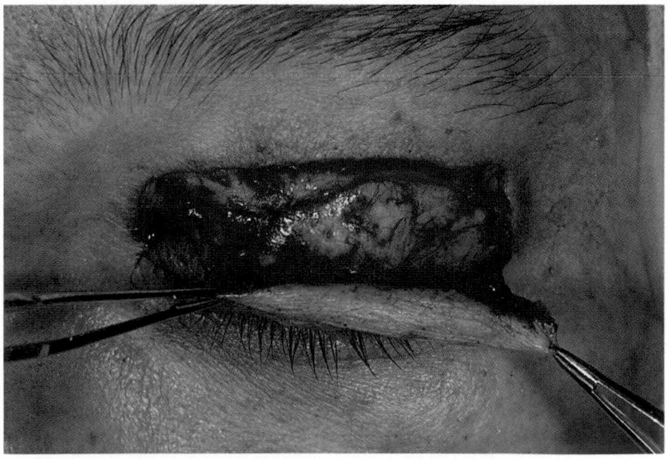

FIGURE 13–3

Figure 13–4. The orbital septum is button-holed and opened along the entire length of the incision.

Figure 13–5. This exposes the medial and preaponeurotic orbital fat pads. If inferior migration of the eyebrow fat pad is present, it is contained by fibrous septa and is located in the plane of the postorbicular fascia, anterior to the orbital septum, and clearly differentiated from the orbital fat. Blood vessels, which can be significantly dilated in thyroid-associated orbitopathy, are prominent in the fat capsule. Many of these can be avoided if the capsule is opened in a favorable line. Excision of the eyebrow and orbital fat in a smooth line with the orbital rim can then be accomplished with high-temperature disposable cautery or sharp dissection with either thermal or electrocautery.

Figure 13–6. Alternatively, gentle pressure on the globe will cause herniation of the preaponeurotic fat, which can first be clamped with a hemostat, then excised with a scissors.

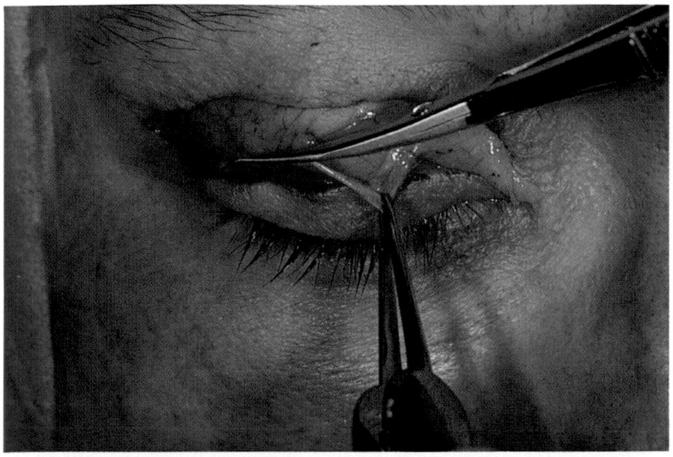

FIGURE 13–4

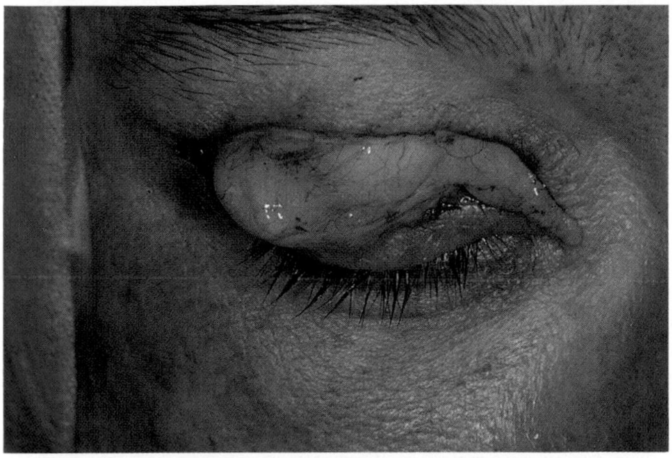

FIGURE 13–5

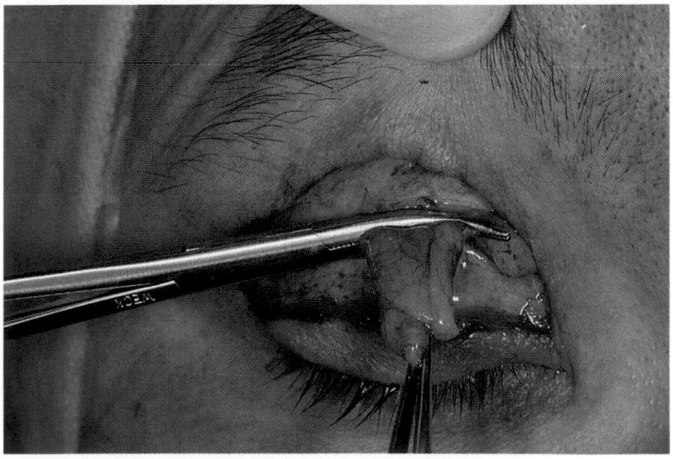

FIGURE 13–6

Figure 13–7. The cut edge of the stump of orbital fat should be cauterized before allowing it to retract into the orbit. Care must be taken in excision of the medial fat pad to avoid the penetrating medial palpebral artery.

After removal of the preaponeurotic fat, the levator aponeurosis is examined for any defects. If aponeurosis disinsertion is apparent, it should be repaired. Temporary knots aid in the fine adjustment of lid height and contour. Anterior displacement of the lacrimal gland may be present and can be repaired by suturing the capsule of the gland to the periosteum of the lacrimal gland fossa.

Figure 13–8. After a final check for hemostasis, the lid crease is reformed with multiple supratarsal fixation sutures using 6–0 plain gut.

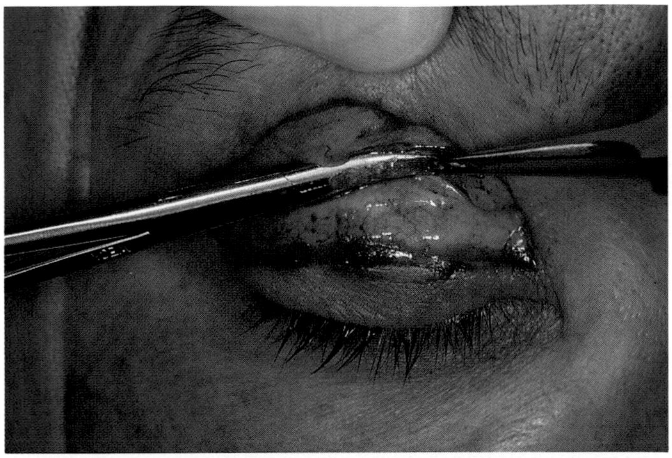

FIGURE 13–7

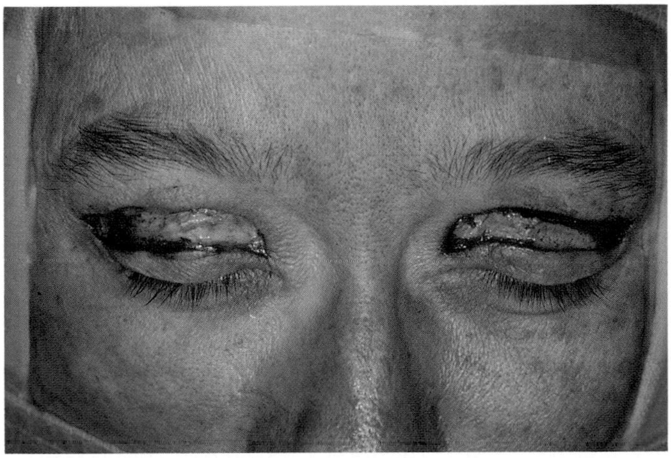

FIGURE 13–8

Figure 13–9. Suture passage for lid crease formation should unite the pretarsal and preseptal orbicularis to the levator aponeurosis below the normal insertion site of the orbital septum, which is never sutured. Thus, the attachment of postorbicular fascia to levator aponeurosis is reconstituted. This will provide support to the pretarsal orbicularis and allow the crease to efface normally in down gaze or when the lid is closed.

Figure 13–10. Finally, a running suture of 6–0 monofilament nonabsorbable or fast-absorbing plain (Ethicon) suture is used to close the skin. Antibiotic ointment is applied. The patient returns to the post-surgical area where their head is elevated and iced compresses are applied for 90 to 120 minutes before discharge.

POSTOPERATIVE CARE

The patient is kept in a postsurgical holding area for 90 to 120 minutes, during which time their head is elevated and iced compresses applied to the wound. These compresses are continued as much as possible until retiring that evening. Antibiotic ointment is applied twice a day, and the patient is instructed to gently cleanse crusting from the lids with warm tap water and cotton balls. The iced compresses can be continued the first postoperative day if they make the patient more comfortable, but after this they can be discontinued.

The patient is seen in a postoperative examination 3 to 5 days after surgery for suture removal if nonabsorbable sutures were used. The antibiotic ointment can be decreased to bedtime use only. Warm compresses are used to hasten resolution of edema. In some patients, particularly those with thyroid-associated orbitopathy, a short course of oral dexamethasone may be used if edema is excessive. Although swimming should be avoided for 2 weeks, the patient can usually shower after 3 days. Eye makeup can be used after 7 to 10 days. Full aerobic activity and contact lens wear can be safely resumed in most patients after 2 to 3 weeks. Sun exposure should be limited for at least a month following surgery.

Some thickening of incised skin, with increased crusting and flaking persists for 3 to 4 weeks after surgery. This can be controlled by gently scrubbing the lid with a cotton ball and neutral soap or lid scrub at bedtime. Some patients may benefit from a short course of topical dexamethasone ointment.

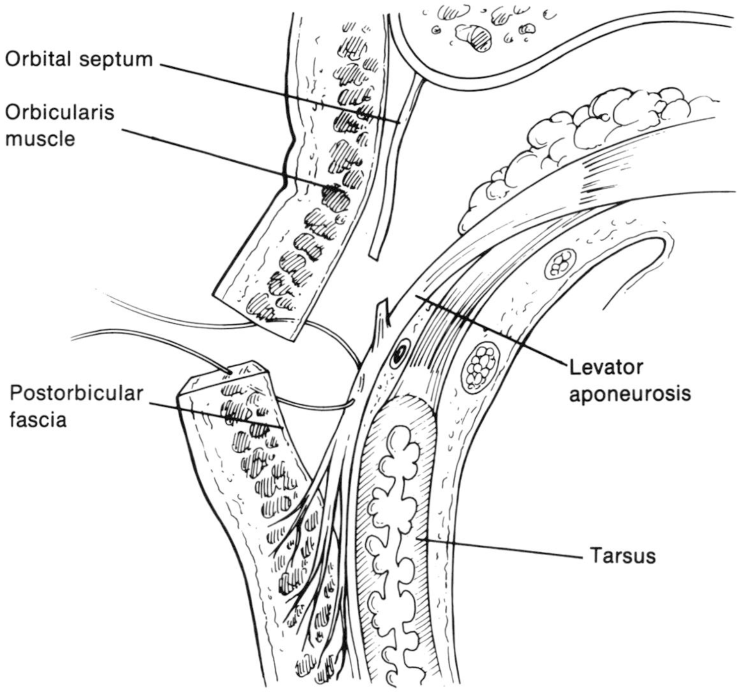

FIGURE 13–9

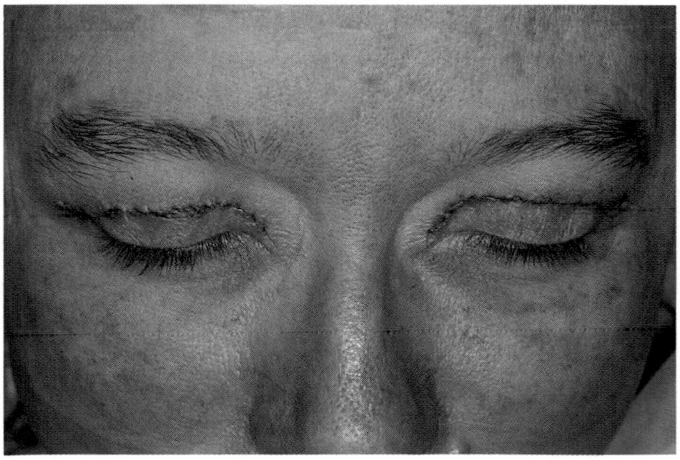

FIGURE 13–10

COMPLICATIONS

Fortunately, the most feared complication of blepharoplasty, decreased vision from orbital hemorrhage, is quite rare. Meticulous attention to hemostasis is mandatory. The use of iced compresses significantly decreases postoperative ooze. The patient should be instructed to seek immediate attention if significant pain or bleeding occurs, or if the vision decreases. If faced with visual loss from an orbital hemorrhage in the immediate postoperative period, the wound should be widely opened when the patient is first seen. High-dose steroids, surgical exploration, or even orbital decompression may be needed.

The most significant complication of upper blepharoplasty is asymmetry, and all patients should be informed of this possibility before surgery. It is not unusual to have asymmetric postoperative edema, and any decision on the need for secondary surgery should be postponed until all edema has resolved. Prolonged redness of the incision line may occur in fair-skinned individuals. This may respond to a 2- to 3-week treatment with topical dexamethasone ointment, but can persist for months.

Minimal transient lagophthalmos may occur when the proper amount of skin and orbicularis has been excised. Care must be taken not to include the orbital septum in the closure, otherwise permanent tethering of the lid may occur. Most cases of minimal lagophthalmos respond to emollient therapy and massage. If they do not, surgical exploration, lysis of septal adhesions, and possible skin graft may be necessary. The most severe form of lagophthalmos occurs when underlying brow ptosis is not recognized. In an attempt to relieve lid fullness, so much lid skin and muscle are excised, that the brow is brought onto the lid. Extensive reconstructive surgery is necessary to relieve this tragic outcome.

Ptosis can occur from failure to recognize levator dehiscence, iatrogenic damage to the levator, or placement of supratarsal fixation sutures too high on the levator aponeurosis. Unfortunately, ptosis other than mechanical caused by transient edema will need surgical correction.

The most difficult complication to deal with is the patient in whom objective results and subjective expectations do not match. Such a situation is best avoided by taking the time preoperatively to obtain a detailed informed consent. However, when it occurs, the surgeon must retain objective surgical judgment, and resist the temptation to either ignore the patient's complaints, or to rush in in an attempt to "touch up" what may not need touching at all. The patient and surgeon are both best served by a frank, open, and attentive response to the patient's concerns.

Chapter Fourteen

LOWER EYELID BLEPHAROPLASTY

Alfred C. Marrone

PREOPERATIVE EVALUATION

As essentially all lower lid blepharoplasties are performed for cosmetic reasons, the most important aspect of the preoperative evaluation is to ask the patient what characteristics of their lower lid appearance they wish to change. If "baggy lids" are of concern, then certainly herniating orbital fat removal will be the principal goal of surgery. If the patient is not concerned about skin wrinkling, then a transconjunctival approach can be considered. If a transcutaneous approach is selected, then there is little reason to risk complication by trying to remove too much skin. Be wary of the patient who expects unrealistic social or occupational rewards from the surgery.

With use of a mirror, one can show the patient what can be expected from skin removal, by pulling down on the cheek to smooth the skin, to approximate the postoperative appearance.

The first physical finding to be evaluated in the lower lid is the presence or absence of fat herniation. Look at the patient from the front and side, make a simple sketch of the three fat pockets and grade the amount of herniation from 1 to 4. Gentle pressure against the globe through the upper eyelid will give an indication of orbital septum tautness to predict whether more fat will herniate forward once the septum is opened.

The next characteristic to evaluate is the amount of excess skin present. Assess the amount of wrinkles present and pull down gently on the cheek skin to approximate the amount of skin that can be removed without displacing the eyelid.

It is important to evaluate the horizontal tone of the lower lid, especially if skin is to be removed. A "snap test" is performed in which the lower lid is pulled downward with the thumb and released without the patient blinking. If the lid snaps back against the globe, the tone is very good. This will allow a prudently aggressive approach to skin removal. If it moves back slowly to its original position, then fair tone exists and judicious skin removal should be exercised. The patient should be advised before surgery of the need for conservatism and its effect on skin removal. If the lid does not return to its normal position until the patient blinks, then the tone is poor and horizontal shortening of the eyelid should be combined with skin removal, or a transconjunctival approach should be used. The lateral canthal tarsal strip method of tightening the lid is preferred (see Chapter 10).

It is also important to evaluate the contour of the orbicularis in the lower eyelid. If the patient has significant redundancy of the pretarsal orbicularis (usually more noticeable when smiling), then a portion of this can be carefully excised during surgery or sutured flat against the tarsus.

If excess rolls of orbicularis are present along the infraorbital rim (so-called orbicularis festoon), then these can also be repaired.

A patient's blinking dynamic and lid closure status are evaluated. Tear film breakup time and results of the Schirmer test are recorded.

Preoperative photographs of the eyelids should be taken. They serve not only as part of the medical record, but patients enjoy looking at them several months later.

A thorough medical history and appropriate physical examination for the type of anesthesia should be obtained. Aspirin intake should be discontinued 2 to 4 weeks before surgery. If a patient uses certain antidepressants, such as tranylcypromine (Parnate) or phenelzine (Nardil), then the use of epinephrine and some sedatives may be contraindicated.

Finally, there should be a thorough discussion of the surgery, type of anesthesia (usually local with mild sedation), and postoperative care, including ecchymosis and swelling.

INDICATIONS

As this is aesthetic surgery, the basic indication is a cosmetically significant excess of lower lid skin or fat herniation that is surgically correctable. Since lower lid blepharoplasty procedures should not be repeated frequently, surgery should result in enough of an improvement to be beneficial to the patient. The surgeon should have good rapport with the patient, and the patient should have a good understanding of what to expect from the surgery.

Most patients are best served with a transcutaneous approach. The transconjunctival approach is best utilized when there is no need to excise skin, a visible scar is very undesirable (as in young male), and the lid is lax enough to permit surgical exposure. This approach requires the surgeon to have more familiarity with eyelid anatomy. This is also a good approach as a reoperative procedure to remove residual fat.

ANATOMY

There are several important points to remember about the lower eyelid anatomy during blepharoplasty.

The pretarsal orbicularis is responsible for lid apposition and blink. Preservation of as much of its function as possible is desirable. Care should be taken not to excise too much muscle or to separate the muscle from its nerve supply.

The orbicularis, particularly the preseptal orbicularis, can become redundant along with the skin and, therefore, should be excised. Marked redundancy of the orbicularis along the infralateral orbital rim is referred to as *festoons*.

The retractors of the lower eyelid consist of the capsulopalpebral fascia and Mueller's muscle. The capsulopalpebral fascia begins as the capsulopalpebral head, with fine fibrous connections to the inferior rectus muscle and tendon. The capsulopalpebral head divides into two portions as it extends around and fuses with the sheath of the inferior oblique muscle. Anterior to the inferior oblique muscle, these two branches rejoin to form the Lockwood's ligament. The fascial tissue anterior to the Lockwood's ligament is the capsulopalpebral fascia. A large portion of the capsulopalpebral fascia ascends the lower eyelid to insert onto the inferior margin of the tarsal plate. The inferior oblique muscle originates from behind the posterior lacrimal crest, several millimeters behind the orbital rim. It can be damaged during lower eyelid blepharoplasty, particularly the transconjunctival approach.

The fat lobules and the orbit are enveloped and interconnected by a series of membranous septae. Overzealous traction on the orbital fat may result in avulsion of fine vessels deep in the orbit.

Because the orbital septum is attached to the inferior orbital rim, an adhesion between the cut edge of the septum and the movable portion of the lid could result in downward tethering of the lid.

SURGERY

Transcutaneous Blepharoplasty

Appropriate oral or injectable sedatives may be given before injection of the local anesthetic. The patient must be reasonably alert to cooperate in assessing the amount of skin for removal.

Ten parts of 2% lidocaine (Xylocaine) with 1:100,000 epinephrine is combined with one part of 8.4% sodium bicarbonate for the anesthetic mixture. The addition of this buffer is to change the pH of the solution to minimize any burning sensation during anesthetic infiltration. After placing a drop of topical proparacaine in the cul-de-sac, an infraorbital nerve block may be given. This is accomplished by directly injecting over the infraorbital foramen, which is located about 1 cm below the midinferior orbital rim. A small amount of anesthetic is also injected along the preseptal region of the lid. Gentle pressure at this point minimizes hematoma formation. Since epinephrine takes 10 to 15 minutes to take effect, the incision should be delayed appropriately. The patient is then prepared and draped. It is essential that surgical drapes do not distort the facial skin, which can result in an over- or underestimation of the amount of skin removal. Slight reverse Trendelenburg positioning is preferred to minimize orbital venous pressure and to more closely approximate the effect of gravity on the cheeks.

Figure 14–1. A short incision is made through the skin in a crease near the lateral canthal area and directed downward.

Figure 14–2. A Westcott scissors is used to dissect the skin away from the pretarsal orbicularis to create an infraciliary incision. The skin flap is continued inferiorly over the pretarsal orbicularis.

Figure 14–3A. A small iris scissors is used to incise the preseptal orbicularis at a point below the inferior tarsal margin and anterior to the septum. The surgeon elevates the skin with forceps and the assistant gently pulls the eyelid superiorly for countertraction. Dissection within this plane is carried inferiorly until the inferior orbital rim is reached.

Figure 14–3B. A cross-sectional view illustrates the path of dissection and point of incision on the orbital rim. Blunt and sharp dissections complete the skin–muscle flap, which is only a skin flap over the pretarsal orbicularis (and a lateral extension to protect its nerve supply). This enhances postoperative function and gives the infraciliary area a more rounded and youthful appearance.

Mild bipolar (wet-field) cautery is used to control bleeding. With the skin–muscle flap elevated and with gentle pressure through the upper lid against the globe, the fat pockets are displaced forward. The orbital septum is incised along its entire length over the medial and central fat pockets and over the lateral pocket separately. Each of the fat pockets is then gently grasped with a forceps and the individual septae are incised with scissors to fully facilitate forward herniation of the orbital fat. Never exert tension on the fat when lifting out of the orbit. This can avulse vessels in the posterior orbit, contributing to the development of orbital hemorrhage.

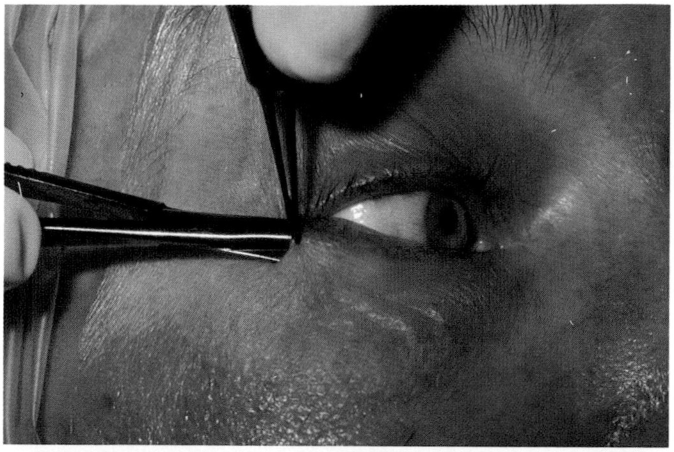

FIGURE 14–1

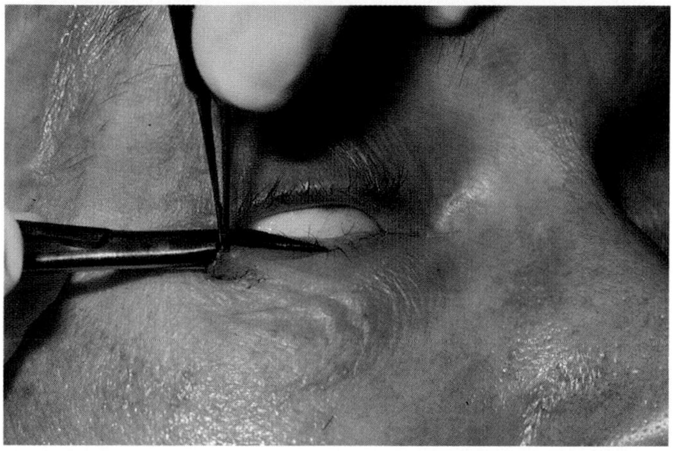

FIGURE 14–2

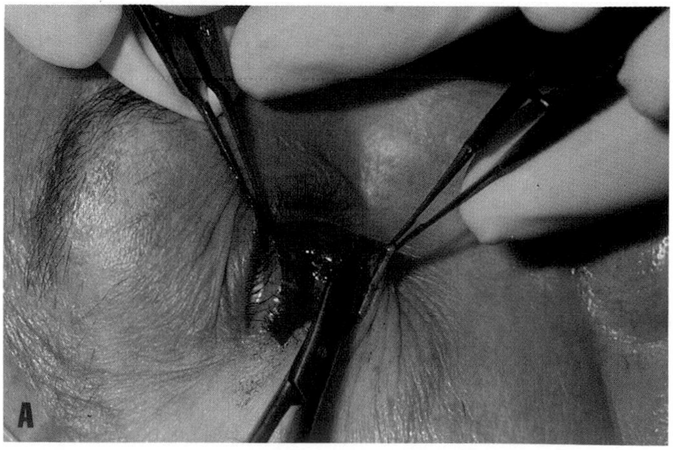

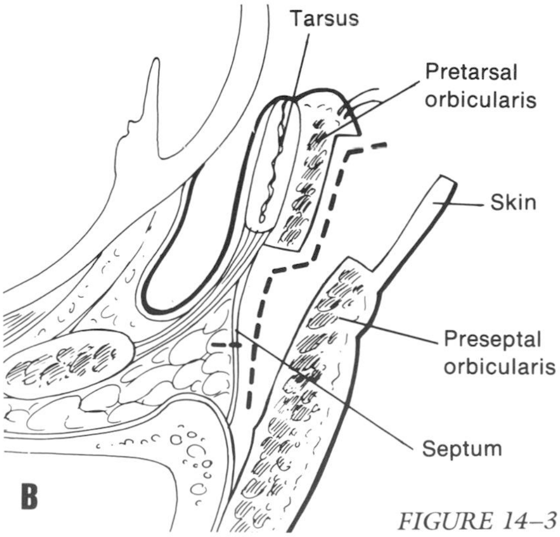

FIGURE 14–3

Figure 14–4. One way to remove fat is to clamp it with a hemostat, cut the excess away with scissors and cauterize the stump with a bipolar cautery. I prefer to gently lift up the excess fat and cauterize the base with a bipolar cautery; then cut anterior to the cautery mark. This minimizes the chance of traction from the forceps on the posterior orbital fat and vessels. Always ensure hemostasis before allowing the fat to retract back into the orbit. Usually the central pocket is removed first. It is important after removing the fat from the lateral area to check for any further fat herniation that may be present and can prolapse after removal of the first pocket.

After fat removal, the contour of the fat pockets is then evaluated by placing gentle posterior pressure through the upper lid against the globe; cauterize or remove any fat that remains forward of the desired plane (usually flush with the orbital rim). Complete and meticulous hemostasis should be obtained at this point. The patient is then instructed to look superiorly to ensure that the lid is not in a depressed position when excising skin.

Figure 14–5. While looking up, the patient is asked to open the mouth which mimics gravity and pulls the cheek downward slightly. The excess skin is draped over the lid by pulling in a superotemporal direction and then is gently released. It is useful to stroke the skin superiorly with the back of the scissors while cutting the excess skin to match the infraciliary portion of the incision.

Figure 14–6. Any preseptal orbicularis on the skin muscle flap that would lie over the pretarsal orbicularis is excised to prevent bulging at the skin margin. The muscle layer should now dovetail naturally. Any folds can be excised while being careful to avoid cutting the external extension of the pretarsal orbicularis, which may impair the normal tone of the muscle.

A variation of this approach can be used to treat *orbicularis festoons*. These are the redundant folds of orbicularis that exist along, and just inferior to, the inferior orbital rim, usually temporally. The repair is identical with the foregoing approach except, after excising the preseptal orbicularis, the lateral edge of the orbicularis is sutured with 4–0 or 5–0 PDS or a nonabsorbable suture to the lateral orbital rim just beneath the lateral canthal tendon. This is done while the orbicularis is pulled superotemporally.

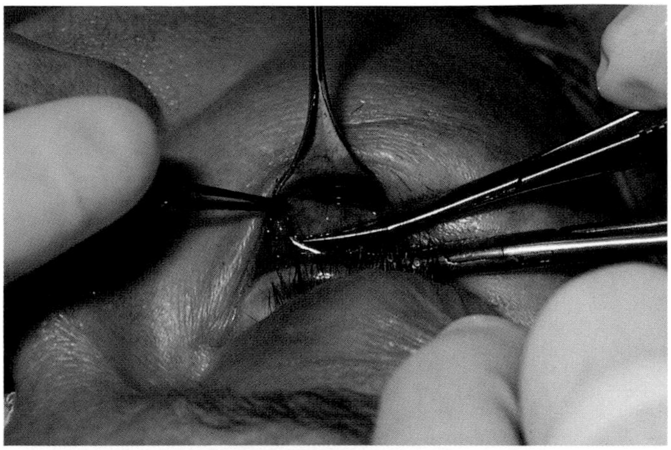

FIGURE 14–4

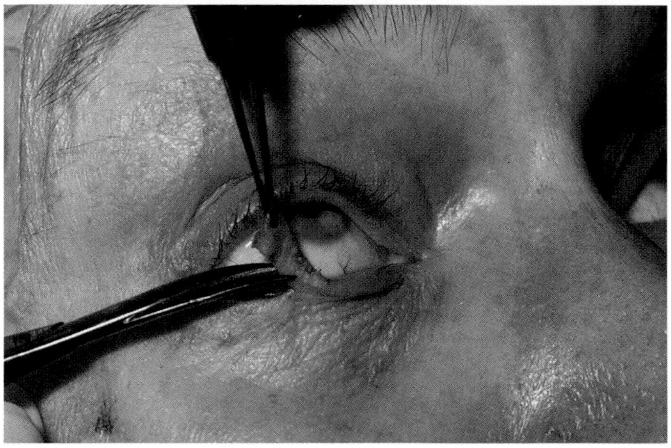

FIGURE 14–5

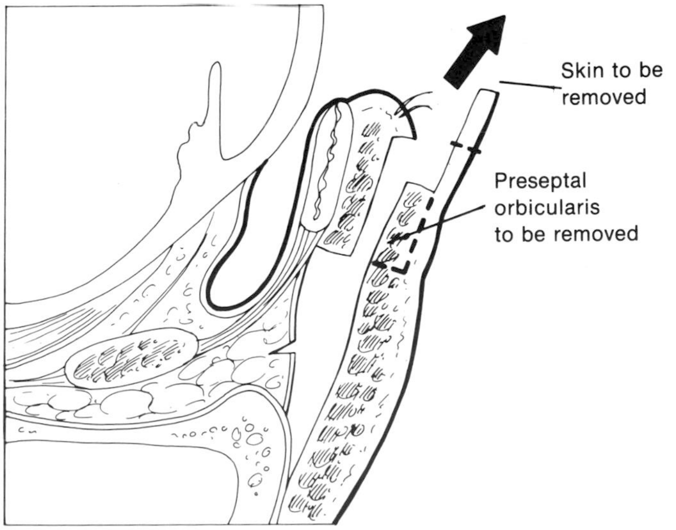

FIGURE 14–6

Figure 14–7. A final check for hemostasis is carefully performed. The skin is then closed with a running 6–0 braided nylon or monofilament suture. An important step at this point is to pass a traction suture through both edges of the wound in the center of the lower lid and tape it above the brow to keep the lower eyelid in upward traction. This prevents a maladhesion caused by the upper lid pushing the lower lid inferiorly, allowing tissue to adhere, keeping the lid in an inferiorly displaced position.

A saline-moistened gauze is placed over the eyelids. A tight dressing should not be used. Observe the patient for bleeding at least until the epinephrine effect has worn off, usually 1 to 2 hours or more.

Transconjunctival Blepharoplasty

A subconjunctival injection of anesthesia is given 5 mm below the lower tarsal border. A small amount of anesthetic is also delivered along the inferior orbital rim to block the infraorbital nerve. Injections are then given into each fat pocket, by directing the needle just behind the inferior orbital rim.

After waiting 10 to 15 minutes for hemostasis, a Desmarres retractor is used to pull the lower lid anteriorly and slightly inferiorly.

Figure 14–8. A hot-tipped battery cautery is used to begin a conjunctival incision about 5 mm below the inferior tarsal border to incise the conjunctiva and retractors just posterior to the inferior orbital rim. This is best done while pushing the globe posteriorly with a finger through the upper eyelid or with a lid plate. The incision should be made in this area because the fat is situated behind the septum, which inserts into the rim, and the fat does not usually extend all the way to the inferior border of the tarsus. A combination of cautery followed by Westcott scissors is used to expose the fat in the middle compartment and then the incision can be extended medially and laterally.

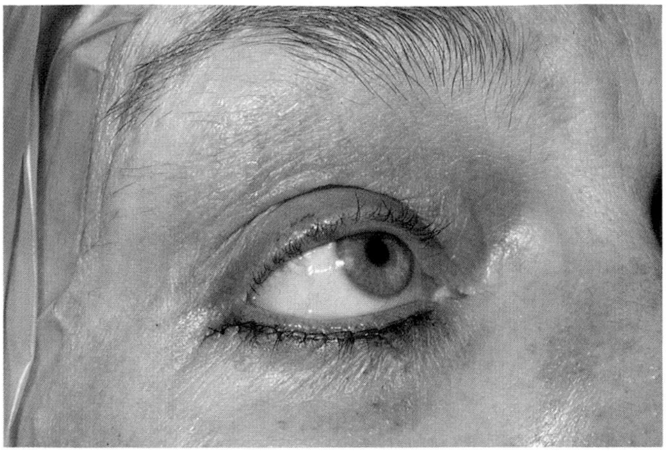

FIGURE 14–7

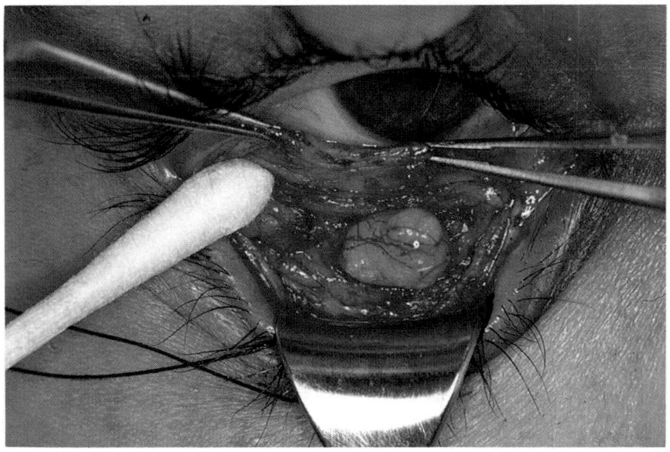

FIGURE 14–8

Figure 14–9. Fat pockets are then isolated in a manner similar to the transcutaneous approach. Careful control of the fat pad to prevent its retraction back into the socket before cauterization is important. The use of a hemostat before cutting is often helpful.

The desired amount of fat to be removed is generally determined by preoperative evaluation in this approach. When this is completed, the conjunctiva is closed with a running 6–0 chromic suture. The retractors are just behind the conjunctiva and will be well reapproximated by the conjunctival closure. Do not take deep bites because the septum may be inadvertently incorporated in the closure.

A traction suture to the brow is also used in this approach, although the chance of a maladhesion is much less than in the transcutaneous approach.

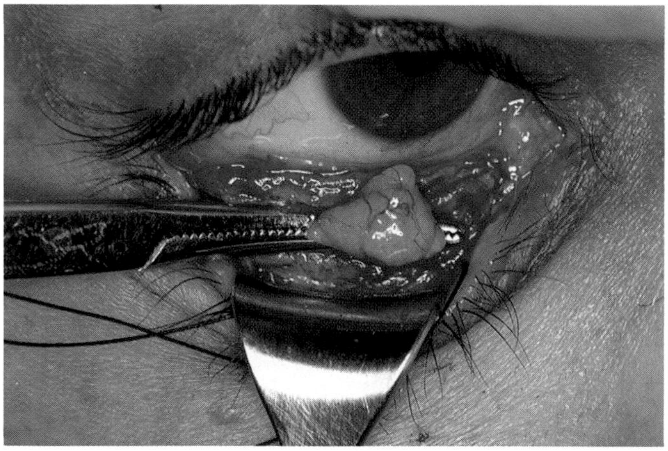

FIGURE 14–9

POSTOPERATIVE CARE

Ice packs are applied over the lids intermittently during waking hours for 2 to 3 days after surgery. Starting on the first postoperative day, the patient is instructed to clean the incision with a cotton-tipped applicator moistened with 3% peroxide or water once a day. Bacitracin ointment is applied to the incision 3 times a day. This is continued for 3 days after the sutures are removed. For the transconjunctival approach, an antibiotic drop is used four times daily for 1 week.

Acetaminophen, with or without propoxyphene (Darvon), may be used for pain relief. A complaint of severe pain should be investigated.

Occasionally, a small amount of exposure keratopathy develops in the postoperative period, even without excess skin removal. This is from orbicularis weakening or swelling. It is easily treated with lubricants and usually resolves within a few days. Sutures should be removed in about 5 days.

COMPLICATIONS AND TREATMENTS

Lower lid blepharoplasty is much more likely to have serious complications than upper lid or most other eyelid surgeries. The best way to treat complications is to avoid them by paying careful attention to the preoperative and intraoperative details.

Inferior Displacement of the Lower Lid

Inferior displacement is the most common complication of lower lid blepharoplasty. It results either from too much skin being removed or a maladhesion of internal tissues caused by the closed upper lid holding the lower lid down during the postoperative period. This results in an unattractive scleral show or ectropion, and if severe enough, can produce exposure keratopathy. In the presence of borderline dry eyes, the patient may have chronic ocular discomfort.

Avoidance of this problem is best accomplished by careful skin removal, especially in the dry eye patients, and by using traction sutures to place the posterior lamella on stretch.

Mild cases will often resolve on their own over a period of a few months. Lubricants or moisture shields may have to be employed. More serious cases of inferior scleral show may require a release of the internal cicatricial band along with a lateral tarsal strip procedure to supraplace and tighten the lower lid. If anterior lamella shortage is also present, a skin graft may be required.

Loss of Vision

Blindness following blepharoplasties is rare, but a definite entity. The mechanism of visual loss is most likely due to an interruption of ocular perfusion and resultant ischemia of the eye secondary to an expanding orbital hematoma. The source of intraorbital hemorrhage is either from surgically cut tissue or from avulsion of posterior vessels by overzealous traction on orbital fat. Hemorrhage usually occurs within the first 12 to 24 hours and is often accompanied by severe orbital pain. The best way to avoid this devastating complication is to avoid excessive traction on the orbital fat and to have meticulous hemostasis. The avoidance of preoperative aspirin and strenuous postoperative physical activity is also helpful.

Treatment of an expanding orbital hematoma must be initiated without delay. Sutures should be removed and the wound opened to evacuate the blood clot. The source of the bleeding should be identified and cauterized. Further treatment may not be necessary if bleeding ceases spontaneously and there is no threat of vascular compromise to the eye. Frequently, increased orbital tension tamponades the bleeder, preventing a progression of proptosis and intraocular pressure elevation. In the interim, the patient's ocular tension and fundus perfusion status should be monitored. In the presence of elevated intraocular pressure, medical therapy should be initiated. Topical timolol (Timoptic, 0.5%), and intravenous mannitol (1–2 g/kg of a 20% solution infused over 20 minutes) may be administered to decrease intraocular pressure and enhance retinal perfusion. If, despite these measures, there is progression of exophthalmos or evidence of a pending central retinal artery occlusion, a lateral canthotomy and inferior cantholysis will permit partial decompression of the orbit. In rare instances, when maximal medical therapy and lateral canthotomy fail to restore retinal perfusion, orbital decompression may be needed. Intravenous corticosteroid may be given to reduce orbital swelling, decrease vascular permeability, and protect the optic nerve from ischemic damage.

Infection

Postoperative infection is very rare in eyelid surgery and should be treated with appropriate antibiotics. Occasionally, a very small localized suture abscess can be seen. These respond well to removal of the suture and application of topical or systemic antibiotics.

Residual Excess Fat

Excess fat can be removed satisfactorily by either completely revising the surgery, a transconjunctival approach, or a limited incision over the fat pocket. There is much greater vascularity and less mobility of the fat in the early postoperative period. It is much easier to reoperate between 6 and 12 months later if possible.

Excess Skin

If an insufficient amount of skin was removed and asymmetry between the eyelids is noticeable, revision through the original skin incision may be necessary.

Chapter Fifteen

ORIENTAL BLEPHAROPLASTY

Don Liu

To perform a blepharoplasty successfully on an Oriental patient, the surgeon must take into consideration the following points: What does the patient perceive as beautiful? Does the patient desire a lid crease? If so, of what type and where should it be located? Furthermore, the surgeon should avoid using terms such as "correction, revision, or westernization" of Oriental eyelids.

To facilitate communication, the surgeon should use terms familiar to the patient. In the Orient, an eyelid that has no crease is termed a *single eyelid*, and an eyelid with a crease, a *double eyelid*. These terms are literal translations from the Chinese idiogram. They are widely used by both the lay public and the medical professions. There are four types of double eyelids: outer, inner, partial, and intermittent. The outer double eyelid, quite similar to a typical lid crease found in an Occidental person, lies 7 to 10 mm above the lash line at the midpupillary line. It is a well-defined lid crease, and the epicanthal fold associated with this type of eyelid is generally minimal. The inner double eyelid is located 3 to 5 mm above the lash margin at the midpupillary line. It is generally the extension of an epicanthus tarsalis, and the fold is fairly prominent. Unilateral double eyelid can be of any type. Intermittent double eyelid can be unilateral or bilateral. It may be present depending upon the presence or absence of lid edema, up or down gaze. A partial double eyelid is present only in portions of the eyelid.

As a rule, do not attempt to remove the epicanthal fold for Oriental patients unless it is noticeably prominent or specifically requested by the patient. Generally, the patient is not bothered by its presence, and Orientals have a greater tendency to form hypertrophic scar than do Caucasians.

PREOPERATIVE EVALUATION

A pertinent medical history should be taken to make sure there are no thyroid, cardiac, or renal disorders. Most importantly, it should be ascertained that there is no psychiatric contraindication. An ocular examination should include recorded visual acuity, fundus examination, slit-lamp examination, and lacrimal function evaluation. The position and the curvature of the eyebrow should be noted. The position of the eyelid should be carefully measured and recorded. The presence or absence of an epicanthal fold and the degree of fullness in the superior sulcus should also be noted. A detailed discussion concerning sculpturing this area with its possible outcome should be discussed with the patient.

To a patient, the particular type of upper eyelid crease with its height, shape, and curvature is often the most important concern. To demonstrate what can be achieved, use a small paper clip, gently pressing on the upper eyelid skin at the desired level. All surgical candidates who are taking aspirin or warfarin (Coumadin) are instructed to discontinue taking these drugs for at least 2 weeks before the scheduled surgery.

INDICATIONS FOR SURGERY

As is true in any cosmetic procedure, the patient's clear understanding and realistic expectation of what can be achieved is of utmost importance. Doing a blepharoplasty or creating an upper eyelid crease will offer an improved appearance to the patient. In most cases, this will make the patient feel good, feel young, and become more active. These procedures, however, will not necessarily help find an ideal companion, restore a failing marriage, find a new job, or get a promotion. Underlying psychosocial factors or hidden desires must be carefully scrutinized. Very rarely, there may be a patient who would like to have his or her entire facial features "westernized." These very rare patients must be carefully evaluated and properly referred.

For a well-suited surgical candidate, there are at least two types of surgery that can be offered. There are many variations on the theme in each of these techniques. If the goal is to simply create a lid crease, the suture technique is excellent for those younger patients with thin, taut skin and minimal submuscular or orbital fat. The incisional technique is for patients in whom skin, subcutaneous tissue, submuscular and orbital fat are to be removed. The suture technique will create a new lid crease or enhance an existing one, but it will not change the contour or the topography of the periorbital region. The incisional technique, depending upon what layers and how much of these tissues are removed, can recontour this area.

SURGICAL ANATOMY

Figure 15–1A, B. The difference between the Occidental's (**A**) and the Oriental's (**B**) upper eyelid appearance is the result of a difference in the fascia layer of the eyelids. This layer consists of orbital septum, orbital fat, and the levator aponeurosis. Typically, in an Occidental person, the aponeurosis layer fuses with the orbital septum a few millimeters above the superior tarsal border. The aponeurotic fibers extend anteroinferiorly beyond the fused complex and interdigitate in the fibrous septa of the orbicularis muscle. The eyelid crease is the result of the subcutaneous insertion of these most superior fibers. In an Oriental person, typically the levator aponeurosis fuses with the orbital septum below the superior tarsal border, with the preaponeurotic fat extending closer to the eyelid margin. In addition, there may often be a submuscular fat pad that extends inferiorly up to the superior tarsal border. Generally, the Oriental patient's upper eyelid tarsal plate is slightly smaller than the Caucasian's. These differences result in a fullness in the upper eyelid, a less developed, somewhat lower, or an absent eyelid crease. The eyelid skin in the Oriental patient also tends to be slightly thicker.

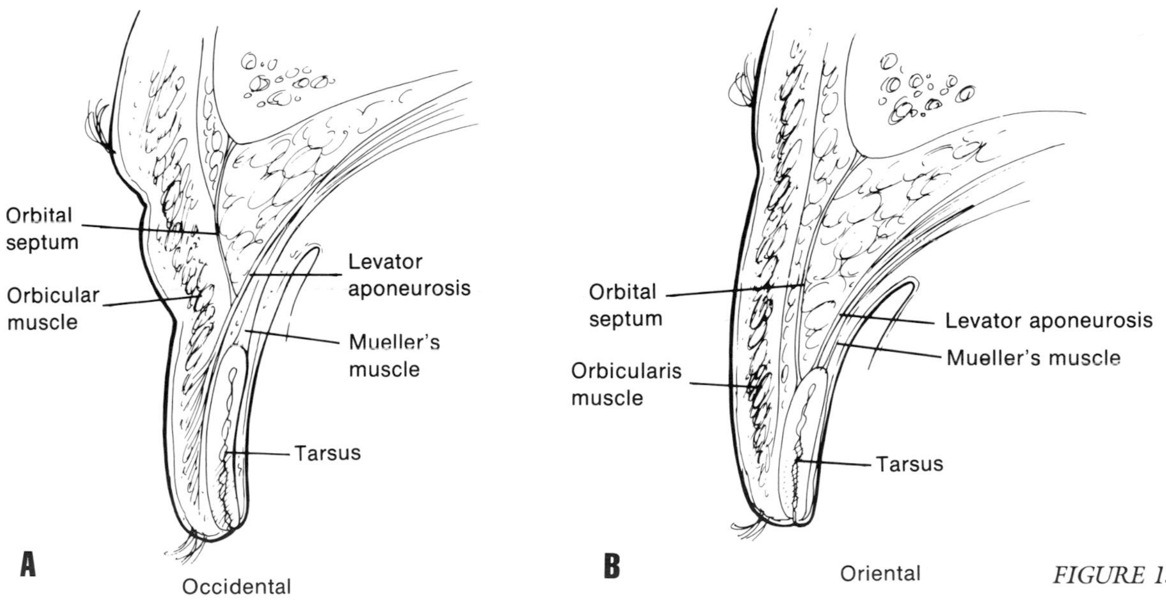

FIGURE 15–1

PROCEDURES

Incisional Technique

Do not attempt to create a new type of lid crease at a new location when there already is one. If the patient has a single eyelid and desires a lid crease, it is best to find out what type of lid crease is desired. Frequently, an Oriental patient will choose the "inner double eyelid." To make sure, we have the patient hold a mirror and look into it.

Figure 15–2. With a paper clip, the eyelid in the superonasal area is gently indented. A lid crease is formed naturally as an extension of the epicanthal fold.

To create an outer double eyelid is oftentimes arbitrary. The new crease is to be located at the level the patient desires.

It is recommended that surgery be done under local anesthesia with intravenous sedation: 2% lidocaine (Xylocaine) with epinephrine 1:100,000 is used. The proposed eyelid crease is marked. A smooth forceps is used to gently pinch the lid tissue with one blade along the lid crease and, the other, superiorly placed. The extent of the skin resection is determined by carefully observing the eyelashes. When the eyelashes begin to evert, the position of the upper blade is marked. Generally, an ellipsoid area is outlined.

Following adequate anesthesia, a skin incision is made with a size 15 blade along the lid crease. The skin is undermined superiorly, but not resected at this time. Dissection is carried deeper and a submuscular fat pad is frequently encountered and removed. This fat pad has the typical subcutaneous fat appearance.

Figure 15–3. A submuscular fat pad is being held by the forceps while the preaponeurotic fat pad is resting in its normal position. It does not have a capsule and it consists of multiple minute globules. It has a harder consistency than the preaponeurotic orbital fat. If a still deeper superior sulcus is desired, the orbital septum is incised and orbital fat is prolapsed. In older patients, make sure when dissecting this orbital fat that dehiscence is not created in the aponeurosis. Frequently, the aponeurosis is infiltrated with fatty tissues. Aim toward the orbital fat superiorly when dissecting, not deep toward the globe. Repair dehiscence if present. Generally, a single interrupted 6–0 nylon suture placed centrally is sufficient.

A small amount of injection superiorly in the fat pad may be necessary before clamping. Direct the needle superiorly toward the orbit, not deep toward the globe. The amount of subcutaneous tissue removed from each eyelid should be set aside for comparison to assure symmetry. Usually, the central fat pad is found along with its smaller medial pad. The lateral fat pad is the smallest of all, and sometimes cannot be found in an Oriental person. When excising the tissue laterally, one should avoid damage to the lacrimal gland. The skin flap is draped over the lid crease incision. Once again the skin redundancy is estimated. Usually, this coincides with the previous marking. Skin resection should be conservative, especially following sculpturing of the periorbital area by the removal of other soft tissues.

Skin closure is achieved with multiple interrupted 6–0 nylon sutures. The lid crease itself is accentuated by three supratarsal fixation sutures. The surgeon may use a different type of suture or cut these sutures long to distinguish them from the rest of the skin sutures. The first lid crease suture is centrally located, with the other two 5 mm on either side. The first suture is placed by taking a bite in the lower edge of the skin flap, followed by a bite in the aponeurosis, and finally, joining the upper edge of the skin flap. Ideally, when the skin edges are brought together, there is no skin redundancy, and there is a palpebral opening measuring 1 to 2 mm upon gentle closure of the eyelids.

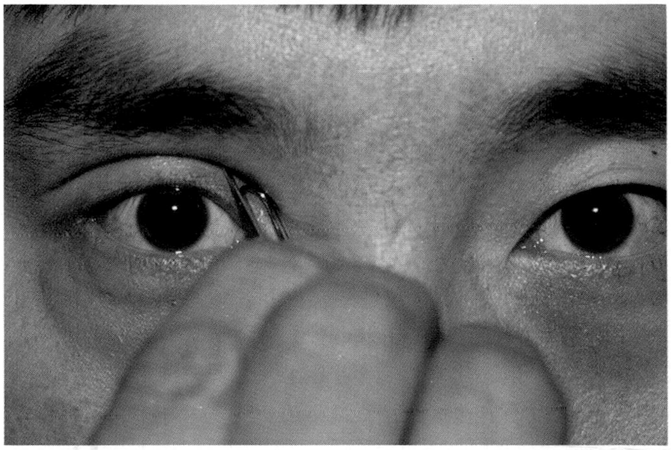

FIGURE 15–2

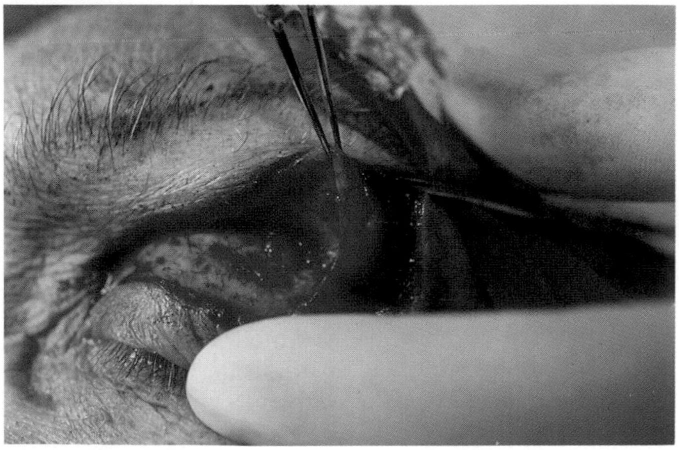

FIGURE 15–3

Suture Technique

To create an eyelid crease without performing a blepharoplasty, the suture technique may be used. The creation of an eyelid crease is based on scar formation between the skin and conjunctiva induced by the absorbable suture. The proposed lid crease is located and marked as described before. Injection is given both on the skin side along the marking and on the conjunctival side just above the tarsal plate. A minimal amount should be used lest the lid tissue be distorted.

Figure 15–4A, B. For this technique, a 5–0 chromic suture is used. Starting laterally, the suture is anchored on the skin surface. The needle is passed full-thickness through the eyelid and is brought out on the conjunctival side at the superior margin of the tarsal plate (**A**). The needle reenters the lid substance through the same conjunctival exit wound. Advancing medially, it takes a bite of the subcutaneous tissue to come out on the conjunctival side again, 3 to 4 mm away from the first exit wound. The needle never exits through the skin. The needle then reenters the lid tissue by this next wound and continues advancing medially (**B**). The process is repeated for six or more bites until the needle reaches the most medial portion of the lid crease. The needle then exits on the skin side and anchors there. The suture is left in place until it is absorbed.

POSTOPERATIVE CARE

Ice-cold compresses are applied to the eye immediately after the operation. Antibiotic ointment is applied over the incision and in the fornix. Before discharging the patient, vision and motility are checked. The skin sutures are removed in 5 to 7 days.

COMPLICATIONS AND HOW TO AVOID THEM

Of special interest to an Oriental patient is the proper type, shape, and height of the eyelid crease. Improper placement or creation of an improper type of lid crease can be avoided by careful preoperative evaluation and good communication with the patient. Technically, make sure repeated measurements and proper markings are made, and lid crease sutures are properly placed. To avoid over- or undercorrection, it is recommended that only the eyelid crease incision be made initially, and resection of the skin be performed last. To ensure contour symmetry, the amount of subcutaneous tissue removed from each eye is set aside for comparison. Intraoperative precautions, such as clamping and cauterizing the fat pedicle will ensure hemostasis and, thereby,

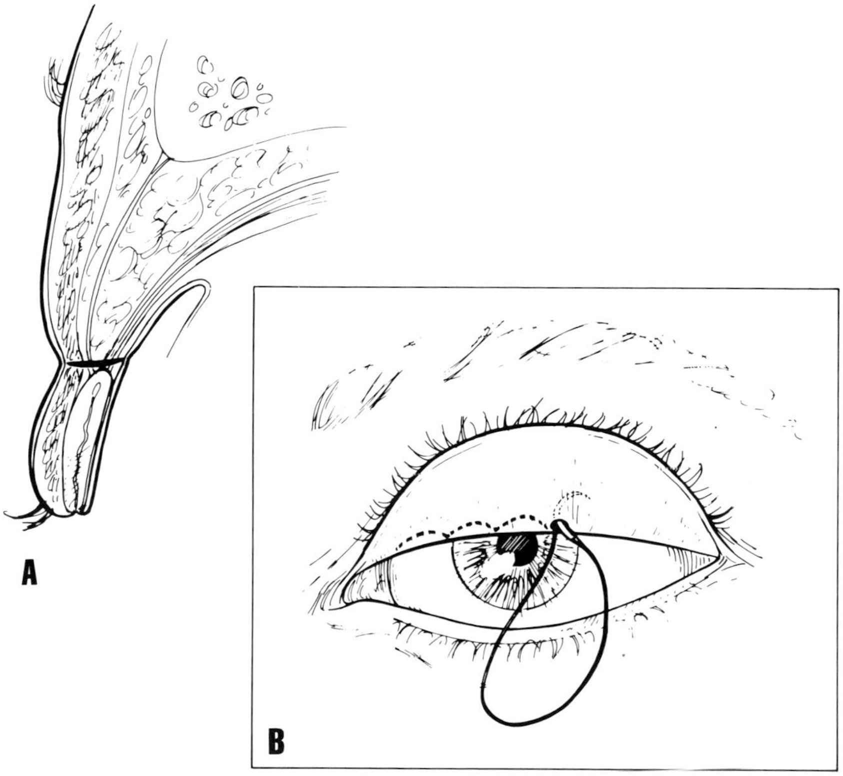

FIGURE 15–4

prevent possible postoperative orbital hemorrhage. An immediate cold compress also helps prevent prolonged edema. Suture tunnels can be avoided by timely removal of sutures. A W-plasty may be necessary to remove skin redundancy medially. Minor bumps and lumps, suture granuloma, or minimal redundancy can be revised easily by a secondary excision.

Care should be taken that orbital fat is not manipulated excessively, all bleeders are stopped, and cautery or diathermy is not used excessively. The surgeon should be careful when removing the submuscular fat pad. The dissection should not extend so far superiorly that the brow anatomy is disturbed, unless a brow lift or fixation is planned. Retraction or ectropion is avoided by not suturing the septum and the muscle layers. Ptosis should be identified preoperatively and repaired. If dehiscence of the aponeurosis is detected intraoperatively, it should be repaired.

When the suture technique is used to create an eyelid crease, corneal abrasion can be avoided by careful and proper placing of the sutures. No suture should be exposed on the conjunctival side. An indistinct or temporary lid crease may be the result of shallow suture passage and unpredictable absorption rate of the suture. A hematoma or edema immediately postoperatively may disinsert some or all of the sutures, thereby preventing formation of adhesion. Suture granuloma and localized infection may occur.

Chapter Sixteen

BROWPLASTY

Robert C. Kersten
Dwight R. Kulwin

Eyebrow ptosis is frequently encountered by the ophthalmologist and must be distinguished from upper lid dermatochalasis. Both will result in the appearance of redundant tissues in the upper lid. The surgeon must determine which of these is present, or if there is a combination of both, before deciding on appropriate treatment.

In women, the brow tends to be higher and more arched in its contour, with the high point over the lateral canthus, whereas the male brow is lower and less arched. The resting height of the brow diminishes with age. The amount of resultant brow ptosis depends upon heredity, history of smoking, sun exposure, and skin thickness, oiliness, and color. The individual patient's pattern of facial animation also contributes to the development of brow ptosis, typically resulting in a more pronounced lateral droop in patients who squint frequently, and in more medial brow ptosis in patients who frown frequently.

Some surgical procedures are directed strictly toward elevating and repositioning the ptotic brow. Others also remove excessive forehead, glabellar, and temporal wrinkles and skin. These latter procedures are more often performed for cosmetic purposes, whereas the former are used to correct functional brow position abnormalities.

ANATOMIC CONSIDERATIONS

Any operation to elevate the brows must be planned to avoid damage to the sensory and motor nerves of the forehead. The supraorbital nerve provides sensation to the forehead and scalp. It lies on the surface of the frontalis muscle in the central third of the forehead and runs vertically from the supraorbital notch toward the crown. The temporal branch of the facial nerve provides motor innervation to the forehead muscles. This branch courses deep to the frontalis muscle in the forehead, running horizontally from lateral to medial. The nerve runs on the superficial temporalis fascia, descending beneath the frontalis muscle at a point approximately two finger breadths above the temporal orbital rim. Skin incisions should be placed either above or below this point to avoid nerve injury. Similarly, dissection must be carried out either superficial or deep to the frontalis muscle to avoid the sensory and motor nerve branches.

DIRECT BROWPLASTY

Direct browplasty involves the excision of tissue immediately above the brow. Closure results in elevation of the brow. The procedure is usually performed under local anesthesia.

Skin Marking

Preoperatively, one must determine the amount of medial, central, and lateral brow droop. Discussion with the patient should determine the desired postoperative appearance of the brow.

The superior several rows of brow hairs should be included with the incision to better camouflage the scar. If there is a large degree of temporal brow ptosis, the incision can be carried temporally beyond the lateral aspect of the brow in an S-shaped fashion. Although the scar lateral to the brow will be fully exposed, the thinner temporal skin results in a less noticeable scar than occurs in the thicker, more sebaceous skin that is present immediately above the brow. If the excision does not extend temporal to the brow, only minimal elevation of the temporal brow can be achieved.

The superior half of the incision should be marked out to approximate the desired height and contour of the brow, as direct closure will result in the brow directly following the superior incision. The amount of skin to be excised is determined by elevating the brow to its desired position and estimating the amount of the excess forehead tissues that results. It is preferable to do this with the patient sitting upright. The desired high point of the brow is marked directly above the lateral canthus. The superior skin line is tapered medially and laterally from this point. The superior incision should be slightly overelevated, as there is usually some decay several months after surgery.

Local anesthetic with epinephrine is then directly infiltrated within the outlines of the proposed excision. It is important to wait 10 minutes, to allow maximum vasoconstriction to occur following injection, before making the incision.

Figure 16–1. A scalpel is used to incise the skin markings, starting with the inferior line. The knife handle is beveled in a cephalad fashion so that it parallels the plane of the emerging superior brow hairs. This prevents transection of underlying follicles, which may result in some hair loss inferior to the healed wound. Beveling of the superior incision must also be done in the same direction so that the wound edges heal properly. The cephalad orientation of the brow incision is less important over the lateral one-third of the brow where the hairs tend to lose their caudad orientation. After hemostasis is obtained, excision of skin and underlying subcutaneous tissue is carried out with Stevens or other curved scissors.

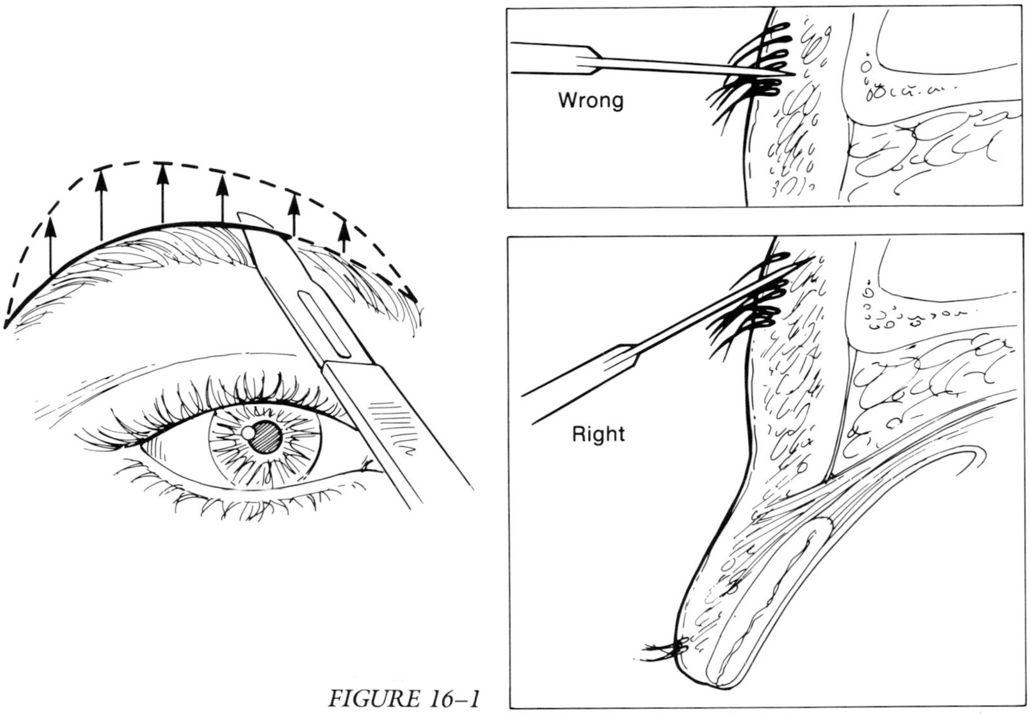

FIGURE 16–1

Excision of Skin

There are two alternative methods of skin and soft-tissue excision in direct browplasty.

Most surgeons favor excision of skin and subcutaneous tissue, leaving the frontalis muscle undisturbed. Others feel that excision of underlying orbicularis and frontalis muscle down to the pericranium is desirable to provide a more permanent result and to avoid "bunching-up" of the frontalis muscle and resulting contour irregularities. If such a full-thickness excision is carried out, care must be taken to remain superficial in the medial portion of the browplasty that overlies the supraorbital neurovascular bundle. In addition to the risk of damage to the supraorbital neurovascular bundle, excision down to the pericranium also tends to give a more depressed scar. Consequently, it is preferred to excise skin and subcutaneous fatty tissue only, staying just above the frontalis muscle.

Resuspension of the Brow

The orbicularis muscle directly beneath the brow (at the inferior edge of the excision) is imbricated to the frontalis muscle at the superior incision border with 4–0 clear nylon sutures. Three to four sutures are placed in an inverted fashion.

Figure 16–2. Subcutaneous closure is performed with 4–0 chromic sutures placed in an inverted fashion. One must initiate the interrupted suture from a deep entry to a superficial exit, and then a superficial entry to a deep exit, to bury the knot. The suture ends must be cut flush with the knot or they tend to migrate through to the surface of the skin. Meticulous approximation of the subcutaneous tissues in superior and inferior incisions is required to avoid an unnecessarily prominent scar. If the subcutaneous sutures are properly placed, the epithelium should be exactly approximated.

After this subcutaneous closure has been carried out, it is important to inspect the two brows for symmetry. If one brow is lower than the other, the additional skin above the lower brow must be marked in a symmetric fashion with a marking pen, the sutures released and additional skin excision carried out with repeated layered closure. Intraoperative asymmetry of the brows will persist postoperatively and must be dealt with directly if it is noted.

Once the symmetry of the two brows is assured, skin closure is carried out in two layers. A running 5–0 Prolene subcuticular suture is left in place for 10 days, and then a 6–0 Prolene running baseball closure of the skin is performed, which is removed on the fourth postoperative day. This provides the benefits of a long-lasting skin closure, yet, the most superficial sutures can be removed before the development of cross-hatching.

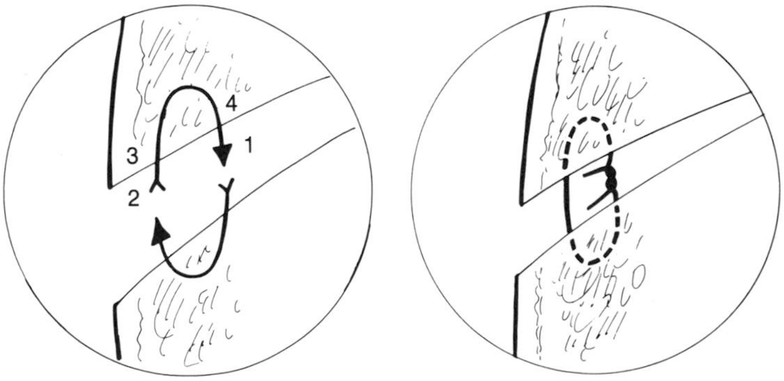

FIGURE 16–2

Postoperative Management

Polysporin (bacitracin–polymyxin) ointment is applied to the incision at the completion of the procedure, and ice packs are used for 48 hours. The patient is encouraged to sit upright and to elevate the head during sleep to reduce edema, which can be substantial.

Problems With Direct Browplasty

The advantages of direct browplasty are its effectiveness and simplicity. The desired contour of the brow can be directly marked on the forehead and effectively achieved. No undermining is required, and bleeding is minimal. Significant disadvantages relate primarily to the contour of the reconstructed brow and the incision placed directly above the brow.

Direct excision of a crescent of skin above the brow will necessarily result in an arched brow. An excision limited to tissue lying within the brow (to hide the scar in the brow hairs) will have no effect on the medial and lateral ends of the brow and its maximum effect at the widest point of excision. The resulting arched or "feminine" eyebrow is not desirable in men. Even in women, when significant brow ptosis exists, an unnatural arch will be created, as a large amount of tissue must be removed centrally above the brow, resulting in a perpetually "surprised" look.

Regardless of the care with which wound approximation and closure is undertaken, the healed incision is frequently more noticeable than one would like. Excision of tissue immediately above the brow results in a wound with thinner forehead skin superiorly and thicker brow skin inferiorly. Closure of these disparate tissues results in some degree of stepoff. In addition, the skin adjacent to the medial brow contains prominent sebaceous elements, and when incisions are made in this thicker sebaceous skin, wound contracture with a depressed scar may result. This depressed scar will be even more noticeable if the incision is not beveled and thus transsects the follicles deep to the skin, causing additional brow hair loss inferior to the incision, leaving it more exposed. If the incision is properly beveled and placed within the brow to include several rows of superior brow hair, exposure of the incision is less of a problem. For these reasons, a full direct browplasty is now infrequently used.

DIRECT TEMPORAL BROW LIFT

For temporal brow ptosis, which is more prevalent and more likely to infringe on the peripheral field of vision, many patients will benefit from direct excision carried out over the lateral 30% to 50% of the brow. This minimizes depressed scarring, maintains a more horizontal brow contour and is very effective in eliminating the more functionally significant temporal brow ptosis. Such a limited temporal elevation is especially helpful in men, as it will prevent formation of an arched brow contour. Because the forehead skin above the brow becomes thinner temporally and has fewer sebaceous elements, depressed scars are less likely to form. This allows the temporal incision to be carried beyond the lateral end of the brow without concern for camouflage by the brow hair. In addition, there frequently are wrinkles in the temple in which the incisions can be inconspicuously placed.

Figure 16–3. The technique is identical with that previously described, except that the skin markings are shifted temporally and sweep to an S-shaped curve temporal to the brow.

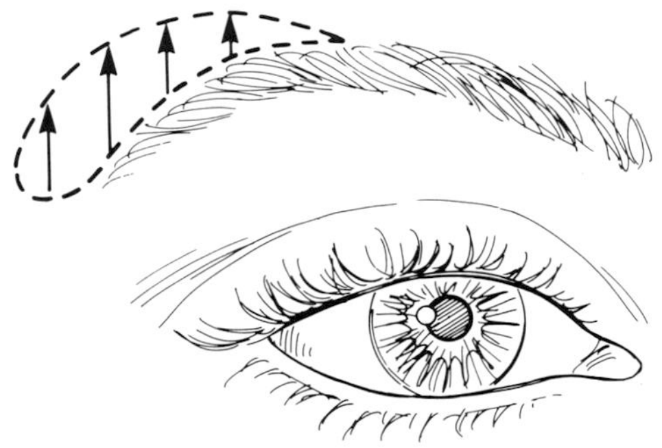

FIGURE 16–3

MIDFOREHEAD BROWPLASTY

Because of the aforementioned problems with direct browplasty, alternative procedures are frequently chosen to elevate the brows. Placement of the incision within the scalp hair and undermining in the subgaleal plane down to the brow region, the *coronal browplasty*, is a recently developed alternative. This is a procedure that is generally outside the ambition of the general ophthalmologist. An alternative approach, which is often more acceptable to the patient and the surgeon, is the midforehead browplasty.

Goals and Principles

In this procedure, the tissue excision is moved to the midforehead region and centered on a transverse forehead furrow. Undermining in the subcutaneous plane is carried down to the level of the brow and the excision site closed.

Marking the Incision

Figure 16–4. The patient is instructed to elevate the eyebrows so that the natural transverse forehead rhytids are apparent.

Figure 16–5. A transverse rhytid is selected on each side above the brow. It is preferable to select these rhytids at a different level on each side to enhance scar camouflage. An excision is then marked out centered on this rhytid and extending above and below it so that closure will then reapproximate the rhytid. The amount of skin to be excised is estimated by raising the brow to its ideal height with the patient sitting upright. Final skin excision is tailored at the time of closure. The excision normally extends from the nasal edge of the brow to a point 1-cm lateral to the brow. The temporal extension depends on the amount of temporal brow ptosis and how much temporal correction is desired. The widest point of the fusiform excision will usually lie over the lateral canthus, but this is adjusted intraoperatively.

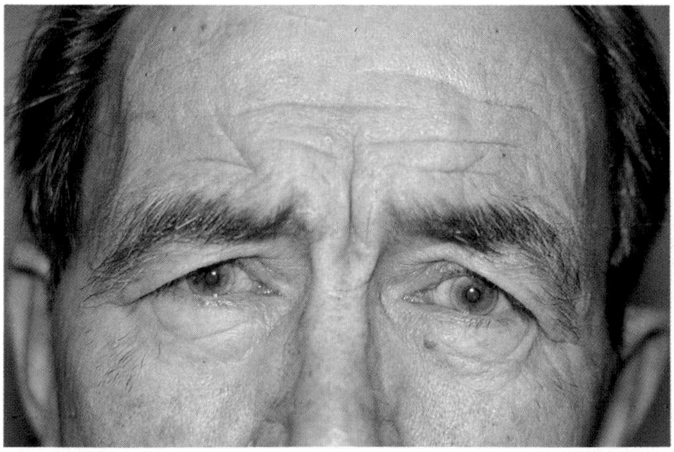

FIGURE 16–4

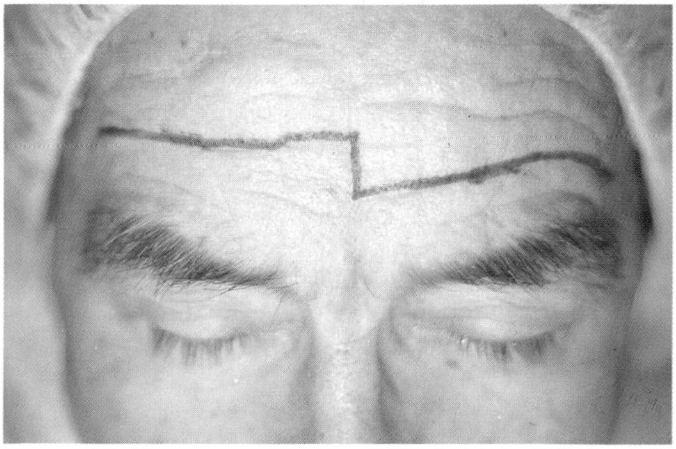

FIGURE 16–5

Anesthesia

Local anesthesia with epinephrine is preferred. The supraorbital and supratrochlear nerves are each anesthetized with 1 ml of anesthetic, injected over the superomedial orbital rim, to provide anesthesia over much of the forehead. Infiltration is additionally carried out across each fusiform excisional site and down the forehead to the brow. This additional infiltration serves to enhance anesthesia as well as to ensure hemostasis.

Skin Incision

Marking and infiltration are performed before the patient is prepared to allow 10 to 15 minutes between injection and incision to maximize the vasoconstrictive effect of the epinephrine. A Blair drape is preferred to a drape taped to the forehead so that no tension is placed on the forehead or the brows. The skin incision is made with a scalpel, taking care not to incise into the underlying frontalis muscle. Particular care should be taken to avoid the supraorbital nerve lying superficially beneath the medial aspect of the brow.

Undermining the Skin Flap

Figure 16–6. After the skin is incised, a fresh scalpel blade or scissors is used to undermine the subcutaneous fat that lies between the skin and the underlying frontalis muscle. This plane may be difficult to establish, as the thickness of the layer of subcutaneous fat varies widely. The depth of the subcutaneous fat can be determined by gently dissecting through the fat until the frontalis muscle is exposed.

As dissection is carried inferiorly, it is important to constantly monitor the depth of the dissection to ascertain that one does not stray into the frontalis muscle and damage the sensory nerves.

At the supraorbital rim the neurovascular bundle should be identified, and care must also be taken that the dissection is not so superficial that the brow hair follicles are damaged.

Hemostasis must be meticulous, as any residual bleeding will result in postoperative hematoma accumulation beneath the skin flap.

Placement of Suspension Sutures

Simple skin excision will not give a permanent result, because the brow will settle as gravity stretches the forehead skin. Therefore, suspension of the brow with nonabsorbable 4–0 nylon or Gore-tex sutures is required. These sutures are used to imbricate the orbicularis muscle immediately beneath the eyebrow to the frontalis muscle. This also permits adjustment of the brow contour.

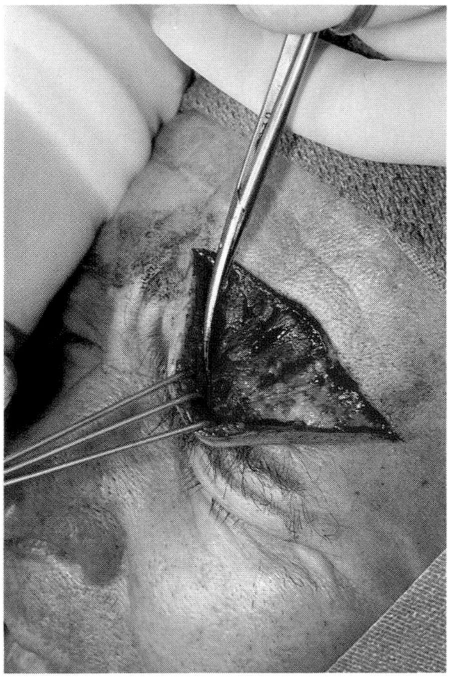

FIGURE 16–6

Usually two horizontal mattress sutures are placed: One medially and one temporally at the junction of the lateral and central one-third of the brow. They are first passed through the orbicularis muscle immediately beneath the brow follicles and then through the frontalis muscle at the level of the superior forehead skin incision. When both sutures have been passed, they are tied with two half hitches, positioning the brow. When the contour and height are acceptable, the assistant clamps the knot as it is tied. Very minimal overcorrection of brow position is the goal, as there is some postoperative downward drift. Once the suspension sutures have been tied, the skin flap is drawn superiorly, overlapped, and any excess trimmed.

Closure of the skin flap is then carried out in two layers. A subcuticular closure, using inverted interrupted 5–0 chromic sutures should bring the skin edges into good approximation. It is important to ensure that all the knots are adequately buried or they may erode through the skin. The epithelium is then closed with a running 5–0 subcuticular and a 6–0 Prolene running baseball suture. This wound is then reinforced with benzoin and Steri-strips.

Wound Drainage

The importance of assuring meticulous hemostasis before closure cannot be overemphasized. Although we do not routinely leave an indwelling drain beneath the forehead flap, occasionally this may be placed if residual oozing persists. A 10 French silicone drain (TLS-Porex Medical, Fairborn, GA) can be placed between the superficial surface of frontalis muscle and the overlying skin flap. This should be positioned beneath the brow, and brought out through a stab incision at the lateral tail of the brow. This is removed once drainage has ceased (usually at 24 hours).

Postoperative Care

Ice compresses are applied over the forehead for the first 48 hours, and the patient is instructed to keep the head elevated for the first 4 days.

Hematoma or seroma formation may occur if a drain is not in place. This can be aspirated with an 18- or 20-gauge needle introduced through the skin incision and directed toward the hematoma site.

The running 6–0 Prolene skin suture is removed at 3 to 5 days after surgery, or noticeable epithelial tracks may result. Following suture removal the wound is again reinforced with benzoin and skin tape.

Figure 16–7. Note the reduction of skin hooding over the lid margin at 2 weeks after surgery (see Figure 16–4).

Patients should be warned that the skin incisions will be noticeable for the first 4 to 6 weeks postoperatively. Patients are advised that if an unacceptable scar does occur, it can be reduced by dermabrasion. Steroid injection to control wound healing in this area is not recommended because atrophy of the subcutaneous fat may produce a noticeable depression that is rendered more obvious because of the flat background of the forehead.

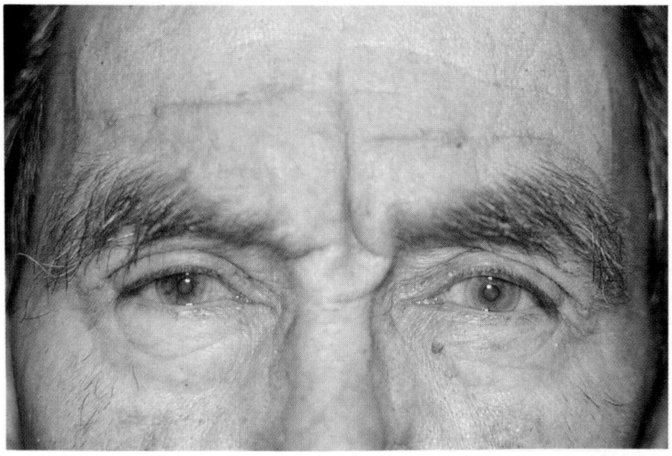

FIGURE 16–7

Chapter Seventeen

TARSORRHAPHY

David T. Tse

Tarsorrhaphy is the surgical fusion of upper and lower eyelid margins to narrow the palpebral fissure. It is usually performed to provide protection to the cornea from exposure in conditions such as proptosis, seventh nerve palsy, neuroparalytic keratitis, indolent corneal ulcer, or tear film deficiencies.

A tarsorrhaphy may be temporary, in which no lid tissues are excised and intermarginal sutures are used for lid closure. It may be a useful adjunct to ptosis repair, eyelid retractor recession, and other procedures for which temporary corneal protection is required. In situations when a permanent bond between the lids is desired, raw tarsal edges are created to form a more lasting adhesion. A tarsorrhaphy may be performed laterally, medially, or both, depending on the clinical situation. Typically, union of the temporal third of the eyelid affords excellent corneal protection and still allows an adequate medial fissure opening for vision. Although tarsorrhaphy is sometimes recommended to narrow the palpebral fissure to produce improved cosmesis in patients with eyelid retraction, such as in Graves' ophthalmopathy, the reader is cautioned that, in patients with progressive exophthalmos, a tarsorrhaphy may exert counterpressure on the orbital contents— preventing autodecompression. Thus, the patient's proptosis and optic nerve functions should be stable before contemplating this procedure. In patients with exposure keratopathy secondary to eyelid retraction, we feel that disinsertion and recession of the eyelid retractors afford a much better cosmetic and functional result (see Chapter 19). The procedure described in this chapter is a simple, permanent tarsorrhaphy technique that does not require bolsters or sutures that need to be removed. It preserves the integrity of the anterior lamella, minimizing the potential problem of lid margin irregularity. In patients in whom the tarsorrhaphy has to be opened, the margins of the posterior lamellae will epithelialize normally without cosmetic or dysfunctional sequelae.

OPERATIVE PROCEDURE

The length of the eyelid adhesion necessary for the desired degree of narrowing is determined by pinching the upper and lower eyelids together with a nontoothed forceps and marking the parallel margins with a marking pen. The temporal portions of the upper and lower lids within the marking are anesthetized with a subcutaneous injection of 2% lidocaine (Xylocaine) with 1:100,000 dilution of epinephrine. A small amount of anesthetic is also injected under the forniceal conjunctiva.

Figure 17–1. The eyelid is gently grasped and stabilized with a nontoothed forceps held perpendicular to the lid margin. A chalazion clamp may also be used. It provides good hemostasis as well as firm support to the eyelid during marginal dissection. The anterior and posterior lamella of the eyelid are split along the gray line with a size 11 Bard–Parker blade. Care is taken not to incise into the tarsal plate or the eyelash follicles. Occasionally, the anatomic landmarks of the lid margin (gray line and meibomian gland orifices) are indistinct. The tarsal plate can be readily identified by gently squeezing the lid margin with a smooth forceps and looking for the oily secretion at the meibomian gland orifice. The gray line is located just anterior to the meibomian gland openings. The blade is passed down along, and held firmly against, the anterior surface of the tarsal plate, and separation of the two lamellae is carried out to a depth of approximately 2 to 3 mm. After the incision in the gray line along the predetermined length has been made, an identical gray line incision is performed in the opposing lid to the same depth and length.

Figure 17–2. The mucous membrane at the margin of the posterior lamella is grasped with a 0.3-mm forceps and excised with a sharp Westcott scissors to expose the edge of the tarsal plate. Care is taken to ensure that the cut tarsal edge is even and minimal tarsus excised. The mucous membrane covering the opposing tarsal plate margin is excised in the same fashion.

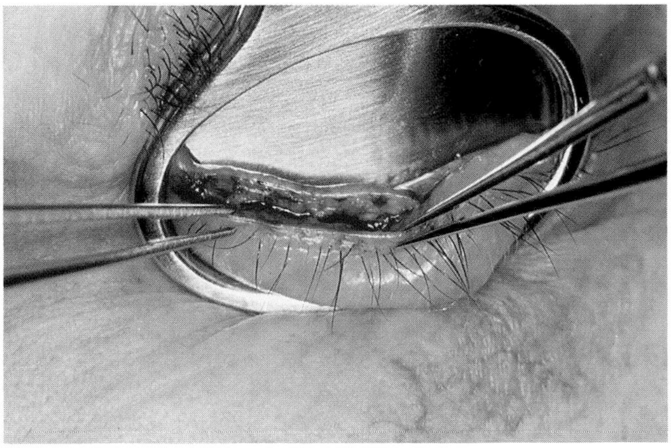

FIGURE 17–1

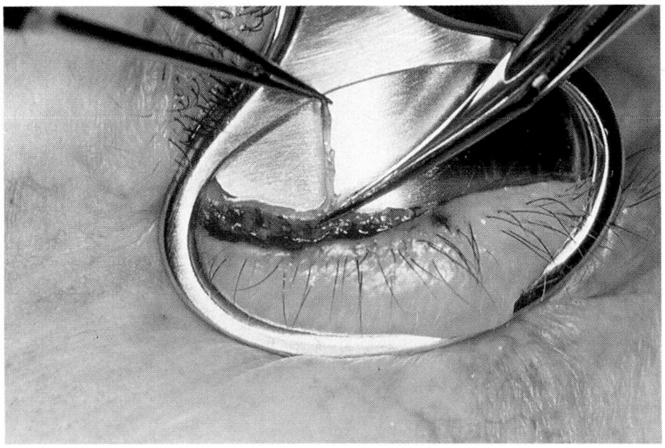

FIGURE 17–2

Figure 17–3A, B. After both tarsal edges are exposed, a 5–0 polyglactin 910 (Vicryl) suture on a spatula needle is passed through the tarsal plates in a lamellar fashion **(A).** The needle first enters through the anterior tarsal surface of the lower lid 2 mm from the edge and exits through a meibomian gland opening at the margin of the posterior lamella.

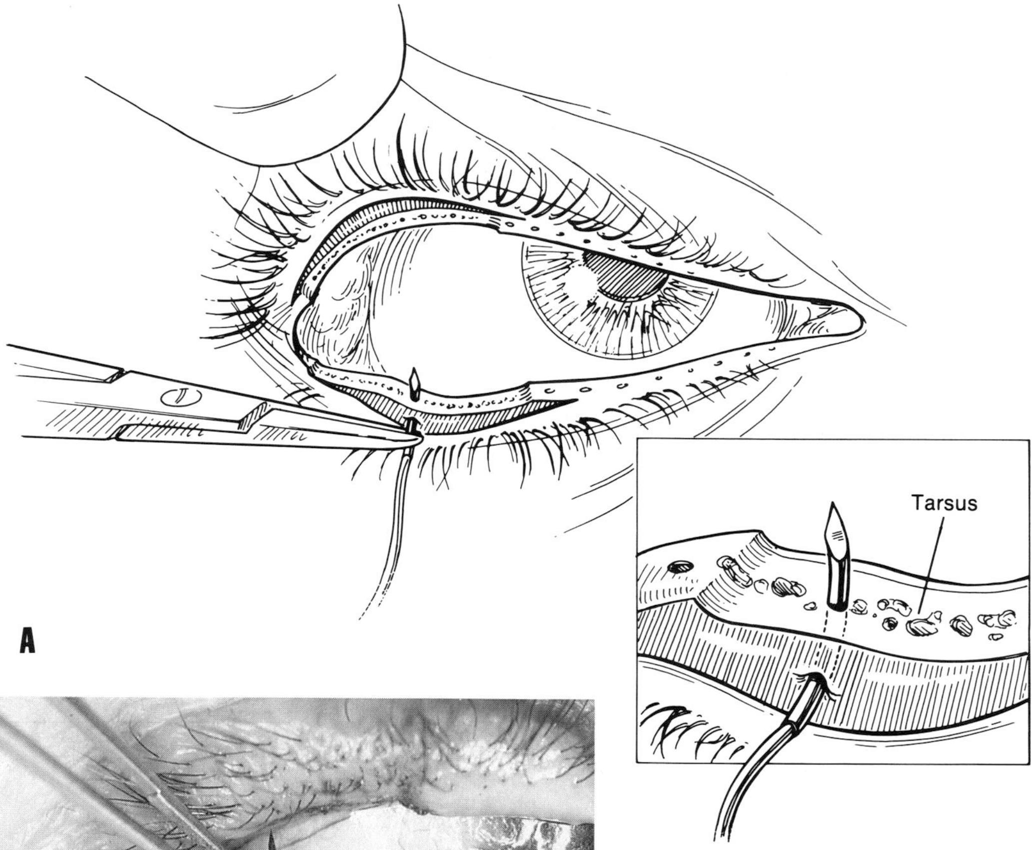

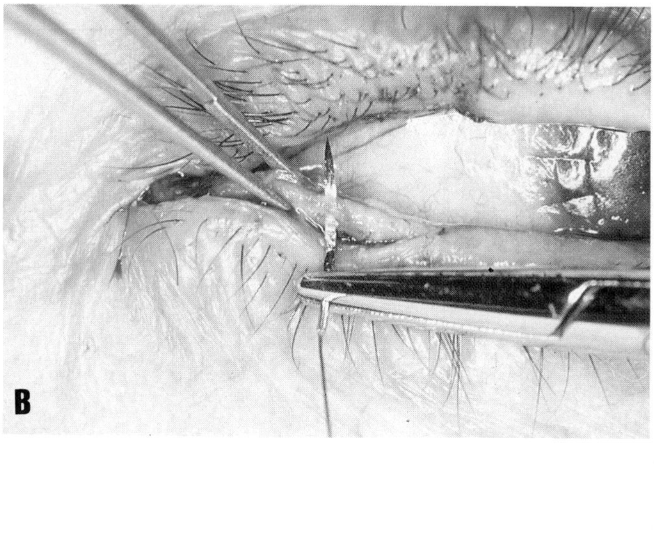

FIGURE 17–3

Figure 17–4. The needle is then passed into the upper lid, entering the meibomian gland opening, and out anteriorly at a point 2 mm superior to the edge of the tarsal plate. It is imperative that the suture is not passed full-thickness through the tarsal plate where it could abrade the cornea. In addition, it is important that these lamellar sutures exit and enter within the meibomian gland orifices at the lid margin, because more anteriorly placed bites are likely to erode through with time.

Figure 17–5. Three or four 5–0 Vicryl sutures are required for the lateral one-third of the lid. All should be passed before any is tied. When the preplaced sutures are tied, the bared edges of the two tarsi will be brought together.

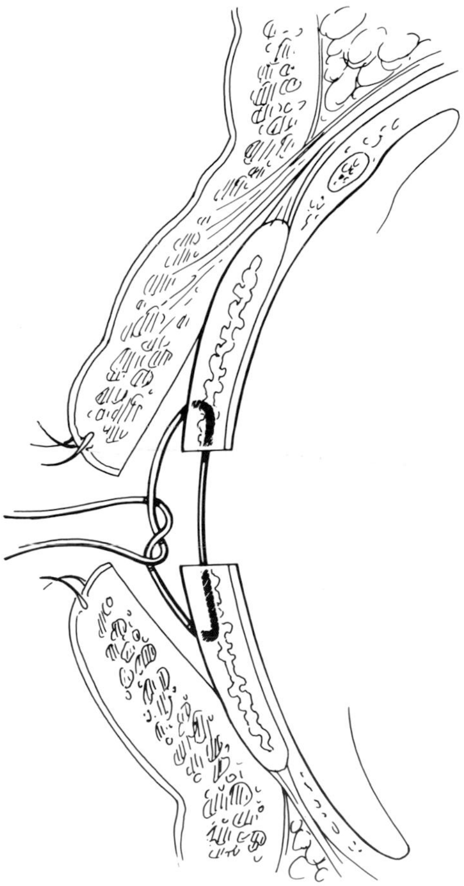

FIGURE 17–4

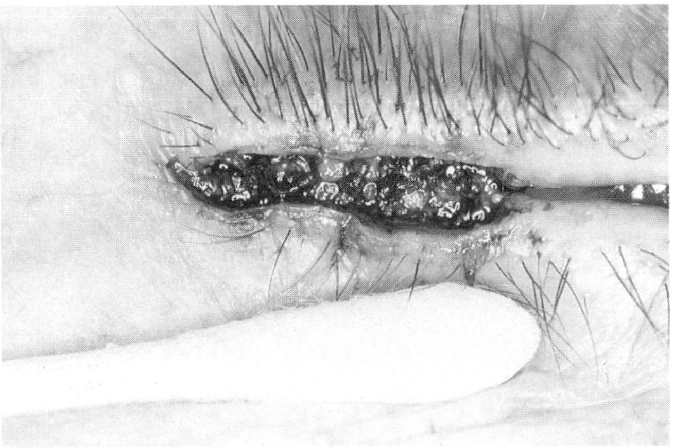

FIGURE 17–5

Figure 17–6A,B. The edges of the anterior lamellae are slightly everted with a 0.3-mm forceps and closed with a running 7–0 Vicryl suture between the lash line and the wound. Care is taken not to bury any lashes in the wound. Manipulation of the anterior lamella should be kept to a minimum to prevent subsequent lash misdirection following take-down of the tarsorrhaphy. The upper and lower tarsal plates will heal together in 3 to 4 weeks, forming a firm adhesion.

POSTOPERATIVE MANAGEMENT

Antibiotic ointment is applied to the wound three times a day for 10 days. Ointment containing corticosteroids should be avoided, because a quick intermarginal adhesion may be impeded. Since only absorbable sutures are used in this technique, there is no need for removal of sutures or bolsters in the follow-up examination.

A tarsorrhaphy can be taken down, if desired, under local anesthesia. A Westcott scissors is used to cut along the lid margin fusion plane. Take down may be done a few millimeters at a time if the status of the exposure problem remains in doubt.

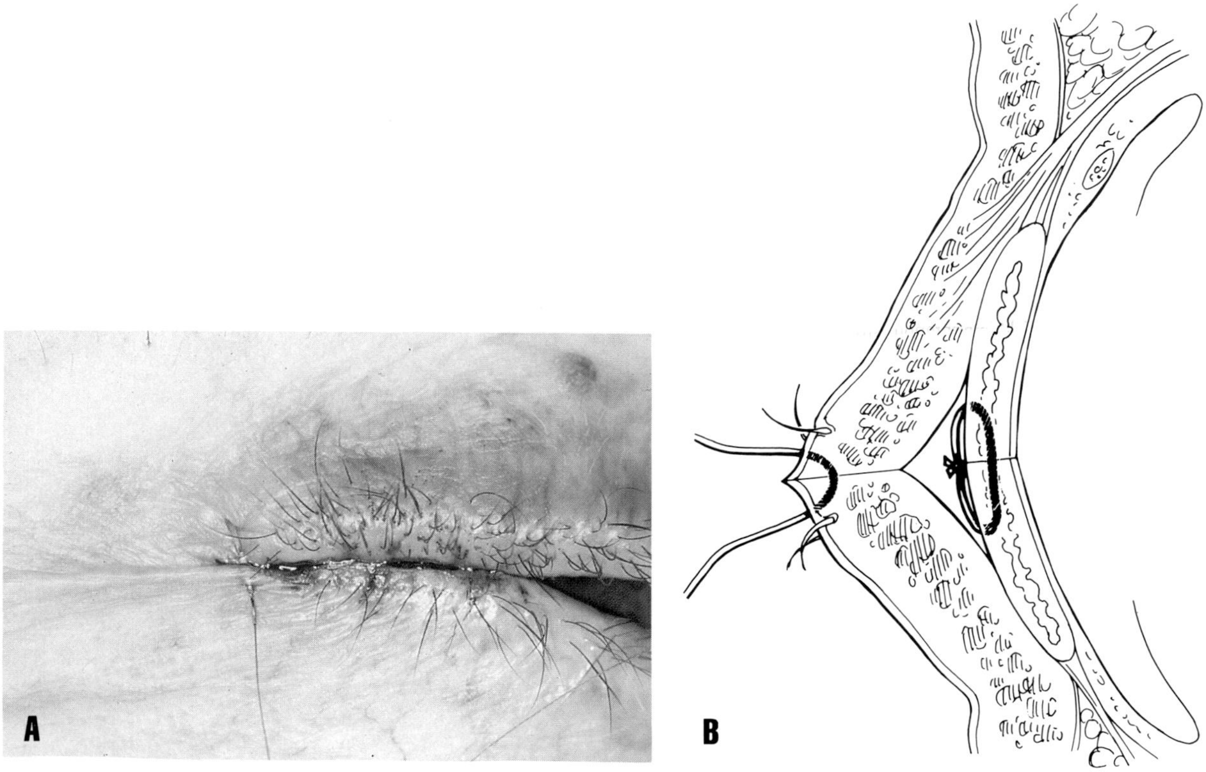

FIGURE 17–6

Chapter Eighteen

GOLD WEIGHT LID LOAD

Don Liu

SURGICAL INDICATIONS

Normal eyelid function may be temporarily or permanently lost owing to trauma, tumor, infection, idiopathic, and iatrogenic causes. An ophthalmologist's concerns are corneal protection and cosmesis. Surgical techniques that accomplish these goals include tarsorrhaphy, the use of a silicone band, a tantalum wire and mesh implant in the upper eyelid, a stainless steel palpebral spring, and gold weight lid load. In addition, there are muscle transfers, muscle grafts, facial nerve repair, cross-face nerve grafting, autogenous nerve grafting, and nerve crossover. All these techniques have their merits, and each has its complications. Gold weight implantation, similar to the palpebral spring or the silicone encircling band, is perhaps one of the simplest to perform. It is also easily reversible and has few serious complications.

Gold weight implantation is indicated in patients with acute, severe loss of normal eyelid function for whom corneal protection is the foremost concern. It is also indicated in patients whose hope of regaining normal lid function is slim and for whom a maximal medical regimen is necessary or barely adequate to maintain the health of the cornea. For many patients, a simulated blink, a good cosmetic result, and the simplicity and reversibility are also reasons for choosing this technique. Furthermore, it can be used as a secondary procedure when other previous procedures have been unsatisfactory; for example, a silicone band or palpebral spring has eroded through the eyelid tissue or has fatigued. These devices need to be removed first before the gold is implanted. A patient may have had a tarsorrhaphy performed, but became dissatisfied with the cosmesis. Finally, in selected patients with dysthyroid ophthalmopathy, this is a possible alternative to many other irreversible eyelid procedures.

Gold weight implantation is contraindicated in patients with an anesthetic cornea. It is relatively contraindicated in patients with very thin and pale skin or with an atrophic orbicularis muscle. In these persons, the color of the gold weight may show through and result in a "discoloration" of the eyelid. The bulkiness of the gold is also more noticeable. Finally, if the patient's incomplete closure or blinking is due to congenital causes or scarring of the eyelid tissue, these causes must be corrected and gold weight implantation is not the solution.

In all patients there will be a postoperative ptosis. The patient must understand this and be willing to accept such an outcome.

The gold weights are commercially available. They come in 1 mm thickness, 4.5 mm width, and in lengths that vary according to the weight. The weight ranges from 0.6 to 1.6 g in 0.2-g increments. They are curved to match the tarsal plate curvature. They are purified and polished so that problems with extrusion and erosion are extremely unlikely. There are three holes for suture fixation superiorly.

PREOPERATIVE EVALUATION

A medical history and a thorough ocular examination are necessary. In addition to recorded visual acuity and slit-lamp examination, lacrimal function should be carefully studied. The blinking reflex, including its frequency and completeness, should be noted, and the basic and total secretion and the tear breakup time should be measured. Asymmetry in the eyebrow, the nasal labial fold, and the forehead wrinkles should be studied. To assess the severity of seventh nerve palsy, the patient is asked to elevate the eyebrow or balloon up his mouth. To assess lagophthalmos, the patient is asked to close his eyes gently and the opening is measured by a millimeter ruler. Following this, the patient is asked to close the eyelids forcefully. If there is an opening, it is measured again. Bell's phenomenon is observed when the examiner digitally opens the eyelid during forceful closure. The orbicularis function can also be assessed subjectively.

For a patient who has never had previous eyelid surgery, determining the weight needed for complete lid closure is a straightforward process. A gold weight is selected and a small strip of tape is used to anchor it to the affected upper eyelid. The upper border of the weight is positioned just below the natural lid crease. The tape is placed horizontally so that it will not mechanically interfere with lid opening. The patient is asked to open and close the eyelid in both the sitting and supine positions. The lid position and completeness of closure are assessed. The ideal outcome is a minimal ptosis in the sitting position with complete lid closure in the supine position. If the weight selected is too heavy, resulting in a severe ptosis, or too light, resulting in incomplete lid closure, it is gently removed from the eyelid and another weight is taped to the lid in a similar manner. This can be done repeatedly and quickly without difficulty. When the correct weight is found, the patient is instructed to wear it for 30 to 45 minutes before rechecking its position. It is frequently found that the next heavier weight is necessary for complete lid closure. Therefore, it is prudent to have at least two weights sterilized and available for the operation.

SURGICAL TECHNIQUE

The patient's natural upper eyelid crease is identified and marked. A small amount, 0.2 to 0.4 ml, of 2% lidocaine (Xylocaine) with 1:100,000 epinephrine is injected subcutaneously along the marking.

Figure 18–1. Only the central 10 to 15 mm needs to be incised. The skin incision is made with a size 15 blade. The skin edges are retracted with 0.5 forceps and the orbicularis muscle layer is opened up with Stevens scissors. A pocket between the orbicularis layer and the tarsal plate is created by blunt and sharp dissection 4 to 5 mm inferiorly. This dissection should stay at least 2 mm superior to the lid margin. This not only avoids damage to the lash roots, but also prevents the gold weight from sinking down to the lid margin. Depending on the size of the selected implant, the pocket is extended 4 to 8 mm in each direction, medially and laterally. Usually there is no need to dissect superiorly. However, to cover the implant completely, 2 mm of undermining along the superior edge of the orbicularis muscle is performed. Care should be taken so that the expansion of the aponeurosis or the aponeurosis itself is not damaged.

The sterilized gold weights are soaked in Neosporin (polymyxin–neomycin–gramicidin) solution.

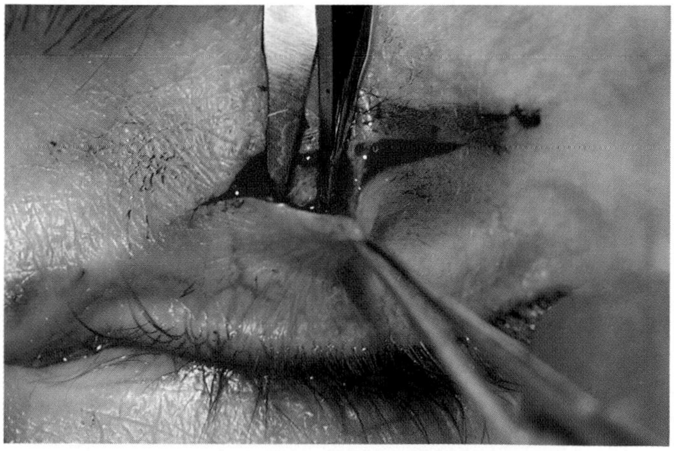

FIGURE 18–1

Figure 18–2. A weight is gently inserted into the pocket.

Figure 18–3. A single 7–0 nylon suture is used either to anchor the weight to the tarsal plate or to close the skin wound temporarily with a slip knot.

The patient is asked to open and close his eyes in both the sitting and supine position to assess the lid closure. If an excessive amount of ptosis is noted in the sitting position, the weight is too heavy. As long as complete lid closure can be achieved when the patient is in the supine position, the lighter weight should be used. Conversely, if incomplete closure is noted when the patient is in the supine position, the heavier weight should be used. To obtain the best lid curvature, the weight can be positioned either slightly medially or laterally. When the curvature is found to be satisfactory, a 7–0 nylon suture is used to anchor the weight. The superior border of the implant should be at the level or slightly lower than the superior border of the tarsal plate. The suture is secured to the expansion of the aponeurosis in the anterior surface of the tarsus, rather than deep in the tarsal plate itself. Two or three holes are used for the fixation. A 7–0 chromic suture is used to close the muscle layer over the implant, and a 7–0 nylon suture is used to close the skin wound in an interrupted fashion.

The patient is given a cold compress immediately following the operation. Maxitrol (dexamethasone–neomycin–polymyxin B) ointment is applied to the wound and to the eye. The patient is seen in the office for suture removal and follow-up examination in 5 to 7 days. The cornea, the lid curvature and height, and the completeness of lid closure and blink are reassessed at this time.

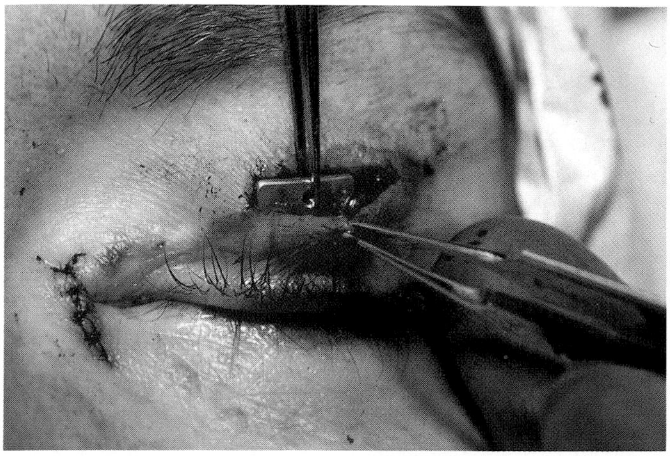

FIGURE 18–2

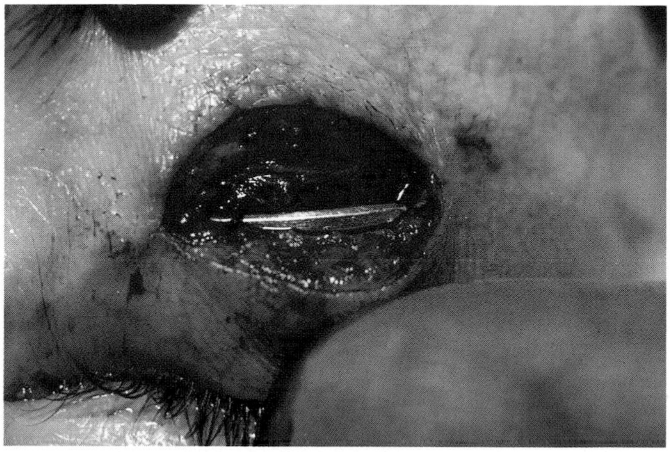

FIGURE 18–3

COMPLICATIONS

Very infrequently bleeding may be a problem. Although epinephrine and local anesthetics help with hemostasis, an injection in the muscle itself or a small vein can result in a hematoma. This may create a mechanical ptosis; therefore, only a minimal amount of anesthetic should be used. A pocket for implant insertion should be created in the central lid, between the muscle layer and tarsal plate. If this is done within the muscle layer, there will be more bleeding. In addition, the implant may be tilted in its position and result in a more noticeable lump externally. Blunt-tipped Stevens scissors should be used so that the tarsal plate and the conjunctiva are not inadvertently penetrated. If this happens, there will be an increased inflammatory reaction, fibrosis, or possible contamination of the wound and implant. All of these can result in infection, implant extrusion, or cosmetic blemish.

The suture holes are designed to be superiorly fixated. The gold implant is designed with a curvature so that it will not be placed upside down or backward. Care should be taken that no foreign material gets into the wound. It is known that extrusion and migration of the implant and erosion through the lid tissue can take place. Undercorrection or overcorrection is rare. They can be easily prevented by careful and precise measurements preoperatively and intraoperatively. Similarly, if the lid curvature is distorted, the lid implant can be repositioned. The most common complaint is the lumpiness in the eyelid that the patient notices. Very rarely, thin-skinned patients may show some discoloration of the eyelid. Theoretically, the weight in the upper eyelid can keep the lid open when the patient is in the supine position. In practice, we have not seen this happen. This possibility can be determined preoperatively and intraoperatively and, therefore, should be preventable.

In summary, gold weight implantation is a simple and effective way to correct lagophthalmos and to simulate blinking in most patients with paralytic eyelid problems. It is easily performed, can be reversed, and has very few complications.

Chapter Nineteen

LID REANIMATION WITH THE PALPEBRAL SPRING

Robert E. Levine

The inability to close the eye (lagophthalmos) or to blink leads to serious corneal complications, including chronic ocular discomfort, corneal ulceration, and loss of vision. In addition, the intensive regimen of frequent drops, ointment during the day, or taping the eye at intervals or at night, that may be required for the medical management of lagophthalmos can add to the disability. It is common to see patients who have recovered well from other aspects of trauma, brain tumor, or other causes of facial paralysis, only to be limited by eye problems in their ability to resume a normal life-style. The treatment of severe lagophthalmos, then, becomes important, not only in preventing visual loss, but also in rehabilitating the patient.

TARSORRHAPHY

The classic surgical answer to lagophthalmos has been tarsorrhaphy, just as the classic surgical answer to cataract was aphakia. Unfortunately, tarsorrhaphy, like aphakia, replaces the original problems with other problems.

Except for patients who had minimal lateral tarsorrhaphies, virtually all were unhappy with the results. Those who had extensive tarsorrhaphies had essentially lost the use of the affected eye. Those with lesser tarsorrhaphies complained of loss of visual field.

The tarsorrhaphy added significantly to the disfigurement and to the difficulty adjusting psychologically to the effects of facial paralysis. In those patients who recovered enough lower facial function so that the lower face looked relatively normal, at least in repose, the tarsorrhaphy continued to be disfiguring. Furthermore, despite the high functional, cosmetic, and psychologic cost of tarsorrhaphy, patients still had chronic discomfort from exposure keratitis.

METHODS OF LID REANIMATION

Because of the limitations of tarsorrhaphy, various procedures have been introduced to reanimate the paralyzed lids. The most physiologic solution is reinnervation of the lids. Unfortunately, even when reinnervation procedures, such as facial–hypoglossal anastomosis, are successful in reanimating the lower face, they may fail to supply enough innervation to the upper lid to restore closure and blinking. Temporalis muscle transplantation into the upper lid also has a low success rate. Closure may be accomplished by conscious "biting down" by the patient, but this has little to do with physiologic blinking and closure. Implanted magnets may hold the lid shut at night, but do not contribute to lid closure during the day.

The most successful reanimation procedures have been those that attempt to create a force in the lids to act against the levator muscle. For example, a small flat gold weight may be implanted into the upper lid and fixated superotarsally, or tarsally. With the patient upright, the weight of the lid acts against the levator to close the eye. The effects of this procedure are limited by the patient's position (since the weight may not act to close the eye with the patient supine), and also by the size of the piece of gold that can be placed in the lid without disfigurement. Gold weights are most successful when lagophthalmos is not severe or when the need for complete lid closure is not critical.

The Silastic (polymeric silicone) elastic prosthesis devised by Arion uses a 1-mm Silastic band as the opposing force against the levator. The band is sewn through the medial canthal tendon. A special introducer is then passed between orbicularis and tarsus in the upper lid. The end of the band is attached to the introducer and brought through the lid laterally, where it is fixated to the periosteum. The other end is similarly passed through the lower lid and anchored. In general, this implant works quite well. Its long-term success, however, is limited by the loss of elasticity in the Silastic, or a loss of tension in the band as it migrates slightly medially through the tendon. The procedure may have a role in patients who are expected to recover normal facial function in 6 months. Unfortunately, in most instances of facial paralysis, it is difficult to predict the exact timing of functional return.

The device that is most successful in providing long-term lid reanimation is the palpebral spring implant. The original concept for this spring was described by Morel-Fatio and Lalardrie (1964). The technique has been modified over the years by Levine (1989).

The spring can provide reliable long-term complete closure of the lid, regardless of patient position. It also provides a simulated blink. Because closing tension is present even in the open position, frequently, there is some degree of pseudoptosis. Nevertheless, the lid can be opened enough to clear the visual axis, and the cosmetic result is generally acceptable. Extrusion or breakage of the spring (e.g., from vigorous rubbing of the eye or from metal fatigue) are uncommon events. Slippage of the spring toward the lid margin can occur, but this is an infrequent problem. If slippage does occur, repositioning the end of the spring is a relatively simple maneuver.

INDICATIONS FOR SPRING IMPLANTATION

The palpebral spring is indicated in any patient with lagophthalmos resulting from facial paralysis that is expected to persist for more than 6 months and in whom the eye problems cannot be readily managed by the use of drops and ointment. It may also be used as a permanent solution to a closure problem that is not expected to improve.

When recovery of facial function occurs and it is clear that the spring is no longer needed, it can be removed. If partial function returns, the spring can be retained and readjusted. If the patient fails to recover upper lid function, the spring can be left permanently.

Patients with coexistent fifth nerve deficits (decreased corneal sensation) or poor Bell's phenomenon may require complete lid closure to protect the cornea. Therefore, in such patients, the presence of even moderate lagophthalmos may indicate the need for spring implantation.

Patients with severe paralysis who are expected to recover function in less than 6 months, but in whom conservative management is impractical, may also benefit from spring implantation. Consider, for example, a patient who could be managed for several months by taping the eye shut. If the affected eye were his only functional eye, long-term lid closure would not be a viable possibility, and a spring implant could be considered.

A decision for placement of a stainless steel palpebral spring should be made cautiously in a patient who is known to need frequent magnetic resonance imaging (MRI) scans, since implant movement or migration could potentially occur when the spring is subjected to the magnetic field of the MRI scanner. In my experience, however, this has not been a problem.

TECHNIQUE OF PALPEBRAL SPRING IMPLANTATION

Building the Spring

The spring is prepared in advance of surgery, not only to save operative time, but also because the configuration of the spring can be more carefully matched to the patient's anatomy in the absence of infiltration anesthesia and lid swelling. In designing the spring, the posterior aspect of the loop is the superior end. Suitable stainless steel, round, orthodontic wire (diameter from 0.008 to 0.011 in.) is selected, depending on the force required to oppose the levator (orthodontic wire may be purchased from Unitek/3M, 3724 South Peck Road, Monrovia, CA). Thicker wire may be used to balance the force of a strong levator, and lighter wire may be used if the levator is weak. The curves of the spring must match the curvature of the lid. Place the spring on the closed lid and make appropriate bends in the wire.

The spring tension preoperatively is set somewhat tighter than will be required, as it is easier to loosen the spring intraoperatively than to tighten it. The spring must also be designed to track well with the upper lid as it moves from the open to the shut position.

Preparing the Patient

The patient is prepared and draped in the usual manner for lid surgery. The eye is protected with a scleral shell. Lidocaine 2% with epinephrine is infiltrated along the lateral two-thirds of the upper lid fold. An additional amount of anesthetic is infiltrated along the tarsus at the junction of the lateral two-thirds and medial one-third of the upper lid. Infiltration is also given along the lateral orbital rim. The amount of infiltration should be limited, to avoid distortion of lid anatomy or levator function. Basal sedation, given preoperatively, should be limited to short-acting agents that will not interfere with the patient's state of consciousness during the procedure, since cooperation is needed to open and close the eyes and to sit up on the operating table.

Implanting the Spring

Figure 19–1. With a protective scleral shell in place, an incision is made along the lateral two-thirds of the lid crease and carried across the orbital rim laterally. Dissection is carried downward at the medial end of the incision to expose the tarsal plate. Dissection is also carried upward and laterally to expose the orbital rim.

Figure 19–2. A 22-gauge blunted spinal needle with the stylette in place is passed from the medial end of the dissection to emerge laterally in the plane between orbicularis and tarsus. The passage should be carried out overlying midtarsus. The needle is angulated slightly downward at its lateral extent. The exit of the needle tract should be close to lateral orbital rim periosteum. The lid is everted to confirm that the needle has not inadvertently perforated the tarsus. The previously prepared wire spring (which has been autoclaved), is passed through the needle and the needle is withdrawn.

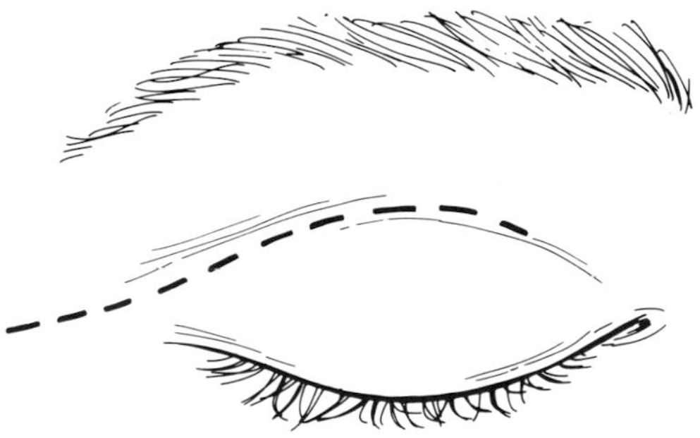

FIGURE 19–1

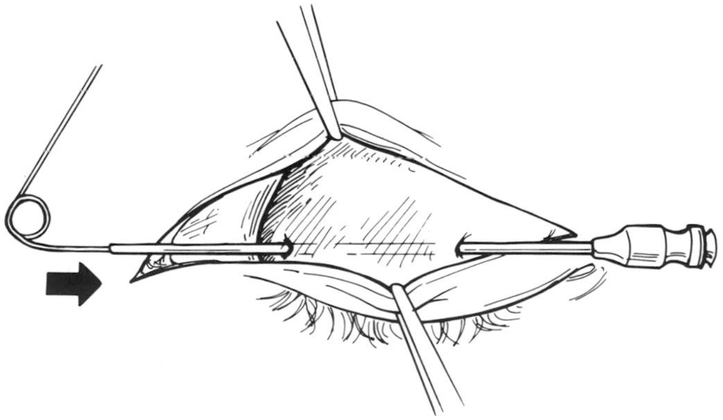

FIGURE 19–2

Figure 19–3. A cross-section of the lid illustrates placement of the needle over the midtarsus in the plane between the tarsus and obicularis. The wire spring should be resting on the epitarsal surface.

Figure 19–4. The scleral shell is removed and the fulcrum of the spring is brought into the desired position along the orbital rim. The spring should be placed in a position where its curves conform perfectly to the eyelid contour. (*Inset*) The fulcrum of the spring is secured to lateral orbital rim periosteum with three 4–0 Mersilene sutures, taking an extra bite of the periosteum with each stitch. The lower limb of the spring should terminate at the point corresponding to the medial limbus in primary distance gaze. Loops are fashioned at each end and the spring is cut to size. The loops should be flat and tightly closed to leave no sharp edges. The medial loop is enveloped in 0.2-mm–thick Dacron patch material, to which it is secured by means of three 8–0 nylon sutures tied internally.

The Dacron patch material is creased in a Gelfoam press before surgery and autoclaved with the other instruments. The folded Dacron envelope is cut to size at surgery. The crease in the patch material should be directed downward so that the spring and patch together provide a smooth inferior surface. The loop at the end of the inferior arm is directed upward for the same reason. Suturing of the loop to the Dacron is facilitated by resting the Dacron on a retractor.

Figure 19–5. The end of the spring with its Dacron envelope is reposited into the lid between tarsus and orbicularis. In time, the end of the spring will become fixed to the tarsus by granulation tissue integrating into the Dacron patch. It is helpful to secure the patch to the tarsus directly with an additional running 8–0 nylon suture, to provide fixation until connective tissue grows into the Dacron. The tension on the spring is checked, with the patient in both the upright and supine positions. The tension can be adjusted by grasping the upper end of the spring with forceps and changing its position. When the correct tension has been determined, the upper loop of the spring is secured to the orbital rim periosteum with a 4–0 Mersilene suture. An extra bite of the periosteum may be taken in the stitch before tying. When placing sutures to secure either the fulcrum or the upper loop of the spring to the orbital rim periosteum, it is safer to sew in the direction away from the globe. Spring tension is again checked with the patient both seated and supine. Additional adjustments can be made by bending the wire or repositioning the loop. When the adjustments are completed, two additional 4–0 Mersilene sutures are placed through the upper loop in a manner similar to the initial suture. Deeper tissues overlying the spring are then closed with 5–0 plain gut suture to assure that the spring and the Mersilene sutures are well covered. Skin and muscle are closed with running 6–0 plain gut fast-absorbing suture.

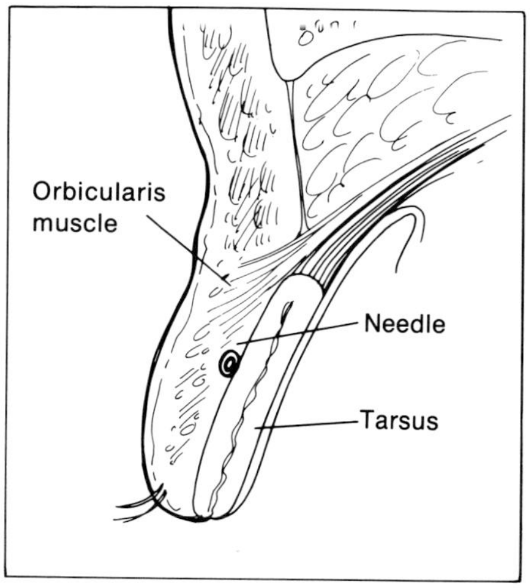

FIGURE 19–3

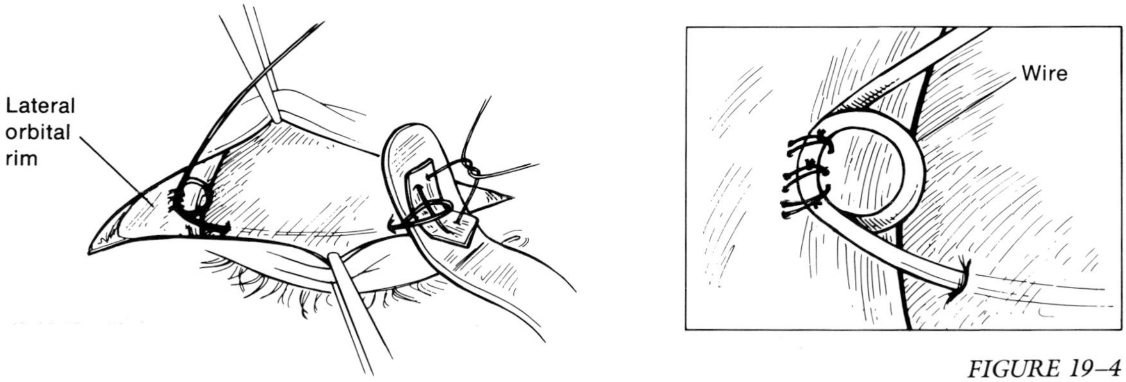

FIGURE 19–4

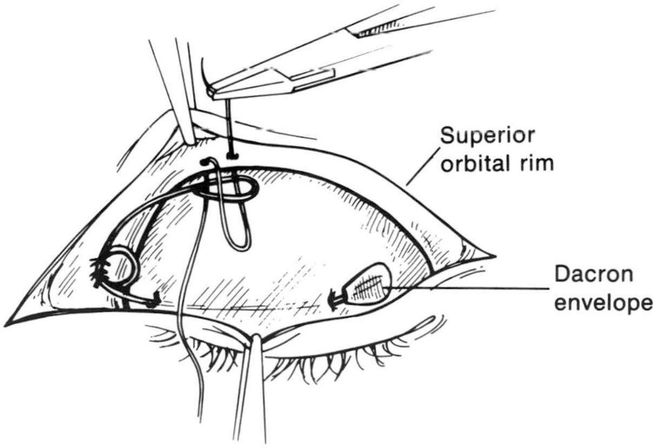

FIGURE 19–5

POSTOPERATIVE CARE

Antibiotic ointment is applied onto the wound twice daily until the wound is healed and skin sutures have been absorbed. Ice packs are applied to the lid during the first 24 hours after surgery. Warm tap water compresses (or some other form of moist heat) are then substituted and continued until lid swelling subsides.

Chapter Twenty

MOHS MICROGRAPHIC SURGERY

Peter B. Odland
Duane C. Whitaker

Mohs micrographic surgery (MMS) is a specialized surgical technique that combines maximal normal tissue preservation with the highest cure rate of any skin cancer treatment. This technique is well suited for periocular cutaneous neoplasms with contiguous growth pattern (i.e., neoplasms with limited metastatic potential). The micrographic (Mohs) surgeon and ophthalmic plastic surgeon (OPS) can combine their skills so that patients can benefit from both specialties. Through this division of labor, the micrographic surgeon can concentrate exclusively on accurate tumor extirpation, and the ophthalmic plastic surgeon can concentrate on restoring function and cosmesis through reconstruction of the resulting defect.

INDICATIONS

Patients may be referred to micrographic surgeons for a variety of lesions. Although basal cell carcinoma (BCC) represents approximately 90% of malignant tumors of the eyelids, other primary eyelid tumors include squamous cell carcinoma (SCC), carcinoma in situ (CIS or Bowen's disease), keratoacanthoma (KA), sebaceous carcinoma, malignant melanoma, and tumors of eccrine, apocrine, or accessory lacrimal gland origin.

In general, any eyelid tumor that can be reliably interpreted by frozen sections and that demonstrates contiguous growth patterns can be treated by MMS. Mohs micrographic excision followed by oculoplastic repair is the accepted method of treatment for periocular BCC, SCC, CIS, and KA. Sweat gland carcinoma, although rare, can generally be interpreted by frozen-section histopathologic methods and, therefore, is also amenable to MMS. Sebaceous carcinoma and malignant melanoma, because of their noncontiguous growth features, metastatic potential, and difficulty of interpretation by frozen sections, present some controversy concerning their suitability for MMS. Basal cell carcinoma and SCC may be classified on their clinical or histologic appearance. On the basis of biologic behavior, morpheaform BCC and poorly differentiated SCC are notorious for their extensive microscopic spread, well beyond the clinically apparent margin. Basal cell carcinoma is much more common on the lower eyelid, but both tumors can be seen on either the upper or lower lid. Sebaceous carcinoma presents special problems because of its multifocal growth pattern, rendering any method of excision with margin control difficult. It may also demonstrate pagetoid spread, a histologic change that can be difficult to identify, even on permanent sections.

PREOPERATIVE EVALUATION

All patients are seen for preoperative evaluation by both the MMS and OPS team. Biopsy, if not already performed by a referring physician, can be done by either the MMS or the OPS. Relevant history and physical examination is done and preoperative laboratory studies are obtained. Once the tumor histopathology is confirmed, the nature of the tumor and the technique of MMS as well as reconstructive options are discussed in detail with the patient. It is important for the patient to understand that the size of surgical defect cannot be accurately predicted, and that is why the surgery is done with microscopic control. Therefore, the OPS will be able to discuss general reconstructive considerations, not precise details. In most centers, MMS and reconstruction by the OPS are scheduled on separate days. In less extensive tumor cases, MMS and OPS reconstruction may be completed in 1 day; however, it is best for patients to plan for a 2-day procedure.

PROCEDURE

The clinically evident tumor is debulked, if necessary, with a curette, scalpel, or a fine tissue scissors. Frequently, the grossly evident tumor is small, and debulking is not necessary. In such cases, or after all the apparent tumor is debulked, a 1- to 4-mm margin (depending on cell type, duration, size, and whether it is primary or recurrent tumor) is marked circumferentially around the clinically apparent tumor or the initial defect. With the scalpel at a 45° angle beveling toward the base of the wound, rather than perpendicular, a shallow incision is made along the mark. From the beveled incision, a saucer-shaped, 1- to 4-mm–thick specimen is carefully excised. The orientation is preserved, and the specimen is placed on a moistened gauze (which is also marked to maintain orientation) in a petri dish. Hemostasis is achieved with bipolar electrocoagulation, and a temporary protective dressing is applied.

A diagram (map) is drawn corresponding to specimen orientation in relation to the defect. The specimen is then subdivided into specimens 5–10 mm in diameter. These subspecimens are carefully colored and number-coded to correlate with the patient diagram (map), so that any tumor subsequently seen on microscopic examination of the specimen can be precisely located from the patient's map. The tissue is then submitted to the histotechnician for horizontal frozen sectioning. The histotechnician assures that the entire deep and peripheral surfaces of the specimen are presented in one plane as the stained sections mounted on glass slides. Close communication and consultation between the physician and technician is essential. The micrographic surgeon then reads and interprets the frozen-section slides for margin determination. If no tumor is present, the patient is referred to the oculoplastic surgeon for repair. If tumor is identified microscopically on any of the slides, the location is color-coded on the map, which serves as a guide for further surgery. The micrographic surgeon then returns to the patient and reexcises tissue only where tumor was identified, preserving all other tissue and anatomic structures. The steps of mapping, color-coding, processing of tissue, microscopic examination, reexcision of tumor foci are repeated until a complete tumor-free plane is achieved.

SPECIAL PROBLEMS

Treating skin cancer of the periocular region is approached with the goals of curing the patient, preserving eyesight, and minimizing deformity or dysfunction. In most cases these goals are achieved, and frequently the patient suffers almost no cosmetic deficit after surgery. However, if tumor extends into the lacrimal drainage system, the deep medial canthal region, deeper orbital soft tissue, or orbital bone, then special risks are encountered.

It is not unusual for the lower lid tumors to be located very close to, and sometimes directly on, the lacrimal punctum. Also, tumors of the medial canthal region are often extensive and deeply invasive, such that the canalicular system must be interrupted or even excised for the eradication of tumor. We tell all such patients about this potential outcome and that reconstruction of the drainage system is not always possible. In an attempt to maintain patency of this system during tumor surgery, some Mohs surgeons have recommended placing a probe through the punctum and into the canaliculus. Our feeling is that such probing may carry with it the risk of seeding tumor deeper into and beyond the canalicular system. Therefore, we do not routinely probe the ducts, but instead, identify the system and meticulously excise the tumor as required at the time of surgery.

Because the periocular skin and subcutaneous tissue is quite thin, cutaneous neoplasms of relatively short duration can invade the orbit through direct extension into the periorbital fat, extraocular muscles, the periorbita, the lacrimal gland, and potentially the globe. Tumors in which orbital invasion is considered should be studied by computed tomography (CT) or magnetic resonance imaging (MRI). Orbital invasion most commonly occurs with medial canthal tumors or radiation treatment failures. Although it is unusual for small, primary lesions to invade the deep orbital tissues, large or neglected primary tumors may. The risk is much greater with recurrent tumors; that is, those that have been treated previously with surgery, radiation therapy, or other destructive techniques. If there is concern that tumor may invade deep into the orbit, the full details should be discussed with the patient and appropriate family members preoperatively. The patient must realize that if cure is the goal, his sight is at risk. Once a tumor has invaded the periorbital fat, even if it has not penetrated the globe or extraocular muscles, a limited, but reliable, removal of tumor cells from within the orbit is usually impossible. A tenet of orbital oncology is that if a tumor has invaded orbital fat, extraocular muscle, the globe, or the lacrimal gland, then exenteration of all orbital contents is the only maneuver that can ensure the entire removal of the tumor.

The presence of tumor in the orbit is not an absolute indication for exenteration. For example, some elderly patients feel they have a limited life expectancy and may understandably refuse orbital exenteration. However, this needs to be discussed in detail so the patient's wishes can be honored, and the option that is most consistent with good medical and humane care can be offered. Such tumors present very difficult management considerations to the surgical team, the patient, and involved family members.

Tumors that invade periorbita (i.e., periosteum lining the orbital bone), but appear to leave the orbital contents unharmed, present management problems as well. In this instance, eradication of the tumor may require surgery of the orbital bones. And although it may be possible to preserve the globe and optic nerve, disruption of the orbital skeleton may be so great that the patient will either have a displaced globe, diminished motion of the globe, or otherwise compromised binocular vision. Once again, the issue of what can be preserved must be discussed in quite simple and straightforward terms with the patient so he or she can understand what the functional status will be afterward.

STANDARD VERSUS MOHS TECHNIQUE

Much of cancer surgery is based on an assumption that tumor growth is spherical, which is not entirely accurate for cutaneous tumors. Many factors probably influence tumor growth, such as genetic predisposition and immunologic status. However, it also appears that physical factors, such as embryologic fusion planes, have an effect. Also, muscle fascia, periosteum, and other tissues may present a temporary barrier to tumor spread, and as a consequence, the growth and configuration of tumor is often asymmetric and irregular. Thus, on a clinical basis, it is not possible to accurately assess surgical margins.

The standard frozen-section technique (SFST) represents the traditional approach to evaluating surgical margins. It is usually employed in an operating room with the patient under either local or general anesthesia, during which an inordinate amount of time cannot safely be devoted to tissue processing. Therefore, practicality has dictated that pathologists receive the tissue and usually vertically section the tissue at the most suspicious areas as indicated by the surgeon. Also, the specimen may be bisected and then "bread-loafed" at intervals to check margins. This type of technique, no matter how carefully done, cannot microscopically examine all tissue margins. Rather, representative checks are done that result in greater potential for residual tumor being left at the surgical margin.

In MMS, the surgeon excises the tumor, orients the specimen, and color-codes the subspecimens. The micrographic surgeon diagrams and maps the surgical defect and surgical specimens so that a histotechnician trained in the Mohs technique precisely cuts horizontal specimens, which will allow the surgeon to examine all surgical margins with the microscope. There are no random cuts, only the most suspicious margins, rather than the entire specimen, are processed and examined. There is no randomness to the MMS technique; rather, its hallmark is the combination of meticulous, precise tumor removal with careful tissue preservation.

LIMITATIONS

Although MMS enjoys a very high cure rate for tumors that grow in a contiguous fashion and without much metastatic potential, tumors that would otherwise not be at risk for spread may, under certain circumstances, recur after this surgery. An example of such a situation would be a recurrent morpheaform basal cell carcinoma. Such a tumor will probably have a very aggressive behavior pattern and may, because of its prior treatment, have a multifocal nature, thereby rendering any margin control surgery difficult. Nonetheless, MMS is still the gold standard of treatment for such tumors.

Because MMS is used, on occasion, to treat aggressive tumors and because this decreases the chances for cure with a single modality, adjunctive therapy may be necessary occasionally. This may also be advantageous in treating tumor not yet clinically recognized as metastatic, but tumor cells that may be "in transit." The need for adjunctive therapy is not a limitation exclusive to MMS, but is required for any tumor extirpation surgery in certain situations.

As mentioned earlier, tumors with a noncontiguous growth pattern are likely to recur with any margin-controlled surgical removal, especially one that is as precise and tissue conserving as MMS. Examples of this are sebaceous gland carcinoma and extramammary Paget's disease.

Extensive tumors arising in the skin are effectively treated with MMS; however, with long-standing, extensive tumors the cure rate drops. Additionally, since the extent of the tumor cannot be predicted with accuracy in such cases, the resulting surgical defect may be too much for the patient to accept.

When MMS is applied to tumors that are difficult to interpret under frozen-section technology (e.g., fibrous tumors; lentigo maligna melanoma), reconstruction may have to be delayed while permanent histologic sections are prepared and read. This type of delay does not defeat the purpose of MMS, but the delays are sometimes difficult for the patient to tolerate and for scheduling.

Dense aggregates of reactive inflammatory cells occasionally obscure the tumor cells present on Mohs frozen sections, and this difficulty in distinguishing reactive from malignant changes can sometimes be limiting to the extent that more layers will need to be taken, thereby enlarging the surgical defect. This may have implications in plans for reconstructive surgery.

MISCONCEPTIONS

A large part of the confusion about Mohs micrographic surgery today stems from the early days of "chemosurgery." The original technique, although used only rarely in modern dermatologic surgery units, included in vivo tissue fixation, days between layers (rather than minutes), tumor extirpation could take up 1 to 2 weeks to complete, and wounds were all left to heal by secondary intention because the fixation resulted in delayed tissue slough. With the development of the "fresh tissue technique" the need for in vivo chemical fixation of the tissues was rarely called for, thus permitting immediate or next-day reconstruction.

Continued use of the term *chemosurgery* causes considerable confusion for some patients and physicians, as they expect the treatment to include chemotherapy and may be concerned that they did not get the proper treatment without it. In an attempt to correct this and other misconceptions, the Mohs surgery governing body was recently redesignated as the American College of Mohs Micrographic Surgery and Cutaneous Oncology.

There are still some surgeons who feel MMS has no advantage over the standard frozen-section–controlled surgery. This thinking may result, in part, from an incomplete understanding of MMS as described in the foregoing. The key to the success of MMS is the combination of horizontally orienting the frozen sections and having the surgeon read his own slides, which is not done with the other techniques.

Chapter Twenty-One

EYELID RECONSTRUCTION

Jan W. Kronish

GOALS AND PRINCIPLES

Loss of eyelid tissues most often results from trauma and surgical excision of neoplasms. Congenital colobomas and necrosis or cicatricial contraction following periocular infections, radiation, cryotherapy, or thermal burns also may cause eyelid defects. The goals of eyelid reconstruction are to reestablish functional eyelids, with an acceptable cosmetic appearance, that provide adequate protection of the globe.

Surgeons who plan to perform eyelid reconstruction must bear in mind the anatomic and functional components of the eyelids. A smooth, mucous membrane internal lining is mandatory to maintain lubrication of the ocular surface and avoid corneal irritation. A rigid support normally provided by the tarsus is essential to retain the eyelid shape and its vertical position, yet it must be flexible enough to mold to the curvature of the globe. A stable eyelid margin is necessary to keep the lashes and skin directed away from the cornea and retain a smooth contour in contact with the eye. Proper fixation of the medial and lateral canthal attachments of the lids will add to the eyelid stability and its proper orientation. A muscle layer is needed to provide enough tone and power to achieve eyelid closure. Finally, the overlying skin has to be thin and supple to accommodate eyelid excursion.

Upper eyelid defects are especially challenging to reconstruct, given the additional requirements for mobility and the upper lid's major contribution to corneal protection. Levator muscle action must be adequate to elevate the eyelid above the visual axis; also, the lid must be of sufficient size and be elastic enough to cover the cornea. Upper lid defects are poorly tolerated by the exposed ocular surface and usually require an expeditious repair. The integrity of the eye protective mechanisms, such as Bell's phenomenon and tear film quality and production, affects the duration that the cornea will tolerate the increased exposure.

The eyelids may be anatomically divided into two layers, both of which must be replaced in the repair of full-thickness defects to satisfy their functional requirements. The anterior lamella, which consists of the skin and orbicularis muscle, partly supports the lower lid position, provides dynamic closure of the upper and lower lids, and contributes to the lacrimal pump mechanism. It may be reconstructed with advancement or rotation myocutaneous flaps or full-thickness skin grafts. The tarsus and its conjunctival lining constitute the posterior lamella and provide structural integrity to the lid with a mucosal surface. Reconstruction of this layer may involve tarsal transposition or rotation flaps, free autogenous tarsal grafts, sliding tarsal conjunctival flaps, or tarsal substitutes, including preserved sclera, auricular cartilage, nasal septal chondromucosa, and hard palate mucosa. When reconstructive methods are utilized to create this bilamellar configuration, at least one of the two layers must have its own inherent blood supply.

Techniques for eyelid reconstruction can be grouped according to the tissues employed. Adjacent tissues used for repair of lid defects, such as direct closure, the Tenzel semicircle flap, and myocutaneous advancement flaps, are ideal because they provide their own blood supply, maintain the same color and surface characteristics as the normal lid tissues, and contract less than a graft. Eyelid tissue from the opposite lid may be transposed, as in the Cutler–Beard and Hughes procedures, which also use tissues similar in character. Contiguous, but more remote, periocular tissues can be used, such as the temporal forehead (Fricke) flap, or glabellar and median forehead flaps. The remaining alternative technique of autogenous grafts, including contralateral eyelid and postauricular skin, tarsus, and nasal or ear cartilage grafts, is usually applied for repair of extensive eyelid defects. The reconstructive surgeon should be familiar with a variety of techniques, given that variations or different combinations of multiple methods may be necessary to properly reconstruct the eyelids.

PREOPERATIVE EVALUATION AND MANAGEMENT

Before deciding which technique to apply, examine the defect, noting its size, location, configuration, and depth, as well as consider the patient's age. Full-thickness eyelid marginal defects are divided according to size into small (<25%), moderate (25% to 50%), and large defects (>50%). Table 21–1 indicates the techniques described in this chapter according to defect size. The availability of tissues utilized in different reconstructive methods is also determined by whether the defect is located centrally, medially, or laterally.

Reconstructive techniques also differ for defects in the medial and lateral canthus (see Table 21–1). When the defect is superficial, only the anterior lamella may need to be repaired, whereas full-thickness defects require re-formation of both anatomic layers. The periocular tissues in elderly patients typically exhibit greater elasticity than those in young patients, allowing them to stretch more easily to reduce the defect size. Finally, if a patient requires lid reconstruction with only one functioning eye on the same side, alternative techniques to avoid a lid-sharing procedure should be considered.

A thorough knowledge of the anatomy and blood supply of the eyelids, lacrimal drainage system, and periocular tissues is essential before performing eyelid reconstruction. Previous radiation, surgery, and chemical or thermal burns may compromise the blood supply to the tissues employed for reconstruction; in such cases, use of tissues that provide their own blood supply is preferable. Methods to salvage the canaliculi might be necessary for repair of defects involving the medial eyelid.

Before reconstruction of an eyelid defect that resulted from the excision of a malignancy, it is imperative that the margins of the remaining tissue are free of tumor. This can be ascertained histologically during the surgical removal of the neoplasm by Mohs micrographic surgical techniques or by frozen-section analysis. This precaution is taken not only to minimize the chance of recurrent tumor, but also to

TABLE 21–1
Eyelid Reconstruction Techniques

Lower Eyelid Reconstruction

- Direct closure (defect size <30%)
- Direct closure with cantholysis (defect size <40%)
- Periosteal strip and myocutaneous advancement flap (defect size <40%)
- Semicircular rotational flap (defect size <66%)
- Hughes tarsoconjunctival flap (defect size <90%)

Upper Eyelid Reconstruction

- Direct closure (defect size <30%)
- Direct closure with cantholysis (defect size <40%)
- Semicircular rotational flap (defect size <50%)
- Free autogenous tarsal graft (defect size <50%)
- Cutler–Beard procedure (defect size <90%)

Periorbital and Nonmarginal Eyelid Reconstruction

- Full-thickness skin graft
- Simple ellipse sliding flap
- Glabellar flap
- Rhombic flap

prevent spread of tumor along newly created surgical planes or transposed tissues, such as from the lower lid to the upper lid following a Hughes reconstruction. Violation of intact bone should also be avoided for at least 1 to 2 years following the initial excision of periocular malignancies, allowing time for monitoring the area for tumor recurrence. Such methods as creating an osteotomy for conjunctival dacryocystorhinostomy with a Jones tube or transnasal wiring create a potential pathway for spread of recurrent tumor into the adjacent sinuses and nasal cavity.

The patient should refrain from taking aspirin or aspirin-containing products for 2 weeks before surgery. The techniques described in this chapter are the author's procedures of choice or are standard procedures with which the reconstructive surgeon should be familiar. These methods singly or in combination should be effective in the repair of most eyelid defects.

SURGICAL PROCEDURES

Anesthesia

Eyelid reconstruction can be performed under local anesthesia, with or without mild sedation, in almost all patients except children and very anxious adults. Subcutaneous infiltration of 2% lidocaine with a 1:100,000 dilution of epinephrine should be administered at the edges of the defect as well as in those tissues that the surgeon anticipates will be manipulated for the reconstruction. If a lengthy procedure is anticipated, 0.75% bupivicaine with a 1:100,000 dilution of epinephrine can be mixed with lidocaine to prolong the anesthetic effect. Once the tissues are infiltrated, the surgeon should wait approximately 10 minutes to allow the epinephrine to achieve the vasoconstrictive effects that facilitate hemostasis. Topical 1% tetracaine hydrochloride drops will provide adequate anesthesia for the ocular surface.

Lower Eyelid Reconstruction

Direct Closure With or Without Lateral Cantholysis

Eyelid defects involving up to one-third of the central lower lid margin can be repaired by primary closure techniques. Depending on the laxity of the periocular tissues, a lateral cantholysis may be necessary to provide sufficient relaxation of the lower lid attachments to directly close the defect without excessive tension. This method of reconstruction is the most commonly employed for lid margin defects and has the advantage of being a single-staged technique that maintains an anatomically normal lid margin with preservation of eyelashes.

Figure 21–1. The edges of the eyelid defect should be trimmed, if necessary, so that the tarsal borders are sharp and perpendicular to the lid margin and the tissues inferior to the tarsus are cut into a wedge, forming a pentagonal-shaped defect. Bleeding should be meticulously controlled with a bipolar cautery. While grasping each end of the defect with a toothed forceps, if the borders of the defect can be approximated without extensive tension on the wound edge, a direct closure can be undertaken; however, if the edges cannot be brought together easily, a lateral cantholysis is necessary.

To perform a cantholysis, a 4- to 5-mm horizontal incision is made with a Stevens scissors from the lateral canthal angle toward the orbital rim through skin and orbicularis muscle (see Figure 21–1). With the canthal tendon split into the superior and inferior division, medial traction is applied to the lateral lid margin, and the tip of Wescott scissors is used to identify the firm lateral attachments of the lower lid.

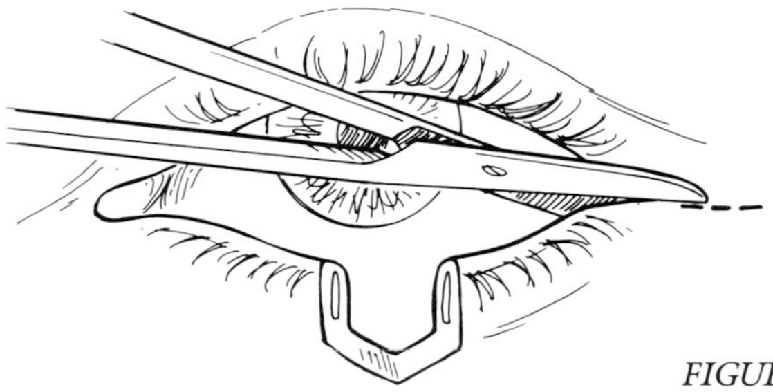

FIGURE 21–1

Figure 21–2. The inferior crus of the lateral canthal tendon is then either partially or completely transected by making a vertical incision with scissors until the lateral margin of the defect can be mobilized medially to close the wound without tension. Disruption of the conjunctiva during the cantholysis should be avoided. The canthotomy incision is closed with interrupted 7–0 nylon sutures.

Figure 21–3. The first and most important step to primarily close a lid margin defect is the approximation of the edges of the tarsus. Exact vertical alignment of these edges is necessary to yield a satisfactory lid margin repair and this layer provides most of the tension-bearing support of the wound.

Some surgeons find it helpful to first place a temporary 6–0 silk suture in the lid margin to properly orient the borders of tarsus. Three interrupted 5–0 Vicryl sutures are passed through the tarsal plate in a partial-thickness fashion incorporating the anterior two-thirds of tarsus. Placement of this suture with a small spatula needle helps to avoid a full-thickness passage of sutures that could lead to corneal irritation. The edges of the subjacent tarsal conjunctiva will be adequately opposed and do not require sutures.

Figure 21–4. Closure of the lid margin is achieved by placing a vertical mattress suture through the lid margin for proper anteroposterior alignment. A 6–0 silk suture enters a meibomian gland orifice 3 mm from the wound edge and exits through the tarsal plate 3 mm from the lid margin; it then enters the tarsus on the opposing edge, 3 mm from the lid margin and exits from a meibomian gland orifice 3 mm from the cut edge. The suture is then passed back through the lid margin in a near-to-near fashion, entering and exiting through a meibomian gland orifice only 1 mm from the wound edge. This suture is tied tightly enough to achieve moderate eversion of the lid margin.

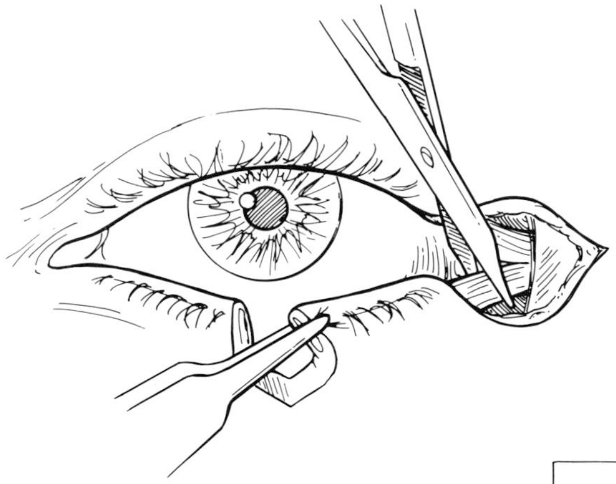

FIGURE 21–2

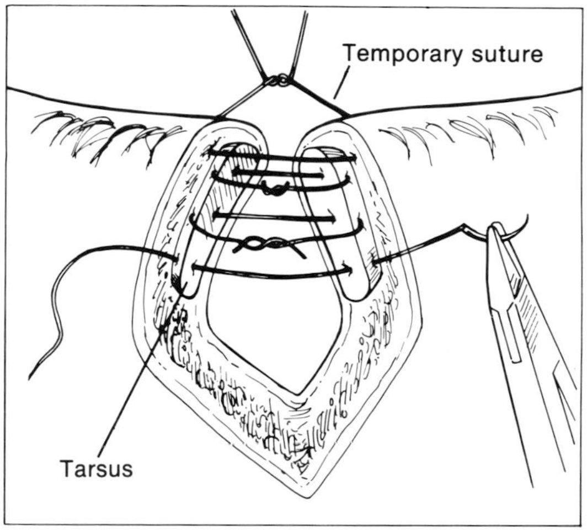

FIGURE 21–3

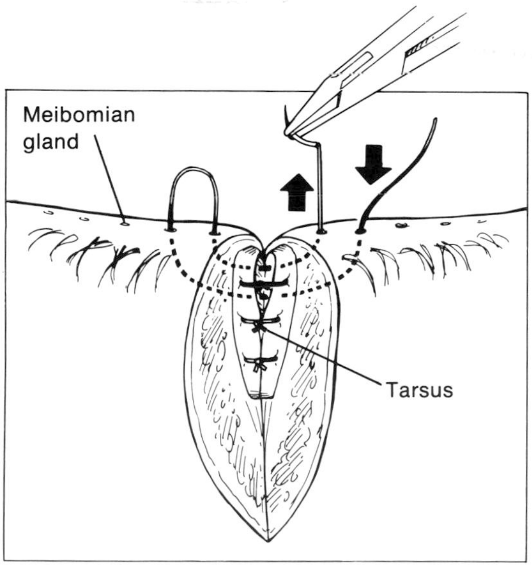

FIGURE 21–4

Figure 21–5. Two additional interrupted 6–0 silk sutures are passed, one just posterior to the lashes and one just beneath the lashes. The ends of these three silk sutures are left long and secured away from the wound on the lower lid skin with a suture or Steri-strip at the conclusion of the procedure to prevent them from irritating the cornea. The anterior lamella is closed in a layered manner by first suturing together the edges of orbicularis muscle with interrupted 6–0 or 7–0 Vicryl sutures with their knots buried.

Figure 21–6. Skin closure is achieved with 7–0 nylon or silk interrupted sutures. A dog ear of redundant skin at the inferior edge of the wound, if present, should be trimmed.

Periosteal Strip and Myocutaneous Advancement Flap

A periosteal strip and myocutaneous flap can be used to reconstruct the lateral one-third of the lower lid when there is no tarsus remaining at the lateral margin of the defect. The periosteal strip can also be used in combination with other reconstructive methods for larger defects. The basic premise of this technique is that the hinged strip of periosteum obtained from the lateral orbital rim provides the posterior lamellar support of the re-formed lateral lower lid with proper posterior fixation.

Figure 21–7. Mobilization of a composite skin and orbicularis muscle flap is first performed by outlining an advancement flap with a marker pen either in a semicircular manner or as a cheek flap extended 1 to 2 cm beyond the lateral commissure. The skin incision is made with a size 15 Bard–Parker blade, and scissors are used to cut through the orbicularis muscle down to the orbital rim. Extensive undermining of the temporal eyelid and cheek skin and muscle is performed with Stevens scissors, as needed, to allow mobilization of the myocutaneous flap nasally.

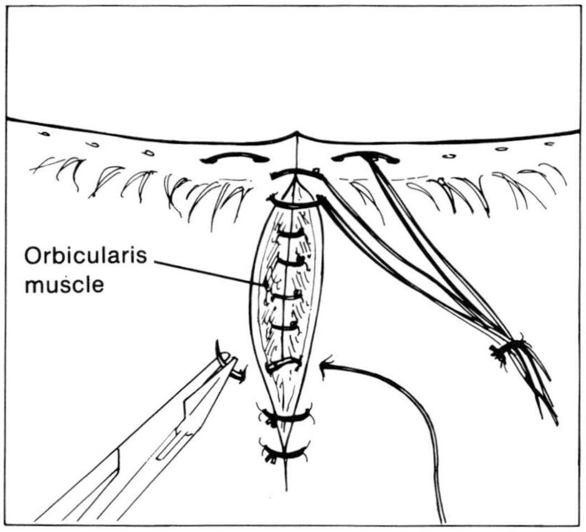

FIGURE 21–5

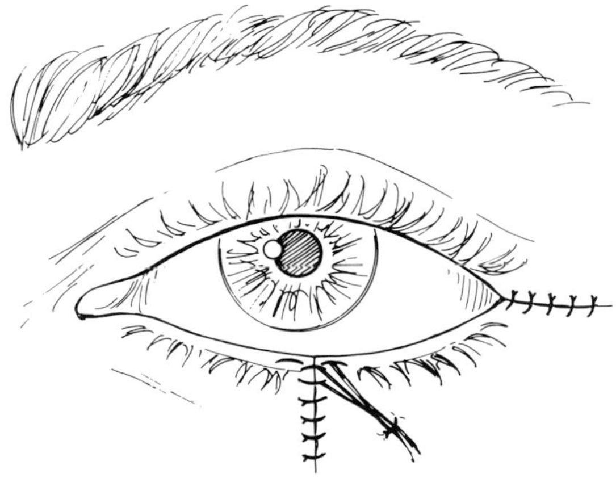

FIGURE 21–6

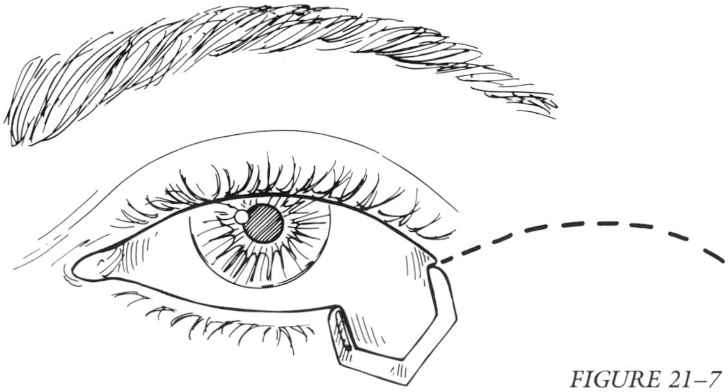

FIGURE 21–7

Figure 21–8. With retraction of the skin–muscle flap, the lateral orbital rim is exposed, and a rectangular strip of periosteum is fashioned, with an intact base at the inner aspect of the rim. The strip is 1-cm wide and is angled superiorly 45° to follow the lower lid contour. The length of the strip is determined by the distance measured from the rim to the lateral edge of the tarsal defect. If the strip needs to be greater than 1 cm in length, the adjacent temporalis fascia can be incorporated by extending the periosteal incisions laterally.

Figure 21–9. The fascia is then bluntly dissected from the underlying temporalis muscle, and the periosteal portion of the strip is separated from the bony rim with a periosteal elevator.

Figure 21–10. The strip is reflected medially so that the anterior surface of the periosteum lies against the globe, and its distal end is sutured to the anterior portion (partial-thickness) of the lateral border of tarsus with 5–0 Vicryl sutures. This provides a posterior lamella and anchors the reconstructed lower lid to the orbital rim.

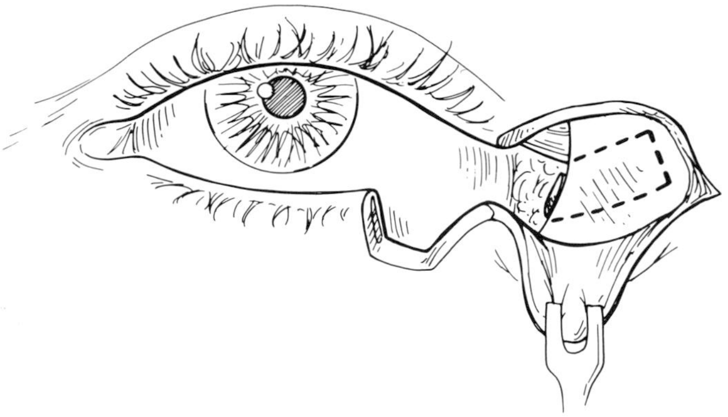

FIGURE 21–8

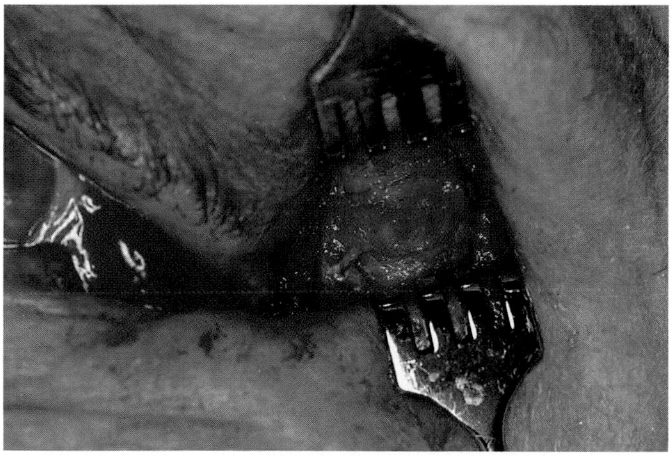

FIGURE 21–9

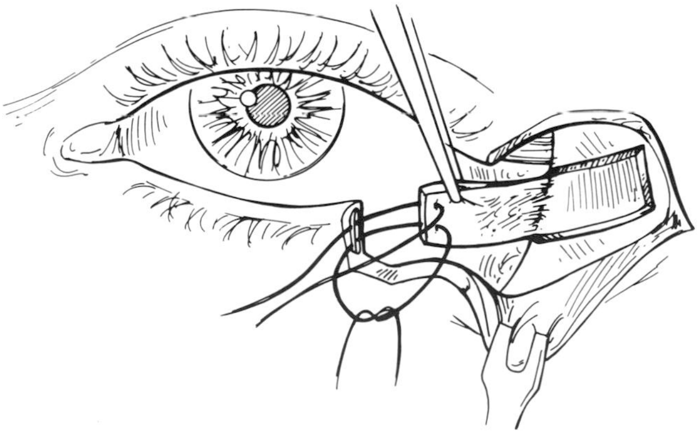

FIGURE 21–10

Figure 21–11. The edge of the inferior forniceal conjunctiva can be secured to the inferior edge of the periosteal strip and the inner surface of the strip will epithelialize. Symblepharon should not develop as long as the opposing bulbar conjunctiva is intact.

The myocutaneous flap is advanced nasally to reestablish an anterior lamella and tension-bearing 6–0 Vicryl buried-interrupted sutures are placed at the level of the muscular layer.

Figure 21–12. The superior skin edge of the myocutaneous flap along the lateral lid margin is joined to the superior border of the periosteal strip with a running 7–0 Vicryl suture. The skin is closed with 7–0 nylon or silk sutures.

Semicircular Rotational Flap

Reconstruction of up to two-thirds of the central lower lid can be achieved by combining the primary closure technique with a lateral semicircular musculocutaneous flap as described by Tenzel (1975). The tarsus must be present on both sides of the defect, and the edges of the wound should be prepared as described earlier for direct closure.

Figure 21–13. A marker pen is used to outline a semicircle, approximately 20 mm in diameter, beginning at the lateral canthal angle, arching superiorly and temporally no farther than the lateral extent of the brow. A skin incision is made along this mark with a size 15 Bard–Parker blade. The skin edges are tented up with forceps, and a Wescott or Stevens scissors is used to dissect through the orbicularis muscle fibers down to the lateral orbital rim.

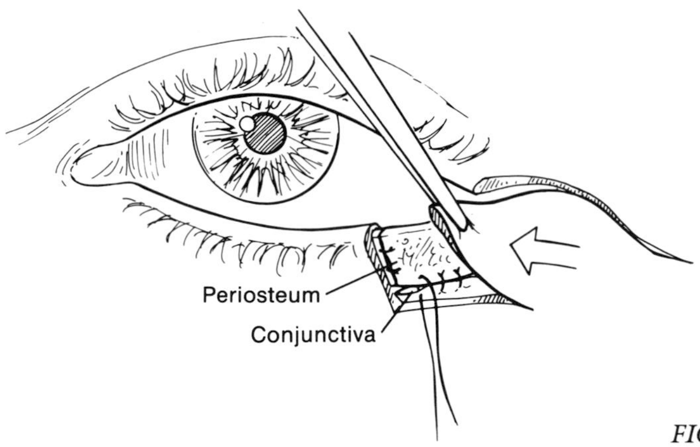

FIGURE 21–11

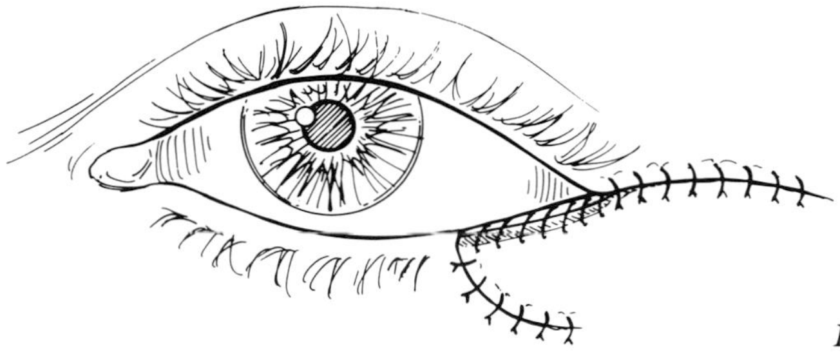

FIGURE 21–12

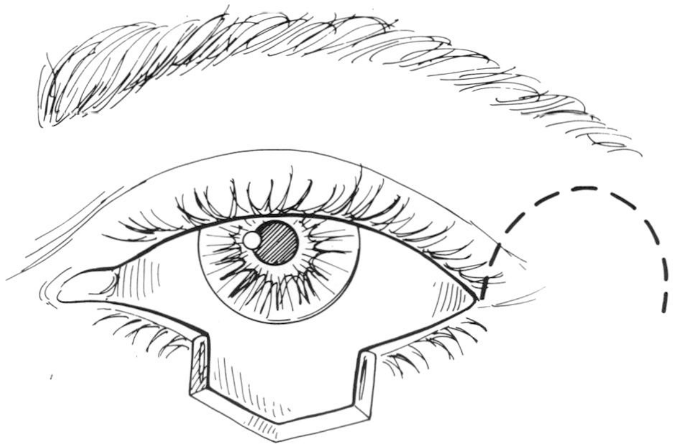

FIGURE 21–13

Figure 21–14. The myocutaneous flap is undermined thoroughly inferiorly to mobilize this tissue medially. All bleeding points should be cauterized with a bipolar electrocautery.

Figure 21–15. With the flap retracted inferiorly, a canthotomy is performed with the scissors extending to the inside of the orbital rim.

Figure 21–16. The inferior crus of the lateral canthal tendon is cut at the rim. The superior crus of the canthal tendon should be left undisturbed. The lateral portion of the lower lid and adjacent flap are rotated medially until the edges of the lid margin defect can be apposed without undue tension, and the defect is directly closed as previously described. If the lateral aspect of the lid cannot be adequately mobilized, its attachments to the orbital septum and lower lid retractors must be severed. Scissors can be introduced just beneath the inferior tarsal border, anterior to the conjunctiva and posterior to the orbicularis muscle, and the septum and retractors are detached from lateral to medial until the lid can be freely rotated nasally.

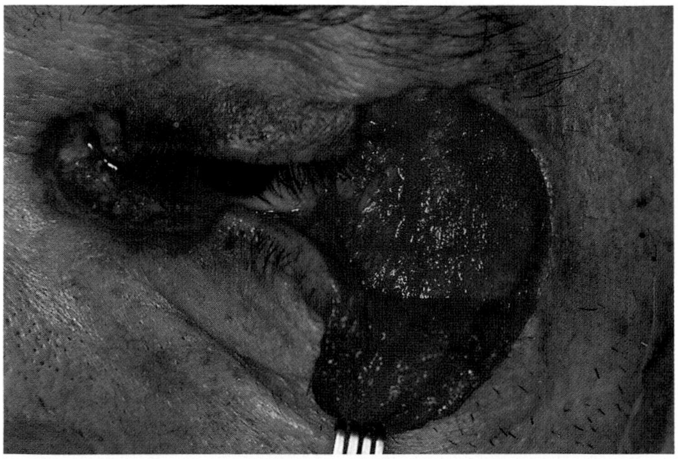

FIGURE 21–14

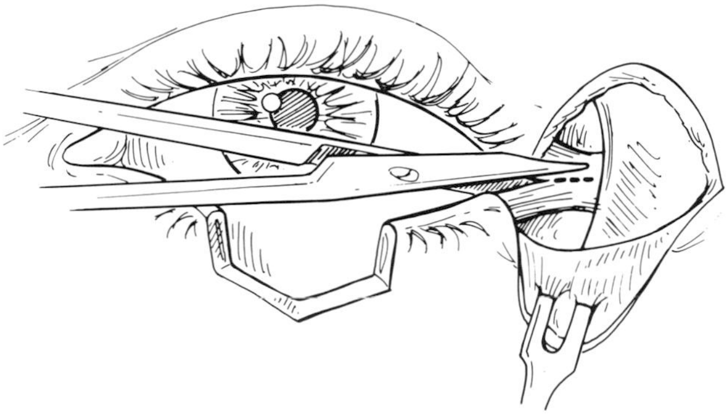

FIGURE 21–15

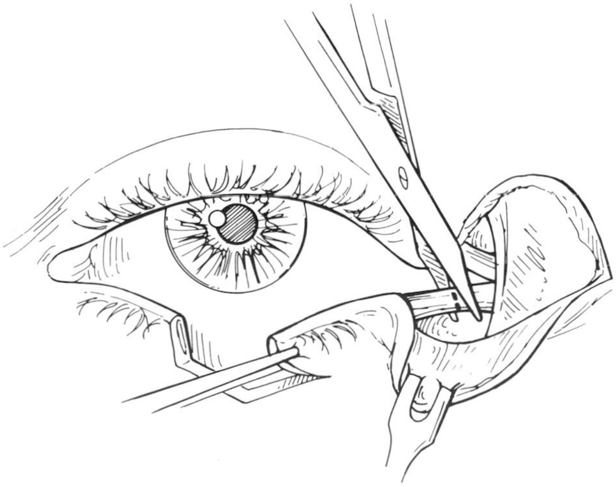

FIGURE 21–16

Figure 21–17. Re-formation of the lateral canthus begins with proper fixation of the lateral aspect of the flap to provide adequate posterior and lateral vector forces so that the reconstructed lower lid lies in apposition with the globe. This is achieved by suturing the deep edge of the myocutaneous flap to the inner aspect of the lateral orbital rim just inferior to the attached superior crus of the canthal tendon with a 4–0 Polydek or Vicryl suture passed on a small semicircle needle.

Figure 21–18. A cross-sectional view of the lateral orbit and lower eyelid demonstrates suture fixation of the deep tissues of the semicircular flap to the inner aspect of the lateral orbital rim to provide adequate apposition of the reconstructed lid with the globe. The lid must be tight and have the proper contour following this suture placement to avoid postoperative sagging or lid margin malpositions.

Figure 21–19. The conjunctival edge previously cut during the canthotomy can be advanced superiorly to the skin edge of the lateral lid margin with a running 7–0 Vicryl suture. The orbicularis muscle layer in the lateral canthal area is closed with interrupted 6–0 Vicryl sutures, and skin closure is completed with interrupted 7–0 nylon or silk sutures. A dog ear often needs to be excised at the lateral extension of the wound, given the unequal lengths of the sides of this defect.

Hughes Tarsoconjunctival Flap

The modified Hughes procedure is a lid-sharing technique in which the tarsus from the upper lid is transposed into the lower lid defect to reestablish a posterior lamella. It is ideal for defects affecting more than 50% of the lower lid margin because it replaces the lost tarsus with the same type of tissue. Its major disadvantages are that it is a two-stage procedure that obligates the patient to a second surgery to separate the eyelids, and it involves temporary occlusion of the affected eye for 4 to 6 weeks between procedures. Alternatives to this method should be considered in children, given the risks of occlusion amblyopia, and in patients who are monocular with their functional eye on that affected side.

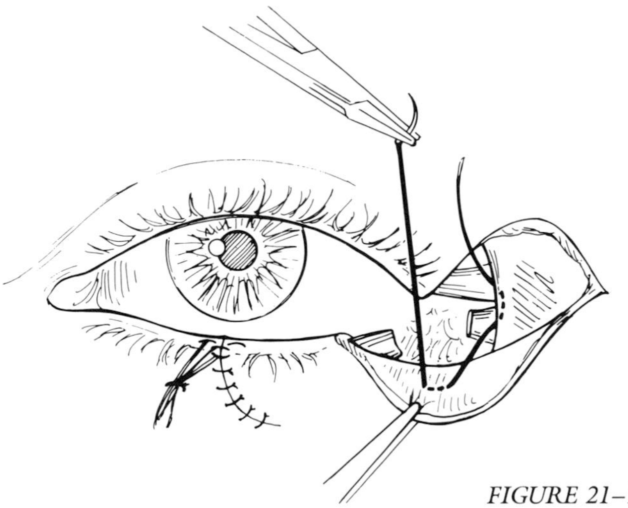

FIGURE 21–17

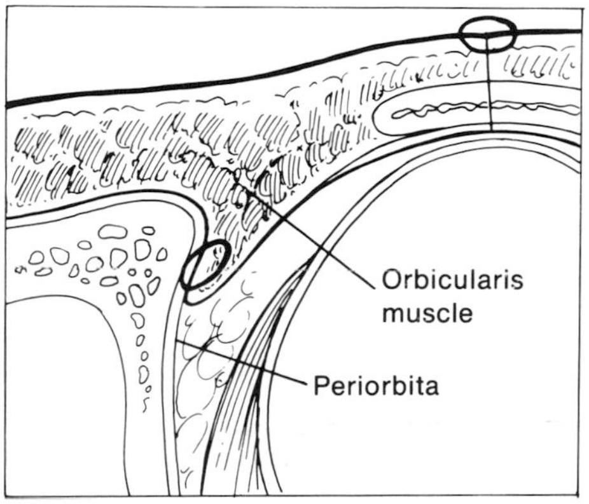

FIGURE 21–18

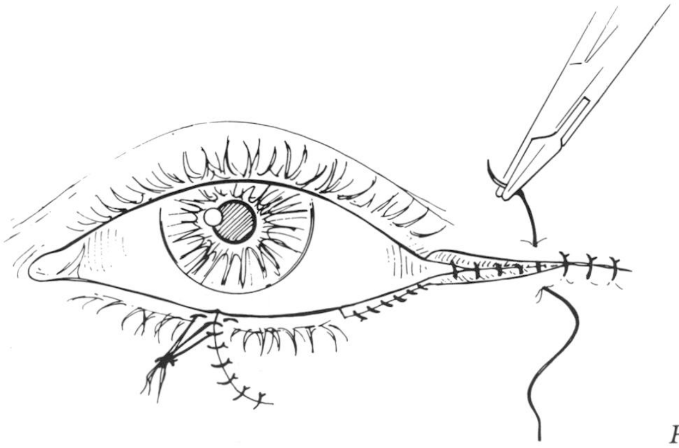

FIGURE 21–19

Figure 21–20. The defect is first prepared by squaring off the inferior border to create a rectangular defect with the medial and lateral edges perpendicular to the lid margin. Hemostasis is achieved with a bipolar cautery. The edges are advanced centrally under moderate tension with forceps, and the horizontal length of the tarsoconjunctival flap to be advanced is measured.

A 4–0 silk traction suture is placed through the central upper lid margin to facilitate eversion of the lid over a lid plate or Desmarres retractor.

A three-sided flap is outlined with a marker pen or light application of cautery on the central portion of tarsal conjunctiva irrespective of whether the lower lid defect is greater laterally or medially.

Figure 21–21. Calipers are used to measure placement of the horizontal incision, which should be at least 4 mm from the lid margin, to avoid the development of upper eyelid entropion, contour deformities, loss of lashes, and trichiasis. The vertical incision marks course perpendicular to the lid margin up to the superior fornix.

Figure 21–22. An incision is made with a size 15 Bard–Parker blade through conjunctiva and tarsus and the flap is easily separated from the overlying levator aponeurosis and orbicularis muscle with Wescott scissors. Blunt and sharp dissection is continued superiorly beyond the superior tarsal border between conjunctiva and Mueller's muscle toward the upper fornix. A small volume of 2% lidocaine with a 1:100,000 dilution of epinephrine injected through a 30-gauge needle subconjunctivally helps to separate these tissue planes and improves hemostasis just before this dissection.

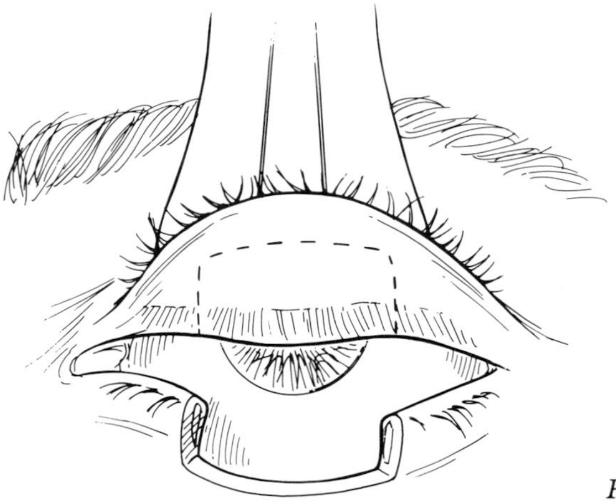

FIGURE 21–20

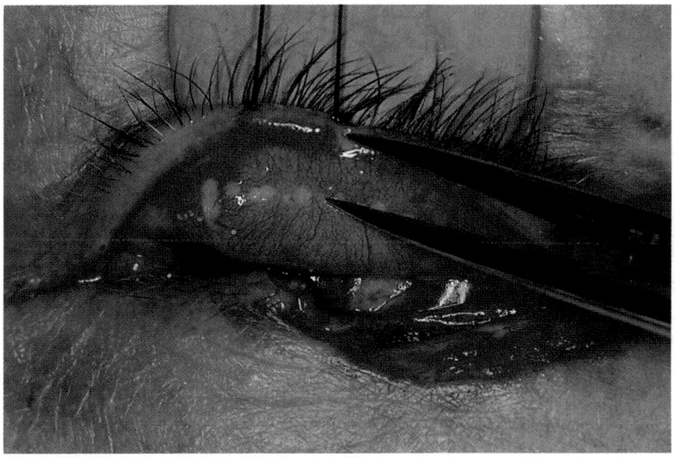

FIGURE 21–21

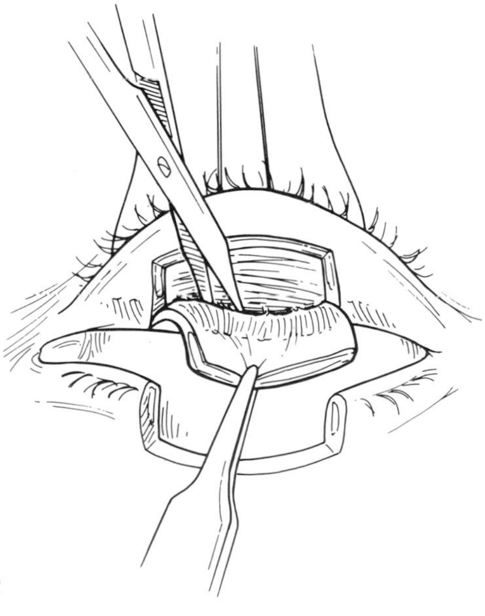

FIGURE 21–22

Figure 21–23. A cross-sectional view of the upper eyelid shows the two alternative planes of dissection to create the tarsoconjunctival flap. Dissection superior to the tarsal plate can be performed between the conjunctiva and Mueller's muscle (**A**) or between Mueller's muscle and the levator aponeurosis (**B**). In most circumstances, the flap receives adequate blood flow from the conjunctiva, and its vascular supply is enhanced when covered by a myocutaneous advancement flap; but when the blood supply is potentially marginal and a skin graft is utilized, Mueller's muscle should be incorporated in the flap. Some authors advocate the advancement of Mueller's muscle with conjunctiva routinely; however, separation of the lids later is more involved and adds to the risk of postoperative upper lid retraction.

Figure 21–24. The tarsoconjunctival flap is mobilized into the lower lid defect so that the advanced upper lid superior tarsal border is in alignment with the remaining lower lid margin.

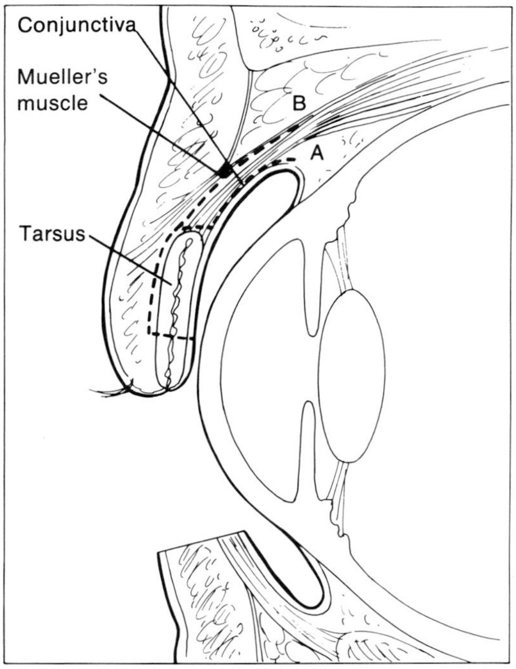

FIGURE 21–23

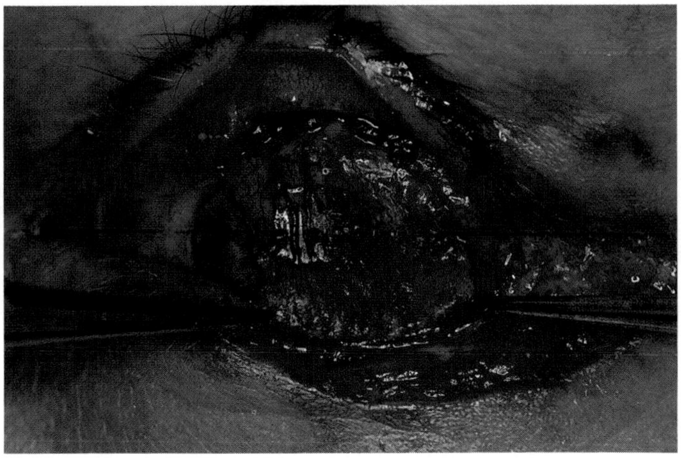

FIGURE 21–24

Figure 21–25A, B. The lateral and medial edges of the flap are secured to the adjacent stumps of tarsus (**A**) with multiple 5–0 Vicryl partial-thickness interrupted sutures passed on a spatula needle through the anterior two-thirds of tarsus so that the sutures do not rub on the surface of the eye (**B**). If no lateral tarsal stump remains, the flap can be secured to the periosteum of the inner aspect of the lateral orbital rim with two 4–0 Polydek sutures. Similarly, if no tarsus is available medially, the tarsoconjunctival flap can be attached to the posterior limb of the medial canthal tendon. The inferior edge of the flap is sutured to the cut edge of inferior forniceal conjunctiva and lower lid retractors with a running 7–0 Vicryl suture. With the posterior lamella reconstructed, the anterior lamella can be restored with a myocutaneous flap or a full-thickness skin graft.

Alternative 1. Myocutaneous Advancement Flap

Figure 21–26. A flap consisting of skin and muscle is designed to be advanced medially to cover the tarsoconjunctival flap by making an infralash incision that extends laterally to the canthus and arches superiorly, as illustrated. The lateral extent of this incision depends on the degree of laxity of the periocular tissues, and it can be extended as far as the ear if greater mobilization is required to repair the defect. A skin incision is made along this outline with a size 15 Bard–Parker blade.

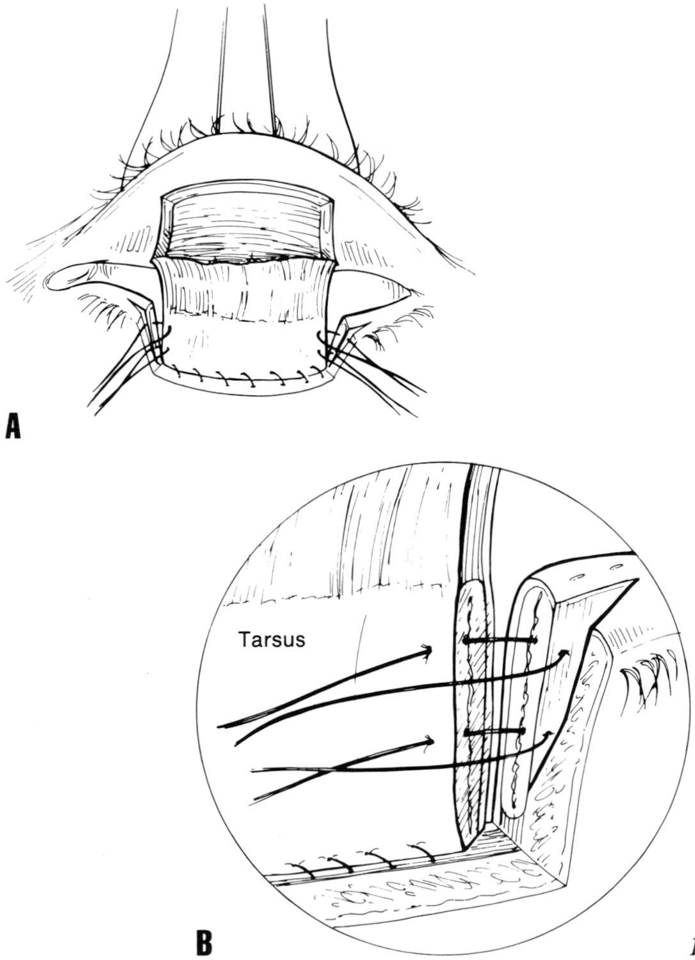

FIGURE 21–25

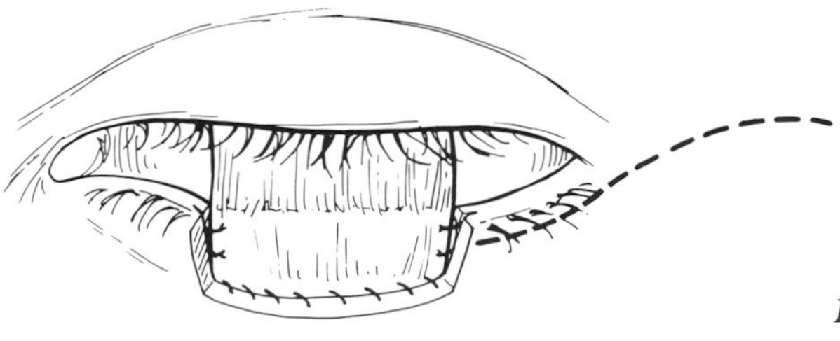

FIGURE 21–26

Figure 21–27. The skin muscle flap is undermined anterior to the orbital septum in the lid with scissors, and this suborbicular plane of dissection is continued laterally into the temporal region and inferiorly toward the cheek. A bipolar cautery is applied to maintain meticulous hemostasis.

Figure 21–28. Sufficient undermining is completed when the lateral border of the myocutaneous flap can be advanced nasally to the medial edge of the defect, under no tension, to provide an anterior lamella with an inherent blood supply. The flap is secured into position by suturing the orbicularis muscle layer together with interrupted 6–0 Vicryl sutures and the skin edges with 6–0 or 7–0 nylon sutures. The skin at the superior border of the flap overlying the tarsoconjunctival flap is sutured to the conjunctiva 1 to 2 mm above the upper border of tarsus with a running 7–0 Vicryl or 6–0 chromic suture.

Figure 21–29. A cross-sectional view shows the upper lid and the reconstructed lower lid following Hughes procedure. Note that the lower lid posterior lamella consists of the advanced upper lid tarsus vascularized by the attached conjunctiva; the anterior lamella is composed of a mucocutaneous flap. Antibiotic ointment and a pressure patch are applied to reduce postoperative swelling and bleeding.

Alternative 2. Full-Thickness Skin Graft

A full-thickness skin graft obtained from upper eyelid or postauricular skin is thinned of subcutaneous fat and connective tissue and placed over the tarsoconjunctival flap (see later section on full-thickness skin graft, under Periorbital and Nonmarginal Eyelid Reconstruction, for harvesting full-thickness skin graft technique).

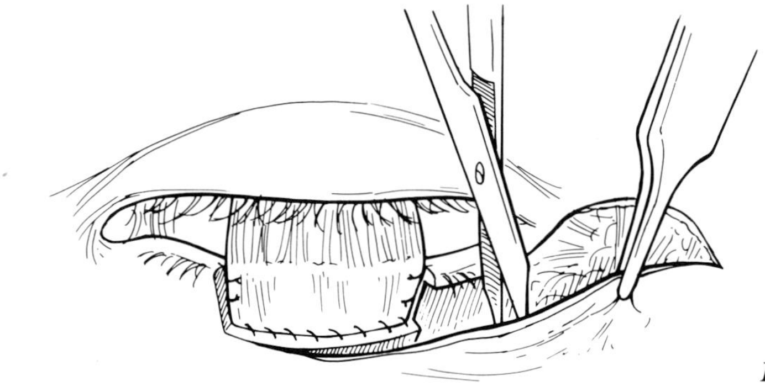

FIGURE 21–27

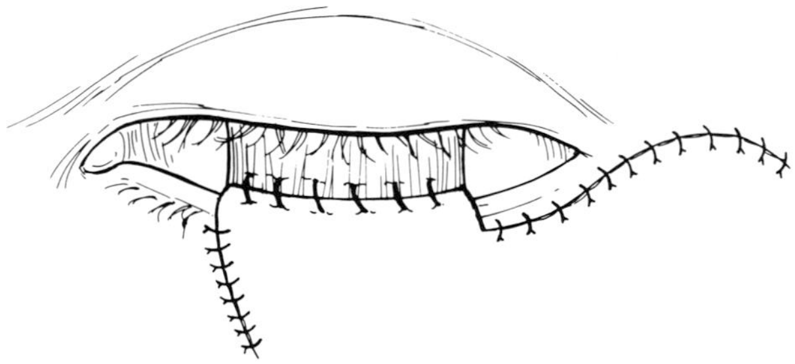

FIGURE 21–28

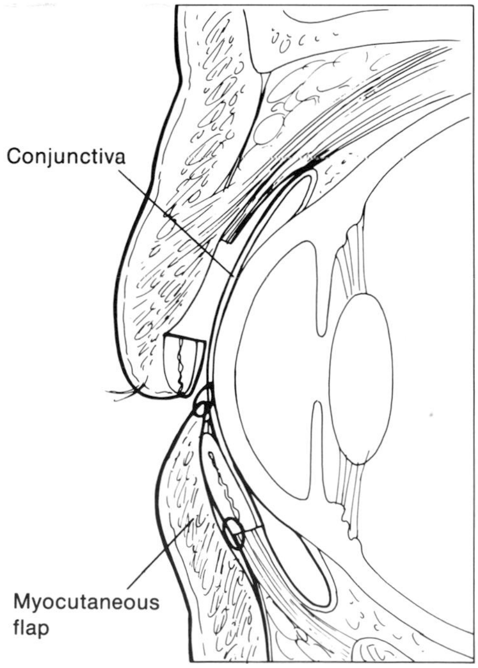

FIGURE 21–29

Figure 21–30. The graft is trimmed to size and sutured to the skin edges of the defect with interrupted 7–0 nylon or silk sutures. The superior edge of skin is sutured to the conjunctiva 1–2 mm above the upper border of tarsus with a running 7–0 Vicryl or 6–0 chromic suture. The full-thickness graft will obtain its blood supply from the tarsoconjunctival flap. Antibiotic ointment, Telfa, and a pressure patch are applied to immobilize the skin graft.

Second-Stage Hughes Procedure

The tarsoconjunctival flap is divided 4 to 8 weeks after the initial surgical repair to allow enough time for the reconstructed lower lid to develop a new blood supply and to counteract the downward contractile forces of scar maturation and gravity.

Figure 21–31. After local anesthesia is administered, a pair of blunt Wescott scissors are used to incise the flap 0.5 to 1.0 mm above the proposed new lower lid margin. During this separation, the blades of the scissors tent the flap away from the ocular surface to avoid abrading the underlying cornea.

Figure 21–32. The redundant mucosa from the lower division of the flap can be left to retract or be sutured to a skin incision made along the new lid margin with a running 7–0 Vicryl suture to reestablish a mucocutaneous border. The upper segment of the flap is allowed to retract under the upper lid and may be trimmed at a later time if necessary. If Mueller's muscle was incorporated in the tarsoconjunctival flap, undermining between Mueller's muscle and the levator aponeurosis toward the superior fornix should be performed in a stepwise fashion until the desired height and contour of the upper lid are achieved to avoid postoperative lid retraction.

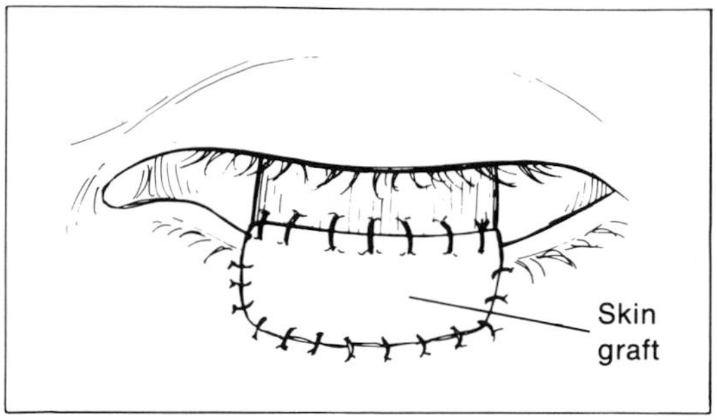

FIGURE 21–30

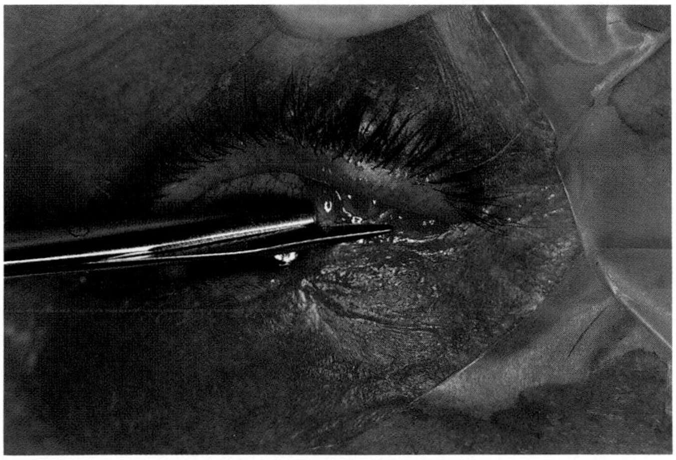

FIGURE 21–31

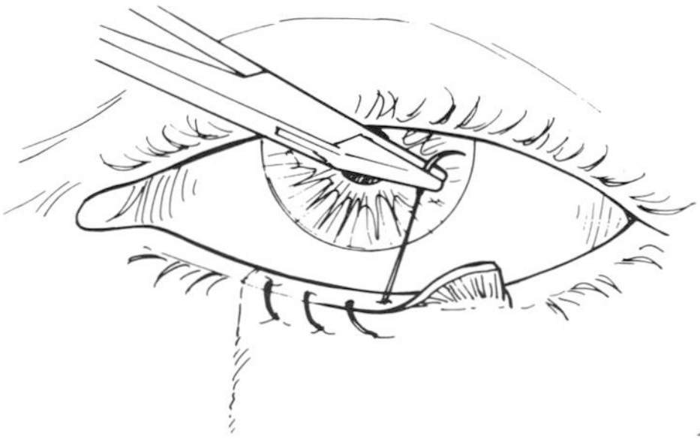

FIGURE 21–32

Upper Eyelid Reconstruction

Direct Closure With or Without Lateral Cantholysis

Central upper eyelid defects affecting up to 30% of the lid margin in younger persons and up to 50% of the lid in older patients can be directly closed using the same technique as described for lower lid reconstruction. One important difference between the upper and lower lid repair is that the tarsus in the upper lid measures two to three times the vertical height of the lower lid tarsus, and it is critical that the tarsal defect extends perpendicularly from the lid margin to the superior tarsal border to result in even wound closure. Approximately five partial-thickness sutures will be necessary to unite the tarsal edges. The levator aponeurotic attachments should be left undisturbed to avoid postoperative ptosis. A cantholysis of the superior crus of the lateral canthal tendon can be performed, similar to that performed on the inferior crus in lower lid repairs, to relax the lateral stump of eyelid and allow the closure of larger defects.

Semicircular Rotational Flap

Reconstruction of up to one-half of the medial or central upper lid can be performed by combining the primary closure technique with a lateral semicircular myocutaneous flap similar to that described earlier for lower lid repair. The differences from lower lid reconstruction include an inferiorly arching semicircle flap and a cantholysis of the superior crus of the lateral canthal tendon.

Figure 21–33. A semicircle, of about 20 mm in diameter, that arches temporally and inferiorly from the lateral canthal angle is outlined.

Figure 21–34. Scissors are directed superiorly toward the orbital rim to cut the superior crus of the lateral canthal tendon.

Figure 21–35. A standard primary closure of the defect is performed with exact approximation of the tarsal edges and the myocutaneous flap is sutured in position according to the steps outlined for lower lid surgery.

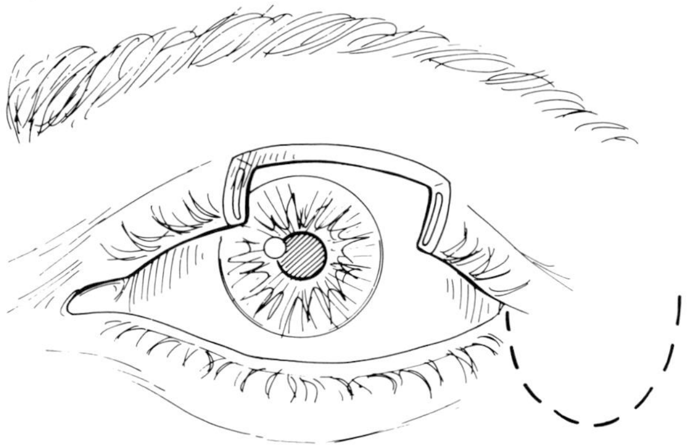

FIGURE 21–33

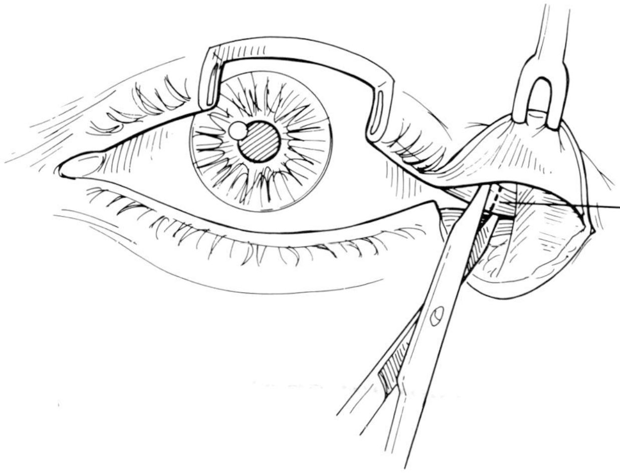

FIGURE 21–34

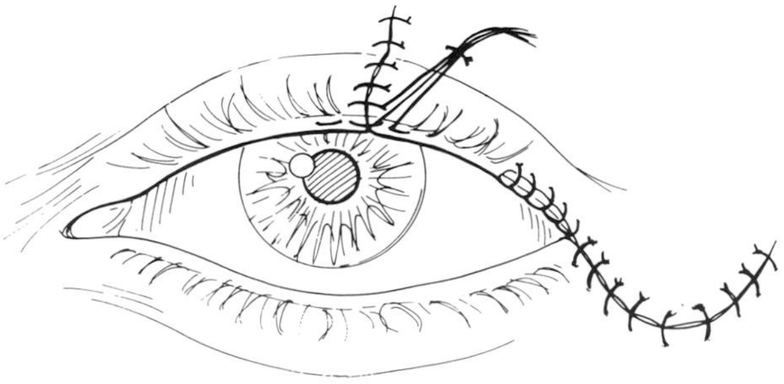

FIGURE 21–35

Free Autogenous Tarsal Graft

Lateral upper lid defects of up to 50% of the lid margin can be reconstructed with a free tarsal graft harvested from the contralateral upper lid. The autogenous tarsoconjunctival graft provides the posterior lamellar support and mucous membrane lining for the reconstructed upper lid, and a myocutaneous advancement flap replaces the anterior lamella and contributes the vascular supply for the underlying graft.

The lateral margin of the remaining portion of upper lid is grasped with a toothed forceps and drawn temporally under moderate tension so that the horizontal length of the defect can be measured. Attention is directed to the contralateral upper lid to harvest the tarsal graft.

Figure 21–36. A 4–0 silk traction suture is placed through the central aspect of the lid margin and the lid is everted over a Desmarres retractor or lid plate to expose the tarsoconjunctival surface. A marker pen or light cautery is used to demarcate the graft, corresponding to the previously determined length of the defect. The inferior edge of the graft is made parallel to and no more than 4 mm from the lid margin, and the superior tarsal border determines the vertical height of the graft. A size 15 Bard–Parker blade is used to make an incision through the conjunctiva and full-thickness of tarsus along the inferior and vertical markings. Blunt and sharp dissection is performed to separate the anterior tarsal surface from the overlying levator aponeurosis.

Figure 21–37. The conjunctival and Muller's muscle attachments are cut from the superior tarsal border with scissors, leaving approximately 2 mm of conjunctiva attached to the graft.

Figure 21–38. A cross-sectional view of the upper eyelid illustrates the full-thickness tarsal graft with a conjunctival "fringe" being removed from the donor site, leaving at least 4 mm of intact tarsus at the lid margin. The graft is placed in a moist gauze pad temporarily. All bleeding points are cauterized with wet-field bipolar coagulation. The donor site is allowed to heal spontaneously without wound closure.

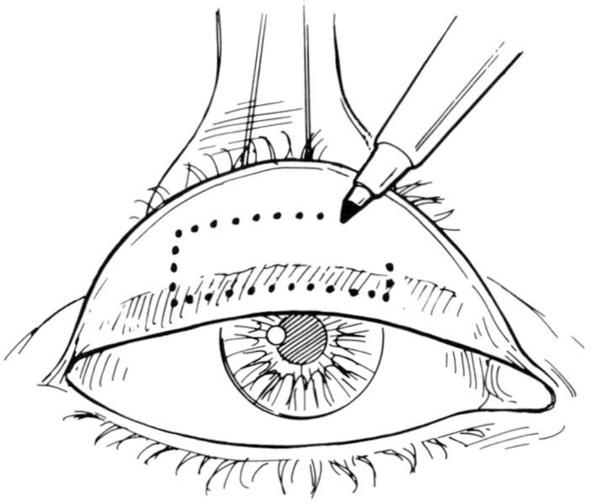

FIGURE 21–36

FIGURE 21–37

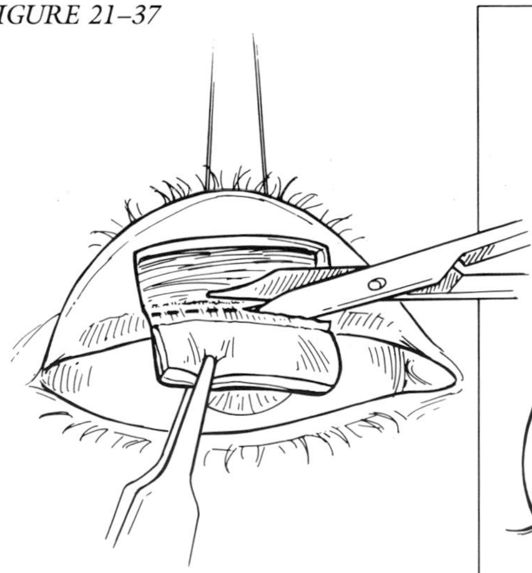

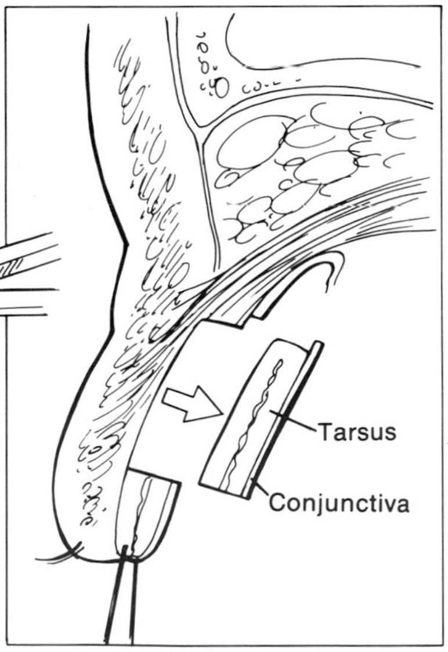

FIGURE 21–38

Figure 21–39A. The tarsal graft is placed into the defect with the conjunctival surface in contact with the globe and the superior edge of the graft with the conjunctival fringe positioned along the proposed new lid margin. The lateral edge of the graft is sutured to the stump of the superior crus of the lateral canthal tendon, if present, or to the periosteum of the lateral orbital rim at the level of the lateral orbital tubercle, with interrupted 4–0 Polydek sutures. The proposed mucocutaneous flap is *outlined* in the lateral canthus.

Figure 21–39B. The medial edge of the graft is sutured to the lateral border of the remnant of upper lid tarsus with partial-thickness 5–0 Vicryl interrupted sutures. Partial thickness sutures are used to avoid suture exposure on the posterior lid surface that could lead to ocular surface irritation. The superior graft border is attached to the superior forniceal conjunctiva and edges of Mueller's muscle and levator aponeurosis with interrupted 6–0 Vicryl sutures.

Figure 21–40. A myocutaneous flap derived from the upper lid or lateral canthal tissues is designed to cover the tarsal graft. If enough redundant upper lid skin and orbicularis muscle is present superior to the defect, it can be undermined and advanced inferiorly over the graft. An alternative is to mark an advancement flap from the lateral canthal angle that arches inferiorly and extends temporally as shown in Figure 21–39**A.** This mucocutaneous flap is rotated into the defect for anterior lamellar reconstruction. A skin incision is made with a blade, and a skin–muscle flap is undermined until it can be transferred to fill the defect under minimal tension.

Figure 21–41. The orbicularis muscle layer is closed separately with interrupted 7–0 Vicryl sutures to reduce the tension on the advanced tissue flap, and the skin edges are united with interrupted or running 7–0 nylon sutures. The conjunctival fringe is then advanced anteriorly and sutured to the inferior skin edge of the flap with a running 7–0 Vicryl suture to reestablish the mucocutaneous junction along the reconstructed lid margin.

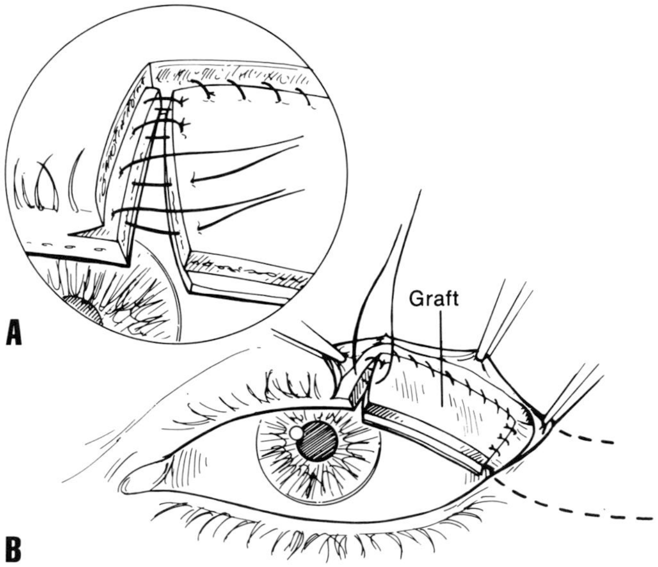

FIGURE 21–39

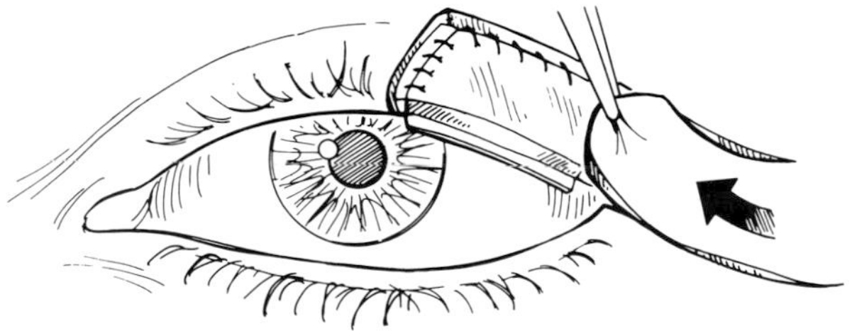

FIGURE 21–40

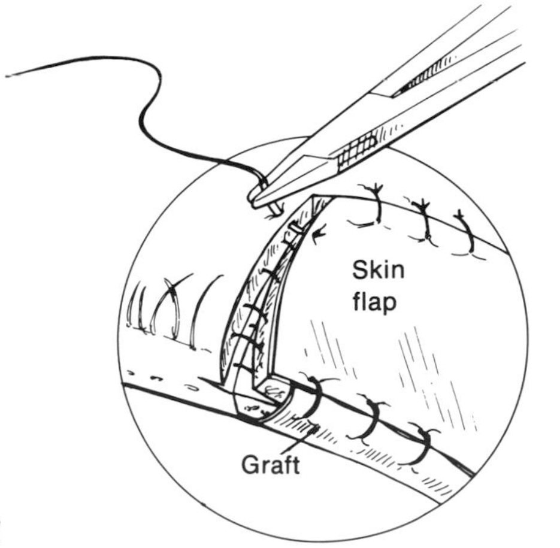

FIGURE 21–41

Figure 21–42. Temporary 4–0 silk tarsorrhaphy sutures tied over bolsters and placed on inferior traction help to immobilize the upper lid and keep it on stretch to counteract postoperative retraction.

Cutler–Beard Procedure

The Cutler–Beard procedure is a two-stage technique used to reconstruct large to total upper lid defects by advancing a composite bridge flap of skin, muscle, and conjunctiva from the opposite lower eyelid. This technique, which does not provide a replacement of the tarsus, can lead to instability of the re-formed lid margin, but is effective for extensive upper lid reconstruction when there are no alternative methods.

Figure 21–43. The full-thickness upper lid defect is trimmed in a rectangular fashion such that the borders are perpendicular to the lid margin. A bipolar cautery should be used to maintain meticulous hemostasis. The width of the defect is measured by pulling the edges together under slight tension.

A marker pen is used to demarcate the superior border of the flap 5 mm below and parallel to the lower lid margin and 1 to 2 mm wider than the upper lid defect. This incision is placed no closer to the lid margin to prevent disrupting the blood supply to the lower lid margin. Vertical markings from each end are made inferiorly approximately 15 mm in length. A 4–0 silk traction suture is placed through the gray line in the central portion of the lower lid and upward traction is applied with a lid plate inserted into the inferior fornix between the lid and globe.

Figure 21–44. With a lid plate protecting the globe, a size 15 Bard–Parker blade is used to make a skin incision along the markings, and then reintroduced to make a full-thickness incision.

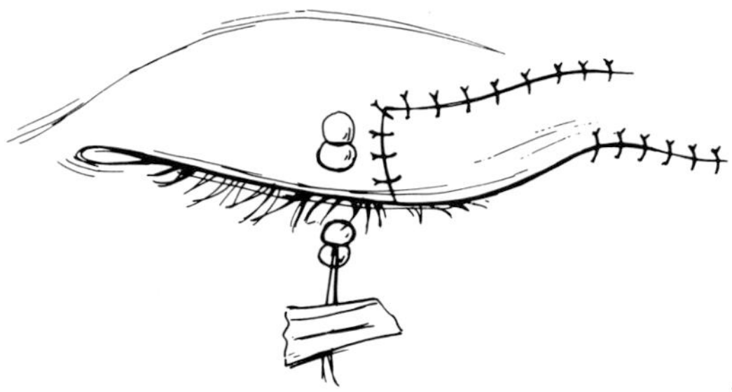

FIGURE 21–42

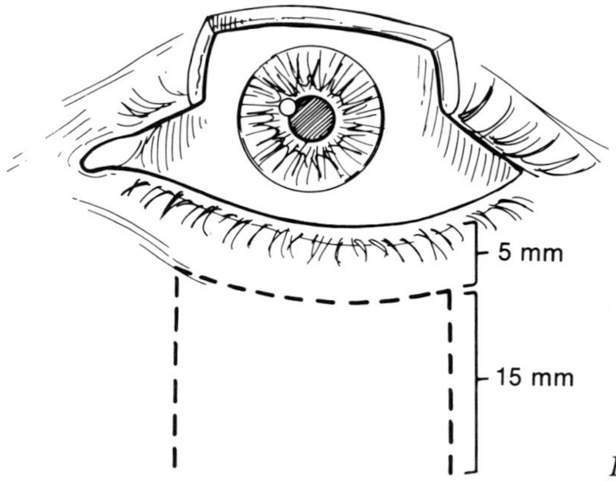

FIGURE 21–43

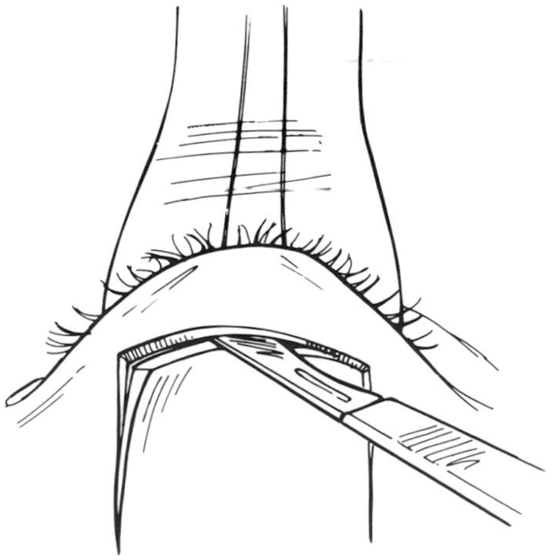

FIGURE 21–44

Figure 21–45. Beyond the inferior conjunctival fornix, a skin–muscle flap is created. The full-thickness cuts are extended horizontally with scissors and then vertically down into the inferior fornix on the conjunctival side of the flap, and the skin and orbicularis should be undermined over the inferior orbital rim. The lid plate and traction suture is removed, and the inferior edge of the marginal bridge is left to granulate.

Figure 21–46. The flap is passed under the bridge of the lower lid margin and is sutured into the recipient bed in layers. If the full vertical height of tarsus is absent in the upper lid, the conjunctival edges of the flap and upper lid are sutured together with a running 6–0 plain gut suture; the lower lid retractors are then sutured to the cut edge of levator aponeurosis with interrupted 6–0 Vicryl sutures. The conjunctiva and lower lid retractors at the medial and lateral borders of the flap are secured to the anterior half of the adjacent tarsal edges with interrupted 6–0 Vicryl sutures; care is taken to pass these sutures only partial-thickness through the tarsus to avoid corneal irritation. If a remnant of tarsus is present along the superior border of the recipient bed, the conjunctiva and lower lid retractors should be sutured to the lower edge of tarsus with interrupted 6–0 Vicryl sutures.

Figure 21–47. Anterior lamellar reconstruction involves advancement of the orbicularis muscle and skin from the lower lid to the reconstructed upper lid. The orbicularis muscle layer is closed with interrupted 7–0 Vicryl sutures and skin closure is completed with interrupted 7–0 nylon sutures.

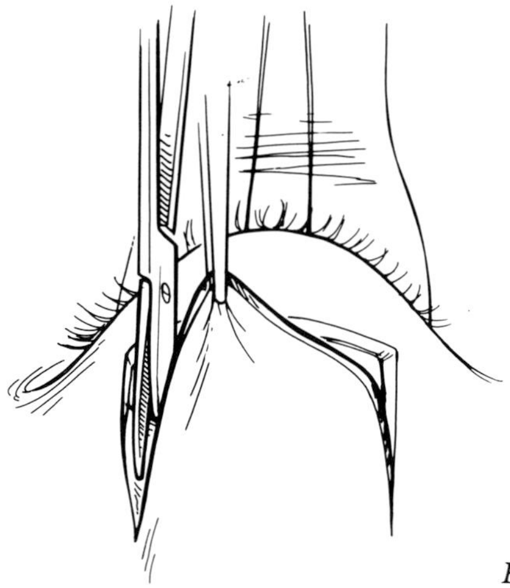

FIGURE 21–45

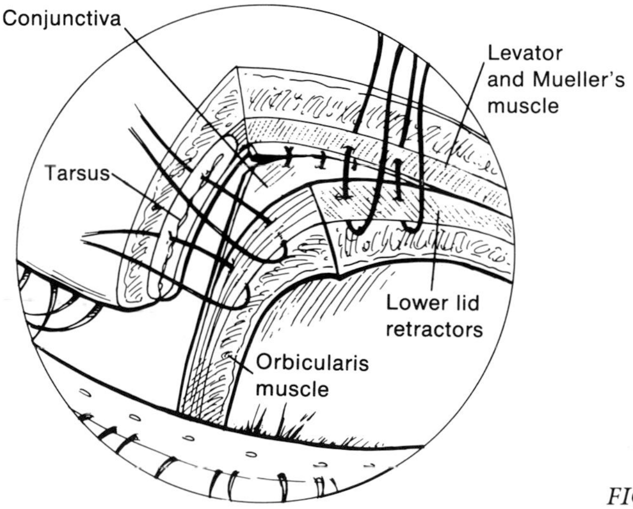

FIGURE 21–46

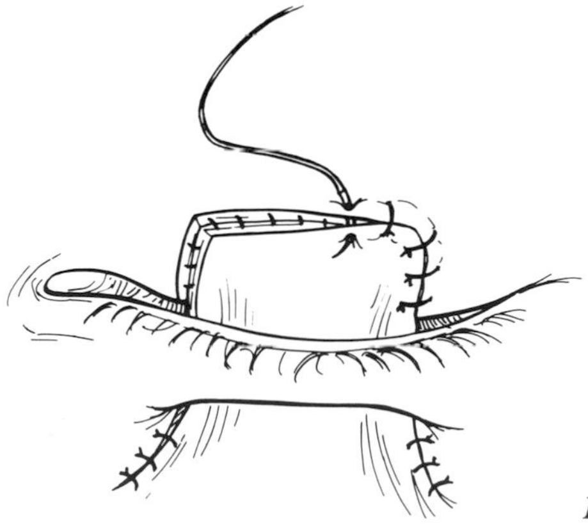

FIGURE 21–47

Figure 21–48. A cross-sectional view of the eyelids at the conclusion of the first-stage Cutler–Beard procedure shows the multiple-layered closure of tissue planes and the marginal bridge of the lower eyelid lying over the composite bridge flap.

Second-Stage Cutler–Beard Procedure

The flap is separated in 6 to 8 weeks after allowing stretching of the advanced tissues and the formation of the new blood supply in the reconstructed upper lid. A longer time interval should be allotted when the tissues are under significant tension or if the periocular vascularity may be compromised from prior irradiation or chemical injury.

A marker pen is used to delineate the incision to divide the flap 2 mm below the proposed upper lid margin. With the lower lid margin retracted inferiorly, a straight horizontal skin incision is made along this mark.

Figure 21–49. A groove director is placed under the flap to tent it away from the globe while a Stevens scissors is used to make a slightly beveled full-thickness incision through the flap leaving the conjunctival edge longer than the skin edge.

Figure 21–50. The beveled cut edge allows lining the reconstructed upper lid margin with a smooth conjunctival surface. The skin and muscle edges can be trimmed by 1 mm so that the extra conjunctiva can be sutured to the skin edge with a running 7–0 Vicryl suture to create a mucous membrane lined lid margin. This step is important to avoid irritation of the cornea from keratinized skin or skin hair.

The inferior border of the lower lid margin bridge is deepithelialized with a blade or sharp Wescott scissors.

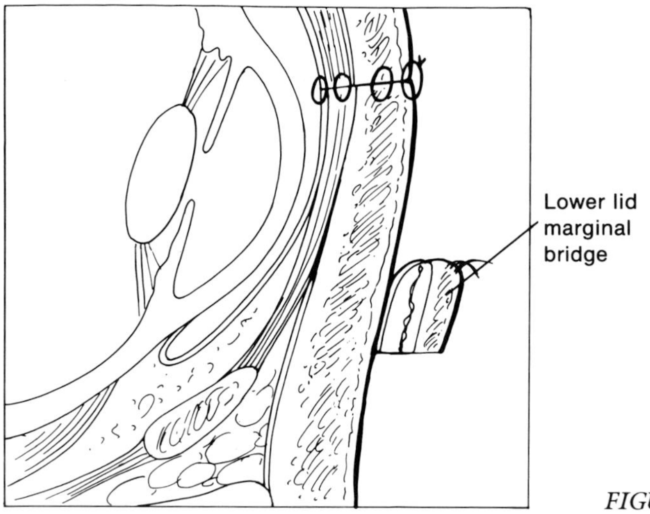

FIGURE 21–48

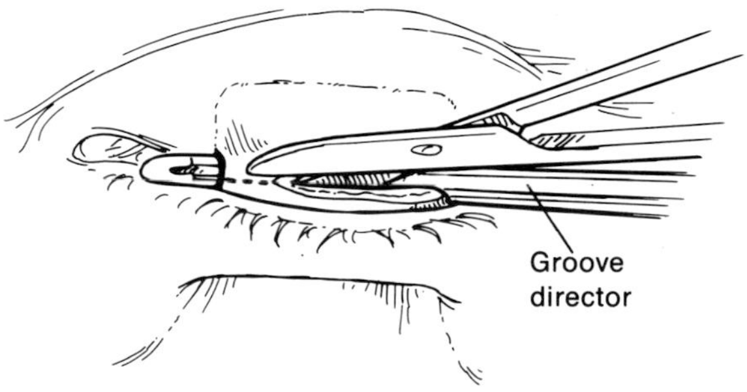

FIGURE 21–49

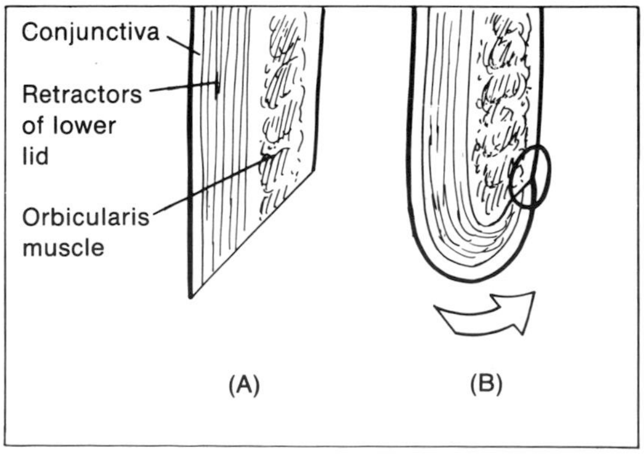

FIGURE 21–50

Figure 21–51. The conjunctiva and retractors of the flap are sutured to the inferior edge of the tarsus with a running or interrupted 6–0 plain or 7–0 Vicryl sutures.

Figure 21–52. The skin is closed with interrupted 7–0 nylon sutures. If lower lid ectropion is induced with this step, the lower lid skin and orbicularis muscle may need to be further undermined to relieve the vertical downward traction. Horizontal tightening with a lateral tarsal strip procedure may also be necessary to properly orient the lower lid.

Periorbital and Nonmarginal Eyelid Reconstruction

Full-Thickness Skin Graft

Skin grafts may be used for closure of periocular defects alone or in combination with other reconstructive methods, such as a Hughes procedure. Full-thickness skin grafts are preferable over split-thickness grafts in eyelid reconstruction because they provide a better color match, undergo less contraction, and result in a more uniform scar. A skin graft obtained from the ipsilateral or contralateral upper eyelid provides the best match for filling an eyelid defect, but when insufficient, skin from the postauricular region is the next best alternative. Also, consider the asymmetry of the upper lids that results from removing redundant skin from only one upper lid. Other sources for lid reconstruction include the supraclavicular area, inner arm, and groin, all of which are hairless, but a poorer color and texture match. Only the techniques to harvest a full-thickness skin graft from the upper lid and postauricular region are described in the following, although the same basic methods can be applied to any donor site.

The defect must be properly prepared to maximize the chances of viability for the graft. The edges of the defect should be clean and sharp, and hemostasis is important to prevent pooling of blood under the graft. Excessive cautery in the recipient bed must be avoided to prevent loss of circulation that eventually will vascularize the overlying graft.

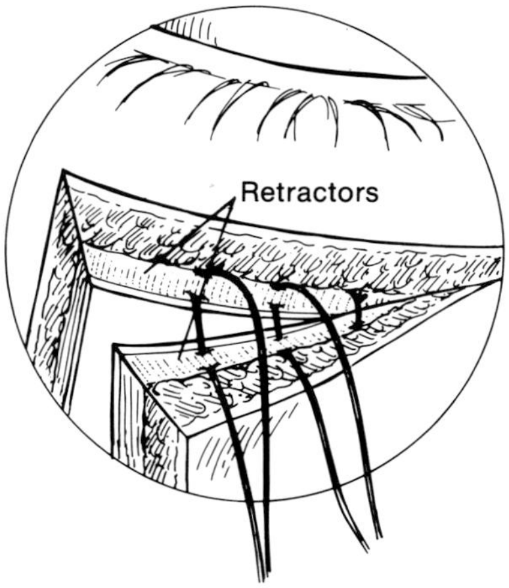

FIGURE 21–51

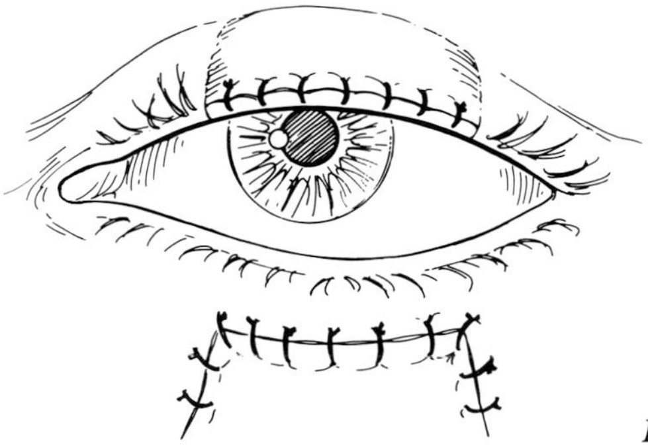

FIGURE 21–52

Figure 21–53. The size of the defect is measured and a template is made using a piece from the transparent plastic surgical drapes.

Figure 21–54. If an upper lid is chosen as the donor site to harvest the full-thickness skin graft, the upper lid crease is marked, and lidocaine containing epinephrine is injected subcutaneously for hemostasis and separation of the skin from the orbicularis muscle. A 4–0 silk traction suture is placed through the lid margin, and while the lid is pulled inferiorly, the template of the defect is placed over the preseptal portion of the lid, with the inferior pole at the upper lid crease, and is outlined with a marker pen. The surgeon should confirm that the vertical height of the skin to be removed will not induce lid margin eversion or lagophthalmos by "pinching" the superior and inferior borders together with a toothed forceps, similar to the technique used for blepharoplasty. The medial and lateral ends should be tapered to prevent dog-ear formation. With the lid on downward traction, a size 15 Bard–Parker blade is used to incise the skin markings. Sharp and blunt dissection with a Wescott scissors is performed to carefully divide the thin lid skin from the underlying muscle, without creating a buttonhole in the skin. Once the skin graft is obtained, it may be placed in saline-soaked gauze while the donor site is closed. Redundant preseptal orbicularis muscle is excised and hemostasis achieved with a bipolar wet-field cautery. The wound is closed with a running 7–0 nylon suture.

When the retroauricular region is the chosen donor site, exposure is gained by passing a 4–0 silk suture in through the helix of the external ear, which is then secured to the preauricular skin. The plastic template is oriented with its long axis parallel and midway between the junction of the posterior aspect of the ear and the scalp. The template is outlined with a marker pen approximately 1 to 2 mm larger than actual size, to compensate for contraction, and the ends are tapered to create an elliptical shape that facilitates wound closure. Local anesthesia containing epinephrine is infiltrated subdermally, and a size 15 Bard–Parker blade is used to make a skin incision along the borders. Sharp and blunt disection with Wescott scissors is performed to undermine and excise the skin graft from the subcutaneous tissue. With the graft set aside in saline-soaked gauze, the traction suture is removed and wound closure is achieved with either a running 5–0 chromic suture with locking bites or interrupted 6–0 silk sutures.

The graft is placed over a moist gauze pad over the surgeons finger and the subcutaneous tissue is meticulously removed with scissors until the white dermis and associated rete pegs are identified. The skin graft is placed into the recipient bed and trimmed to size or left slightly oversized to allow for shrinkage. It is anchored to the adjacent skin with interrupted 6–0 silk sutures approximately every 5 to 10 mm, leaving two to three sutures long at opposite poles. In addition, a running

7–0 nylon suture is placed around the entire border of the graft to secure the skin edges. Two or three small slitlike perforations with sharp Wescott scissors may be made in the graft to prevent serous fluid or blood from accumulating under the graft. If the skin graft has been placed in the pretarsal or preseptal area, the lid should be maintained on traction postoperatively for 1 to 2 weeks to help counteract contraction of the graft. After antibiotic ointment is applied to the graft, a roll of Telfa cut to the appropriate size is secured as a stent with the long ends of the anchoring sutures. Alternatively, a piece of Telfa and a pressure dressing are applied to immobilize the graft for 1 week.

Simple Ellipse Sliding Flap

Many eyelid and periocular defects can be repaired by undermining surrounding tissues and primarily closing the advanced edges. Since most defects are circular or ovoid in configuration, conversion of the defect to an elliptical shape helps prevent dog-ear formation. The ellipse should be oriented to lie parallel to relaxed skin tension lines to lessen deformity of surrounding structures and minimize the resultant scar. Exceptions to this rule are eyelid defects near the lid margin that would cause excessive tension perpendicular to the lid margin and lead to ectropion or retraction.

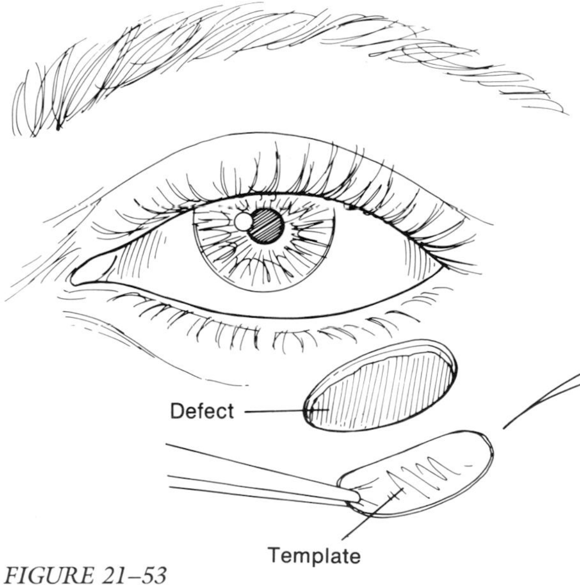

FIGURE 21–53

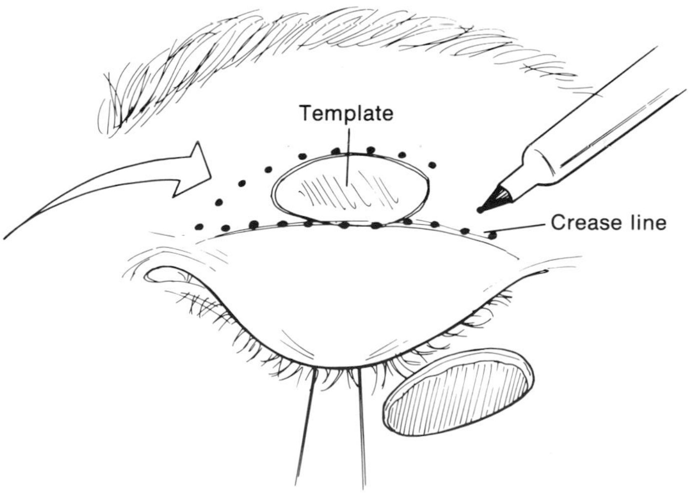

FIGURE 21–54

Figure 21–55. An ellipse is designed to incorporate the defect with its long axis parallel to lines of dependency or wrinkle lines. Ideally, the long axis is made four times longer than the short axis, with an ellipse angle of approximately 30°. A blade is used to incise the skin and subcutaneous tissue along the edges of the flap, and the ends of the ellipse are undermined and excised.

Figure 21–56. The tissues adjacent to the defect are undermined until the edges can be united free of tension.

Figure 21–57. Interrupted 6–0 or 7–0 Vicryl sutures are placed for subcutaneous layer closure, and the skin is closed with interrupted 6–0 or 7–0 nylon sutures. The deeper subcutaneous sutures support the wound edges so that skin closure is achieved without tension.

Glabellar Flap

A glabellar flap is a modified V- to Y-rotation flap of skin from the glabellar region of the midforehead that is used to repair medial canthal defects. The skin and subcutaneous tissues of the flap are thicker than that of the medial canthus and may require a second procedure for debulking.

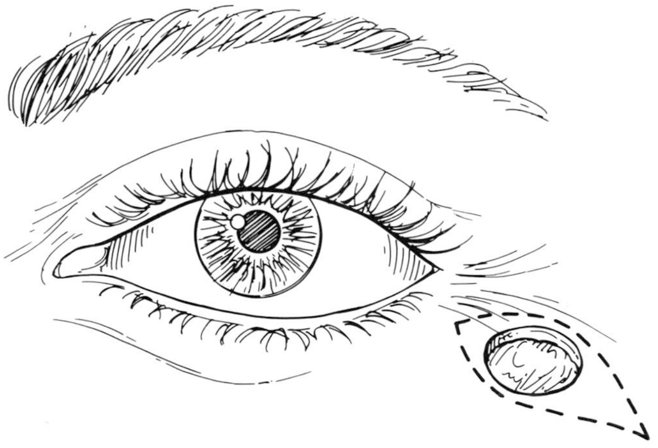

FIGURE 21–55

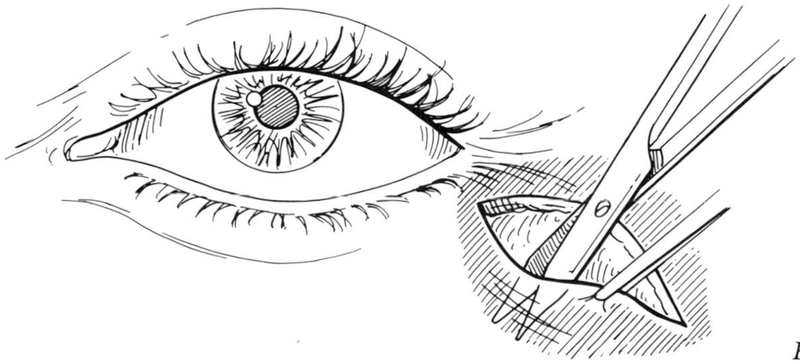

FIGURE 21–56

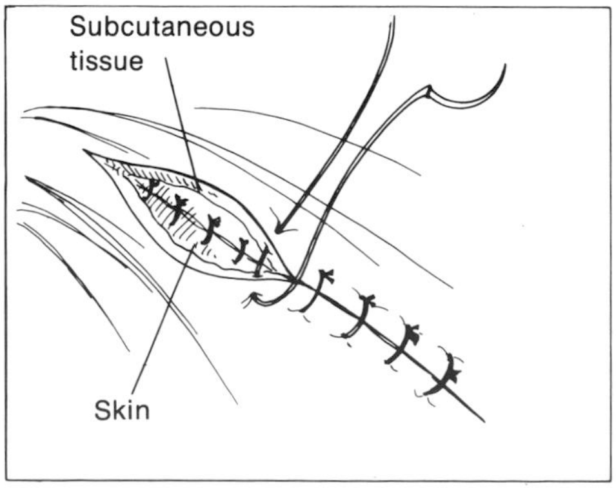

FIGURE 21–57

Figure 21–58. An inverted V is marked from the midpoint of the glabella just above the brow with an angle less than 60°. Both arms of the flap are designed to extend below the brow with the longer arm joining the lateral aspect of the defect. An incision is made along this mark with a size 15 Bard–Parker blade. The skin and subcutaneous tissue of the flap and surrounding area are extensively undermined with Stevens scissors.

Figure 21–59. The flap is rotated into the defect such that the apex of flap *A* is positioned at the lateral edge and the point *B* of the flap is positioned at the inferior tip. The flap's tip is then trimmed to fit the defect. The flap is sutured in place with anchoring 6–0 Vicryl buried subcutaneous interrupted sutures and the skin edges are united with interrupted 6–0 nylon or silk sutures. The donor site is sutured in a V-to-Y closure, which may result in foreshortening the distance between the eyebrows.

Rhombic Flap

The rhombic flap, also known as the rhomboid or Limberg flap, is a transposition flap of great versatility that is useful in the closure of medial canthal and lateral canthal defects. Most defects can be converted into a rhombic configuration sparing very little normal tissue with angles of 60° and 120° and all sides of equal length. The flap should be designed to avoid distortion of the eyelid margins and eyebrows and reduce tension along the vectors of closure of the donor area by proper orientation along lines of maximum tissue elasticity.

Figure 21–60. The defect is converted into a rhombus by first marking two lines parallel to the lines of maximum extensibility (*LME*) and adjacent to the edges of the defect. The LME are oriented perpendicular to the relaxed skin tension lines (*RSTL*). One of two rhombic figures is made by demarcating two more parallel lines equal in length and tangential to the defect at either 60° or 120° to the first set. Flap *A–B* (*shaded*) exemplifies this technique. Minimal tissue excision is performed, as needed, to fashion a rhombic defect. A line is drawn from each end of the shorter diagonal bisecting the 120° angle equal in length to the sides of the rhombus. Additional lines are marked from the end of the previous mark at a 60° angle parallel to the sides of the rhombic defect.

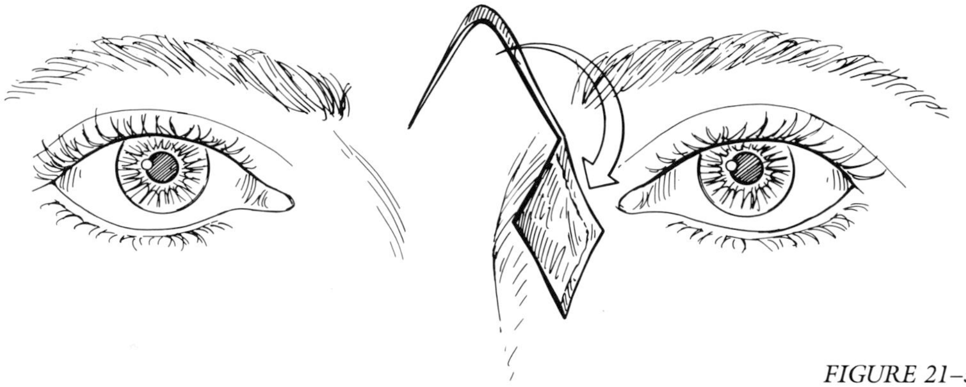

FIGURE 21–58

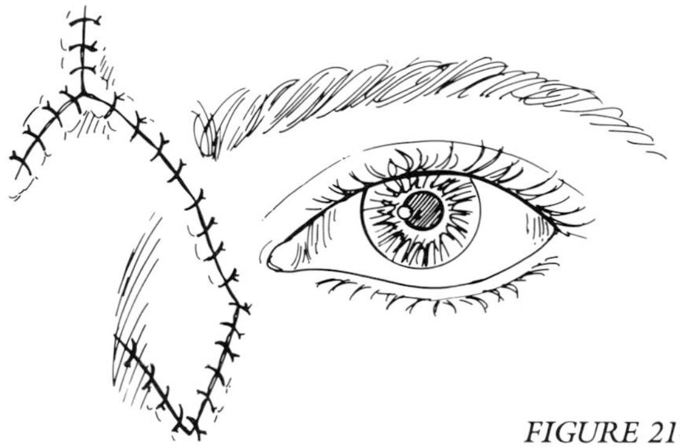

FIGURE 21–59

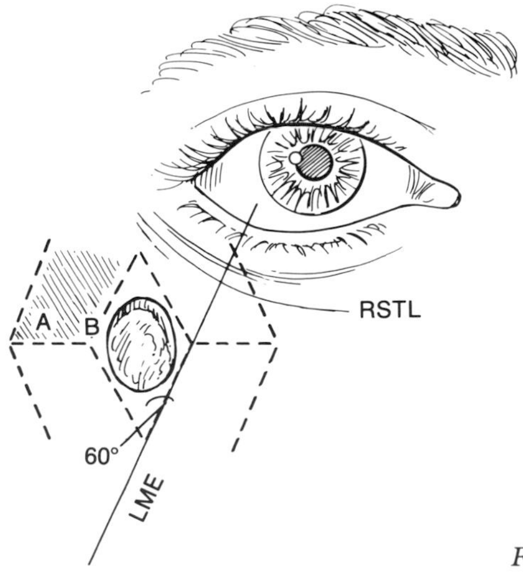

FIGURE 21–60

Figure 21–61. Four possible flap designs are created for closing the defect, but only one of the two flaps oriented to close the donor site along lines of maximum extensibility, and that interferes least with surrounding structures, should be chosen. The edges of the defect and the flap to be transposed are extensively undermined with Steven's scissors. All bleeding points should be cauterized with a bipolar cautery.

Figure 21–62. The flap is advanced into the defect by rotating medially such that point *B* aligns with the medial point of the defect, and point A is positioned at the inferior apex. The subcutaneous layer is closed with interrupted 6–0 Vicryl sutures to reduce tension on the skin edges. Skin closure is completed with interrupted 6–0 nylon sutures for thinner skin and 5–0 nylon vertical mattress sutures for areas with thicker skin.

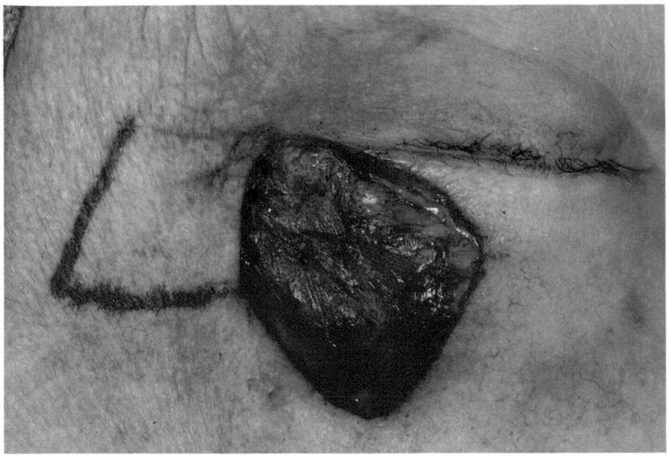

FIGURE 21–61

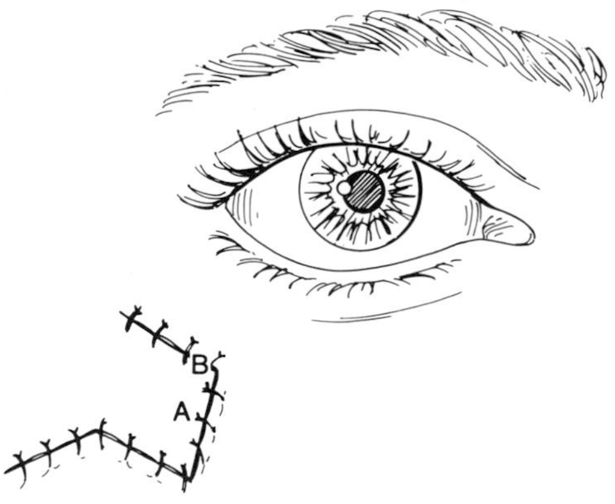

FIGURE 21–62

POSTOPERATIVE CARE

An ophthalmic antibiotic ointment should be applied to the operative site at the conclusion of surgery, and a pressure patch is typically applied. Pressure bandages are useful to reduce postoperative edema and bleeding and to immobilize the advanced tissue flaps or skin grafts. In addition, 4–0 silk traction sutures are useful in selected cases when placed in the eyelid margin to pull the reconstructed lid on stretch to help reduce retraction of the tissues. The pressure patch, traction sutures, and stents for skin grafts are removed 5 to 7 days after surgery, and antibiotic ointment is placed on the healing tissues for an additional 2 weeks three times a day. Oral antibiotics, such as a first-generation cephalosporin, are prescribed for patients who are immunocompromised (e.g., diabetics), have poor hygiene, or undergo skin grafting.

Most sutures are removed from the skin approximately 1 week following the reconstructive surgery. If during suture removal the wound is noted to slightly dehisce, the remaining sutures are left in place for another week. The silk lid margin sutures used to primarily close marginal defects should be left in place for 10 to 14 days. The running suture placed to secure skin grafts is removed after 1 week; however, the interrupted sutures are not removed for an additional week.

SURGICAL COMPLICATIONS

The most common complications following lower lid reconstruction are lid margin deformities and malpositions. A lid notch at the junction of direct lid margin closure may develop because of excessive tension on the wound or inadequate alignment; this can be revised with excision and direct closure. Ectropion or sagging of the lower lid may result from excessive laxity or improper fixation of the medial or lateral canthal tissues; horizontal shortening or refixation of the canthal tendons to the orbital rim periosteum with a nonabsorbable suture is usually corrective. Frost traction sutures help prevent retraction or cicatricial ectropion. Blunting of the canthal angle may occur after cantholysis or a semicircle flap technique and be repaired with a canthoplasty. Symblepharon may develop if a raw surface on the inner aspect of the reconstructed lid is allowed to epithelialize, but often, this requires no intervention; lysis of symblepharon, a Z-plasty, or a mucous membrane graft may be necessary if it is functionally significant.

Upper lid abnormalities can develop following a Hughes reconstruction of the opposite lower lid. Design of the tarsoconjunctival flap such that at least 4 mm of vertical height of tarsus from the lid margin is preserved prevents the development of entropion or contour deformities. Retraction of the upper lid rarely develops if Mueller's muscle is not advanced with the tarsoconjunctival flap, but when included, it must be recessed after the flap is separated. If retraction remains after these measures, recession of the levator aponeurosis may be necessary.

Patients are usually more symptomatic from complications in the upper lid after reconstruction because of its important role in corneal protection. Trichiasis at a primary closure site or from the skin hairs at the margin following a Cutler–Beard procedure can be eliminated with cryotherapy and epilation. Ptosis could develop if the levator aponeurotic attachments are significantly disturbed, although repair with a levator aponeurosis advancement should be delayed at least 4 to 6 months after the initial surgery. Lagophthalmos may result from upper lid retraction or inadequate orbicularis muscle tone. Topical lubricants may be adequate to treat mild lagophthalmos, but surgical correction of the lid retraction or a partial tarsorrhaphy may be necessary if the corneal exposure is not tolerated. Lid notching, canthal angle blunting, and lid malposition may also develop and are treated as just described for lower lid complications.

Skin grafts and myocutaneous flaps may become necrotic owing to insufficient blood supply, hematoma formation, or infection. Meticulous technique is essential, with adequate hemostasis and pressure patching to minimize postoperative bleeding; however, excessive cautery that could compromise the circulation to the site of reconstruction should also be avoided. Infections should be treated aggressively with systemic and topical antibiotics after appropriate cultures are obtained. Nonviable tissue should be debrided, and the areas of necrosis allowed to granulate before secondary repair is considered.

Epiphora may result from inadequate tear drainage because of punctal malposition; loss of components of the lacrimal drainage system, such as the canalicular portion of the lid; or deficiency in the lacrimal pump mechanism. Also, reflex lacrimation secondary to entropion, trichiasis, dry eyes, or exposure keratopathy must be considered as etiologic factors in the tearing patient. Punctal and eyelid ectropion should be corrected as described elsewhere in this text (see Chapter 10). If the epiphora is caused by loss of the lacrimal excretory system or an insufficient lacrimal pump, a conjunctivodacryocystorhinostomy with a Jones tube can be considered. It is emphasized, as stated previously, that secondary lacrimal drainage surgery should be deferred for at least 1 to 2 years after a periocular cutaneous malignancy is excised to allow an observation period to monitor the patient for tumor recurrence.

Chapter Twenty-Two

SOCKET RECONSTRUCTION

Jan W. Kronish

PREOPERATIVE EVALUATION

A functional anophthalmic socket that permits the wear of a comfortable and mobile ocular prosthesis requires (1) a centrally positioned orbital implant of adequate volume, (2) a conjunctival or mucous membrane-lined socket with adequately deep fornices, (3) a correctly positioned lower eyelid of normal length and tone to support the weight of the prosthesis, and (4) an upper eyelid with good levator function that is properly oriented, in apposition to the prosthesis, and with symmetric height and contour with the opposite side. A lack of or disturbance of one or more of these parameters may lead to the inability to retain a prosthesis and severe disfigurement and psychologic distress of the patient.

A thorough history is important in an evaluation of the anophthalmic patient, including determination of the ocular condition leading to enucleation or evisceration, type and size of the orbital implant, previous surgery or therapy (e.g., volume augmentation, eyelid malposition repair, radiation), antecedent periocular trauma and associated orbital fractures, prior sinus disease, and past management of the ocular prosthesis. Examination of the socket should begin with an assessment of the eyelids and periorbital region, with the best-fitting prosthesis properly positioned in the socket. Excessive lower lid laxity and malposition may develop because of its support for the weight of the prosthesis, requiring assessment of its medial and lateral canthal tendon attachments. Measurements should be obtained of the vertical and horizontal palpebral fissures, as well as of the upper eyelid crease and fold and levator function. Notation of the degree of a superior sulcus defect and Hertel exophthalmometry can provide information on orbital volume. The excursion of the ocular prosthesis on vertical and, especially, horizontal eye movements should be noted. A history of previous trauma mandates palpation of the orbital bony rim and evaluation for asymmetry of the malar eminence and lateral and medial canthal positions.

Upon removal of the prosthesis, the socket should be assessed for adequacy of the superior and inferior fornices, presence of symblepharon, integrity of the conjunctival lining, position of the orbital implant, and signs of infection or inflammation. Palpation of the socket cavity can reveal migration of and shape and size characteristics of the orbital implant, as well as space-occupying orbital masses. If the possibility of a significant orbital fracture or recurrent tumor exists, radiographic studies with computerized tomography (CT) are indicated.

Finally, careful evaluation of the ocular prosthesis is important and includes searching for protein deposits, scratches, and irregularities, aided by the use of a magnifying loupe or slit-lamp biomicroscope. An excessively large and heavy prosthesis may aggravate lower lid laxity and result in a dropped socket appearance. Close interaction with an ocularist is critical, as modification or replacement of a prosthesis can correct upper lid ptosis, superior sulcus defects, eyelid malpositions, poor motility, and mild socket contraction in selected cases. Nonsurgical management of sockets in children with congenital anophthalmos is also performed by an ocularist using a progressively enlarging series of conformers until maximum socket and eyelid development is reached.

SURGICAL INDICATIONS

Appropriate management of anophthalmic socket disorders initially requires individualized consideration of a patient's symptoms and goals. Certain clinical conditions responsive to surgical intervention, such as upper lid ptosis or superior sulcus defects, may be considered a minor cosmetic blemish by some patients who prefer no treatment, but a major disfigurement by others who request corrective measures. On the other hand, such problems as implant extrusion and socket contracture require surgical intervention to maintain a functional socket that can retain a prosthesis and prevent secondary complications such as infection or chronic pain. The disorders of the anophthalmic socket are amenable to surgical therapy.

Implant Extrusion

Extrusion of orbital implants can occur in the early postoperative period or develop months or years after enucleation or evisceration. Inadequate wound closure, insertion of oversized implants, and rarely, infection may be responsible for early extrusion. Patients usually present within days or weeks of surgery with mucopurulent discharge, conjunctival inflammation, and evidence of a wound dehiscence. Management involves treating infections with appropriate antibiotics, possibly replacing the implant that is too large with one that is smaller in diameter, and performing a meticulous closure of the overlying Tenon's capsule and conjunctiva.

Late extrusions are usually caused by cicatricial contraction of orbital tissues or the breakdown of tissues covering the implant owing to prolonged pressure by the prosthesis. Such orbital implants as wire mesh implants, Allen implants, and exposed integrated implants are notorious for late extrusions because of their configuration and relation with the central socket conjunctival surface, and their use should be abandoned. Delayed extrusions, which may be partial or complete, might be manifested by irritative symptoms, discharge, and the inability to retain an ocular prosthesis. Small fistulas between the implant and conjunctival lining are typical of partial extrusions, and these fistulas will gradually enlarge, with associated thinning of the adjacent tissues covering the implant. When identified at an early stage, partial extrusions can be effectively managed with a patch graft that uses donor sclera, autogenous fascia lata, or temporalis fascia. Complete extrusion of an orbital implant, however, requires the introduction of a secondary implant if there is adequate mucous membrane present, or a dermis–fat graft in patients for whom there is a deficiency of conjunctiva.

Implant Migration

Migration of the orbital implant from its central location to a peripheral position in the anophthalmic socket may result in difficult prosthetic fitting and wear, poor motility, foreshortened fornices, and eventual implant extrusion. Contractile scar tissue formation, gravitational forces, and differential forces of extraocular muscles when imbricated over the implant are some of the etiologic factors leading to a malpositioned implant. This condition is best corrected by removal of the migrated implant, which is then replaced with either a secondary implant or dermis–fat graft more centrally positioned in the orbit.

Enophthalmos and Superior Sulcus Deformity (Orbital Volume Deficiency)

A reduction in the volume of orbital contents always results following enucleation or evisceration at least partly because of the replacement of the globe with an orbital implant smaller in diameter. Other factors attributed to this deficit include coexistent orbital fractures, lack of an orbital implant, redistribution of the orbital soft tissues, radiation-induced fat atrophy, and contractile fibrosis of connective tissue elements. One or more of these factors lead to anophthalmic enophthalmos and superior sulcus defects. Gravitational effects and loss of support of the superior transverse ligament and superior rectus–levator muscular complex are also thought to play a role in the development of the sulcus deformity.

Surgical correction of these clinical entities may include one or more volume augmentation procedures. If an orbital implant is absent, the preferred method of volume replacement is the insertion of a spherical implant or dermis–fat graft. In a socket in which the primary alloplastic implant is too small (i.e., less than 16 mm diameter), exchange with as large a secondary implant as the socket will allow is recommended. When the original implant is of satisfactory size and is centrally located, or when the foregoing procedures have been performed with inadequate volume augmentation, placement of a subperiosteal implant along the orbital floor may be corrective. Numerous materials for such implants have been utilized including autogenous or lyophilized bone, Teflon or glass beads, Proplast, and bone cement; however, my preferences are prefabricated wedge-shaped soft medical grade silicone, methyl methacrylate resin, or room temperature vulcanizing silicone implants. Not only do these implants provide additional intraorbital volume, but they also yield a mechanical displacement of the orbital implant and soft tissues in an anterior and superior direction that helps to further correct the enophthalmos and superior sulcus defects.

Upper Eyelid Ptosis

Ptosis of the upper eyelid associated with anophthalmos is a common problem. Similar to the pathomechanical alterations causing a deepened superior sulcus, ptosis usually results from stretching and laxity of the orbital tissues caused by gravity, enophthalmos, disturbance in the suspension of Whitnall's ligament, and excessive anterior advancement of the superior rectus muscle over the implant. Foreshortening of the superior fornix by closing Tenon's capsule and conjunctiva under excessive tension, or direct damage to the levator muscle during enucleation surgery, might also contribute to the development of ptosis. If the upper lid malposition cannot be improved by altering the prosthesis, then surgical correction is indicated. External levator surgery is performed when levator function is fair to good (greater than 6 mm of excursion). When there is poor or no levator function, frontalis suspension may be considered. These surgical techniques are described elsewhere in this text.

Lower Eyelid Laxity and Inadequate Inferior Fornix

The lower eyelid provides much of the support of the orbital implant and bears all of the weight of the ocular prosthesis. Over a period, gravitational forces and the weight of the prosthesis loosen the supporting elements of the lower lid. Laxity of the eyelid is accentuated as the orbital tissues migrate inferiorly and the prosthesis is enlarged in an attempt to improve the resultant superior sulcus deformity or upper lid ptosis. Sagging of the lower eyelid contributes to the disfiguring dropped socket appearance and, eventually, may lead to the inability to maintain a properly positioned prosthesis. Horizontal lid shortening and tightening with a lateral tarsal strip procedure is effective in correcting the lower lid laxity and is described in detail in a previous chapter.

Dehiscence of the lower lid retractors, development of scar tissue in the cul-de-sac, and anteroinferior migration of the orbital implant may result in foreshortening of the inferior fornix. Particularly when an inadequate fornix is combined with lower lid laxity, retention of the prosthesis may be compromised. Re-formation of the inferior fornix is achieved with refixation and stenting of the fornix and lower lid tightening when there is sufficient socket conjunctiva. In patients in whom the fornix is deficient of conjunctiva, a free mucous membrane graft that is stented into position is required.

Socket Contracture

Acquired contraction of the socket represents the most serious disorder of anophthalmos and the most difficult to manage. Precipitating factors include chronic infection or inflammation, trauma, radiation therapy, surgery, and migrating or extruding implants. Once the etiologic factors leading to socket contracture are identified and eliminated, surgical and prosthetic management can begin. The spectrum of socket contracture has been divided into mild, moderate, and severe forms.

Mild socket contracture refers to cicatricial entropion of the upper or lower eyelids caused by fibrotic contracture of the posterior lamella. The entropic lid margin and eyelashes result in irritative symptoms and ocular discharge. A transverse blepharotomy and marginal rotation procedure, which is discussed elsewhere in the text, effectively repositions the eyelid and lashes to a normal position.

Contracture of the superior or inferior fornices leading to the inability to retain an ocular prosthesis is categorized as moderate socket contracture. Its development may occur in the early or late postoperative period and is associated with chronic discharge and irritation, poor prosthetic motility, and enophthalmos. Foreshortening of the inferior fornix with inadequate conjunctiva is the most common form of this condition. Reconstructive surgery involves the re-formation of a fornix and placement of a partial- or full-thickness mucous membrane graft, usually obtained from the lip or buccal mucosa, which is held in position with a Silastic (polymeric silicone) stent secured to the inferior orbital rim periosteum or a conformer. If the superior fornix contracts, changes in the upper eyelid position, crease, fold, and levator function may develop, as well as extrusion of the prosthesis. Reformation of the superior fornix is achieved in the same manner as that for the inferior fornix except that a conformer is preferable to a Silastic stent to maintain the configuration of the mucous membrane graft, as it is less likely to damage the levator muscle. Moderate socket contracture is difficult to correct, may require multiple surgical procedures, and often results in an unsatisfying outcome.

The severe form of socket contracture typically manifests marked vertical forniceal contracture, horizontal shortening of the palpebral fissure, and in certain patients, obliteration of the lid margins. Active cicatricial processes and multiple previously failed surgeries may be contraindications to attempt reconstruction. Partial or full-thickness mucous membrane grafts are stented into position with specially designed conformers that often require fixation to the orbital rims to prevent extrusion. Four to six months later, the conformer is removed, and an immediate prosthetic fitting is undertaken. The goal of creating a socket cavity that can retain an ocular prosthesis is often not achieved, however, and, even when successful, the final appearance is often only fair with an immobile prosthesis and eyelids.

TIMING AND PREFERENTIAL ORDER OF SURGICAL PROCEDURES

Surgical management of anophthalmic socket disorders may require multiple, staged operations for a functional and cosmetically acceptable result. Most reconstructive procedures should be delayed at least 4 to 6 months following the initial enucleation or evisceration to allow the orbital tissues to heal and scar tissue to mature. If the fornices are foreshortened or the socket is contracted, preventing the retention of a prosthesis, re-formation of an adequately deep socket, with or without an oral mucous membrane graft, is the first priority. Correction of orbital implant malposition and size or a disturbance of the integrity of overlying tissues is the next goal. Volume replacement procedures may be considered to correct superior sulcus defects and enophthalmos. Severe lower lid laxity can be corrected at the time of volume augmentation or later. Finally, ptosis surgery of the upper eyelid may be undertaken following the revision or replacement of the ocular prosthesis after the completion of any of the foregoing procedures.

SURGICAL ANATOMY OF THE ANOPHTHALMIC SOCKET

The anophthalmic socket comprises a complex unit of orbital fat and connective tissue, extraocular muscles, vessels, nerves, Tenon's capsule, and a conjunctival lining. The pathomechanical changes that develop following the surgical removal of the eye are largely dependent on the type of primary surgery and positioning of the orbital implant within the orbit. For example, if an evisceration has been performed, the orbital tissues are not disturbed and the conjunctiva and Tenon's capsule maintain their anatomic configuration, minimizing the potential for development of socket contracture and implant migration. On the other hand, when enucleation has been undertaken, major alterations in the structural and functional elements of the orbit develop. A deficit in orbital volume, loss of support of the superior rectus–levator muscular complex, retraction of the extraocular muscles, scarring and contracture of the orbital fibrous connective tissue septae, redistribution of the orbital fat, and stretching of the lower lid supporting tendons by the weight of the prosthesis all contribute to the clinical disorders of the anophthalmic socket. Recognition of these anatomic changes is essential to establish the proper management and surgical approaches for these patients.

SURGICAL PROCEDURES

Patch Graft Technique for Extruding Orbital Implants

Repair of partially extruding implants with a patch graft can be performed under local or general anesthesia. Temporalis fascia is the preferred patch graft material because it is easily accessible, the scar at the site of graft harvesting remains hidden by the hairline, and it will result in minimal reaction and shrinkage and maximize viability because it is autogenous. The donor site is located just above the anterior aspect of the helix of the ear and superior to the palpable superficial temporal artery which should be avoided. A disposable razor can be used to trim the hair in the proposed surgical field and lidocaine (Xylocaine) 2% with 1:100,000 epinephrine is injected subcutaneously. The socket conjunctiva in the area of dehiscence is also infiltrated with the same local anesthetic solution to minimize bleeding. An alternative to temporalis fascia for patching material is preserved sclera which, if selected, should be placed in antibiotic solution at the beginning of surgery.

Figure 22–1. A lid speculum is inserted to expose the central socket cavity and the site of implant exposure. Dehiscence of the conjunctiva and Tenon's capsule is seen in the socket.

Figure 22–2. The edges of the fistula are freshened and the conjunctiva is undermined from the adjacent scar tissue and Tenon's capsule with scissors.

Figure 22–3. The plane of dissection is depicted by the dotted line in this cross-sectional view of the socket. The size of the patch graft necessary to cover the exposed orbital implant and overlap the edges of Tenon's capsule by at least 2 to 3 mm is measured.

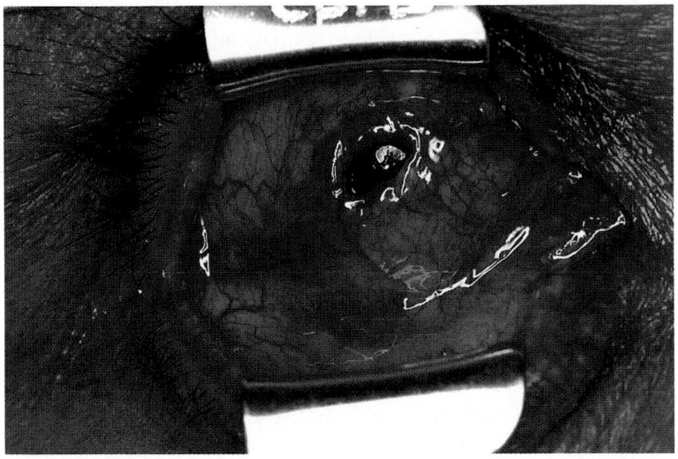

FIGURE 22–1

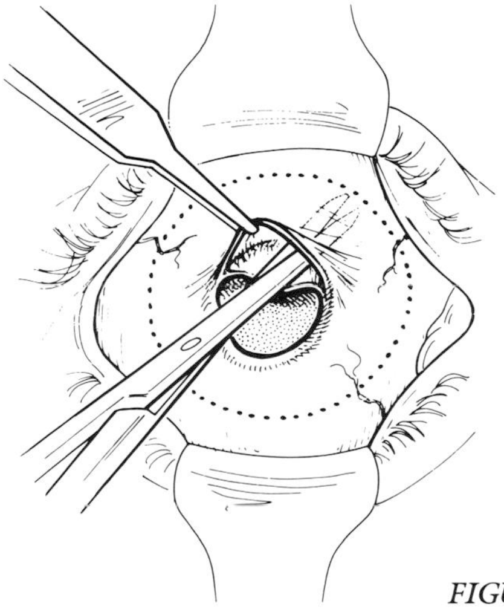

FIGURE 22–2

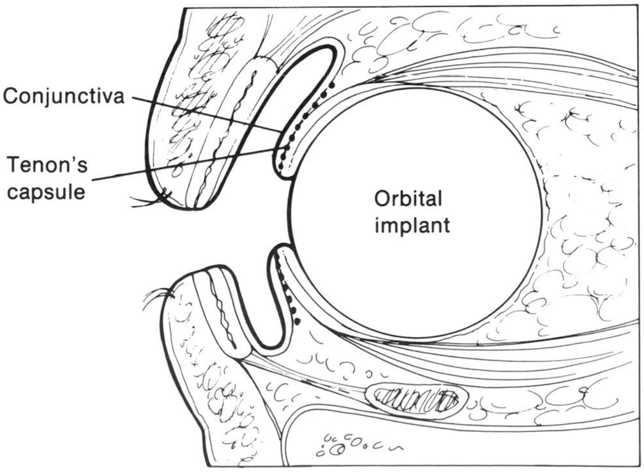

FIGURE 22–3

Figure 22–4. Harvesting of the fascia involves making a 4-cm incision with a Bard–Parker size 15 blade in the temporal scalp. The superficial temporal artery should first be identified by feeling for its pulsations and the incision is made posterior to this landmark to avoid cutting the vessel. Sharp dissection with scissors through the subcutaneous tissue is performed until the temporalis fascia is exposed.

Figure 22–5. With the edges of the scalp incision retracted, a Bard–Parker size 15 blade is used to outline the fascial graft to be harvested. Blunt and sharp scissor dissection is used to separate the fascia from the underlying temporalis muscle, and the graft is set aside in saline-soaked gauze. Hemostasis is maintained with a bipolar cautery. The fascial defect is not repaired. The scalp incision is closed with deep interrupted 4–0 Vicryl sutures and skin closure is achieved with interrupted 6–0 nylon sutures.

Figure 22–6. The temporalis fascia graft (or preserved scleral graft) is trimmed to size and placed into the defect in the socket between Tenon's capsule and conjunctiva. The graft is oversized so that its borders overlap the edges of the defect when it is secured into place with multiple interrupted 6–0 Vicryl sutures passed between the edges of Tenon's capsule and the overlapping edges of the graft.

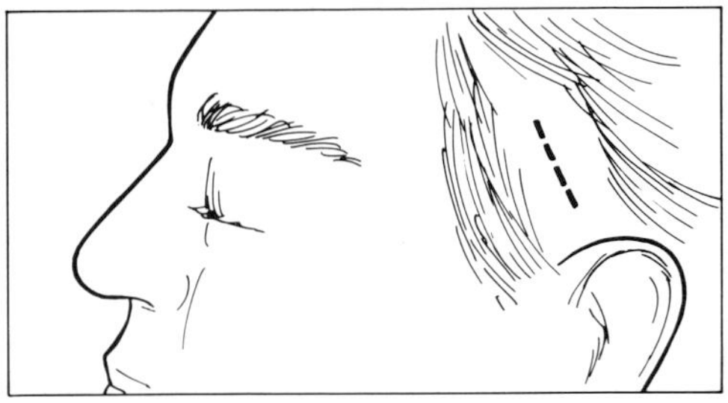

FIGURE 22–4

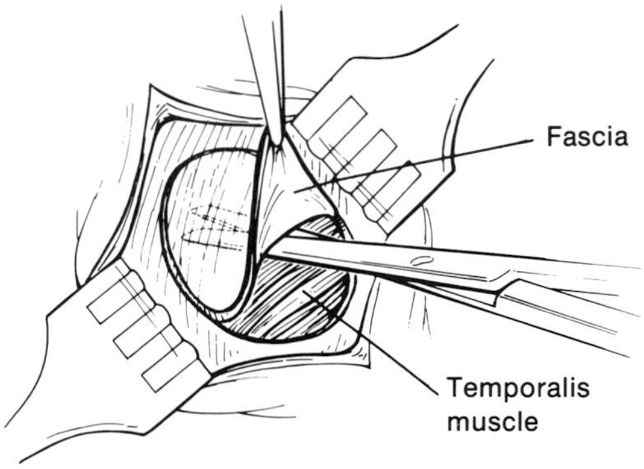

FIGURE 22–5

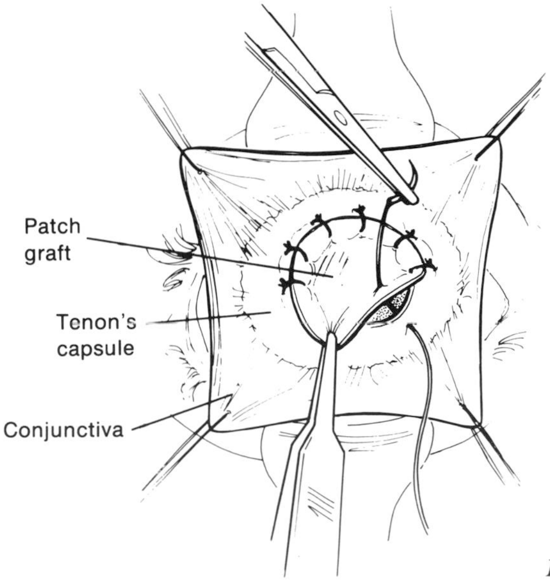

FIGURE 22–6

Figure 22–7. The temporalis fascia patch graft is shown sutured into position to cover the exposed orbital implant.

Figure 22–8. The conjunctival edges are then sutured together with a running 6–0 plain gut suture over the graft to provide its blood supply.

Figure 22–9. A cross-sectional view demonstrates the patch graft borders overlapping and sutured to the edges of Tenon's capsule and the conjunctival closure over the fascia graft.

An antibiotic ointment and conformer are placed in the socket. A pressure patch is most effectively applied by first rubbing benzoin over the central forehead and cheek skin, placing an eye pad and a single fluff of an unrolled 4 × 4 gauze over the closed eyelids, and securing these tightly with paper tape.

Secondary Orbital Implant Placement

The indications for the insertion of a secondary orbital implant include an extruding implant that cannot or should not be repaired with a patch graft, insufficient orbital volume owing to lack of a primary implant or one that is too small, and migration of an implant preventing the comfortable wear of a prosthesis. This type of surgery is usually performed under general anesthesia; however, local anesthesia is an option in selected cases. For local anesthesia, a 50:50 mixture of lidocaine 2% with epinephrine 1:100,000, bupivicaine 0.75% with epinephrine 1:100,000, and hyaluronidase (Wydase) provides vasoconstriction and prolonged analgesia. Administration of this mixture subcutaneously along the length of the lids, subconjunctivally in the socket, and in the retrobulbar space with a 1½ in. (3.7-cm) 27-gauge needle provides sufficient anesthesia for most forms of socket surgery.

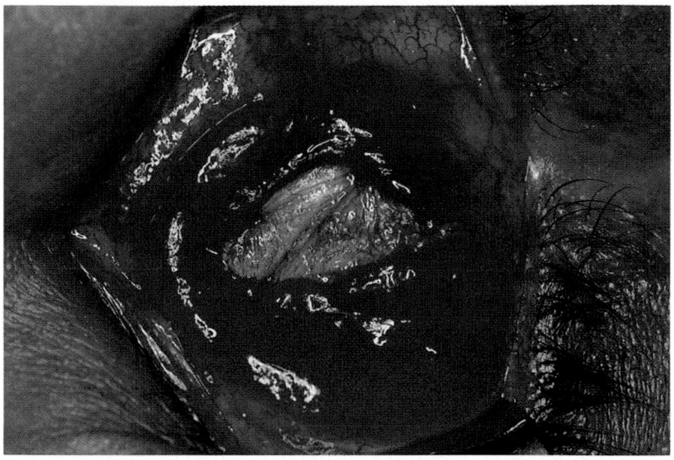

FIGURE 22–7

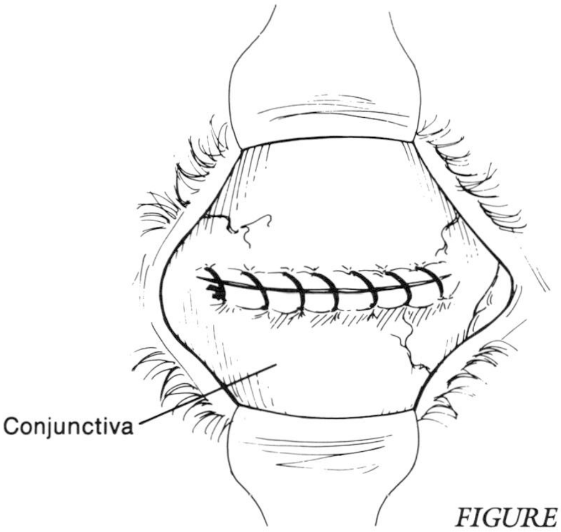

FIGURE 22–8

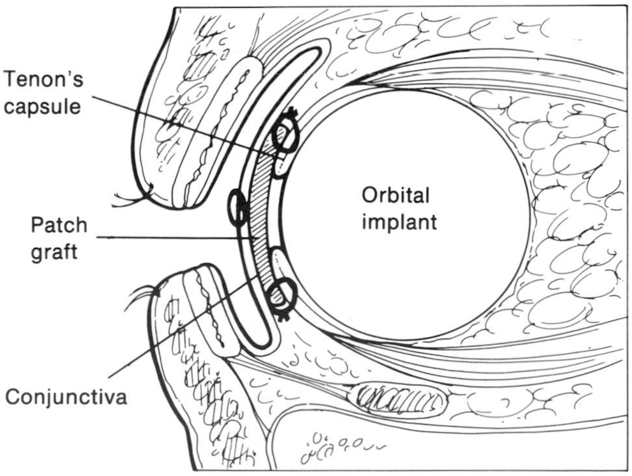

FIGURE 22–9

Figure 22–10. A lid speculum is positioned to expose the central portion of the socket. To remove a partially exposed implant, a horizontal incision through conjunctiva, scar tissue, and Tenon's capsule is made with scissors to enlarge the wound.

Figure 22–11. If the extruding implant is mesh-covered, sharp dissection with Wescott scissors may be necessary to free it from adhesions to surrounding orbital tissues.

Figure 22–12. Curved scissors cut the tissues adherent to the posterior pole of the orbital implant. Care should be taken to spare as much conjunctiva as possible. When an implant of inadequate volume or one that has migrated is to be replaced, the same horizontal incision is made in the center of the socket and dissection carried out posteriorly until the primary implant is identified.

The implant is removed and a fibrous pseudocapsule often remains. If the rectus muscles can be identified, each one is tagged with a double-armed 6–0 Vicryl suture, and the sutures with the needles are set aside temporarily.

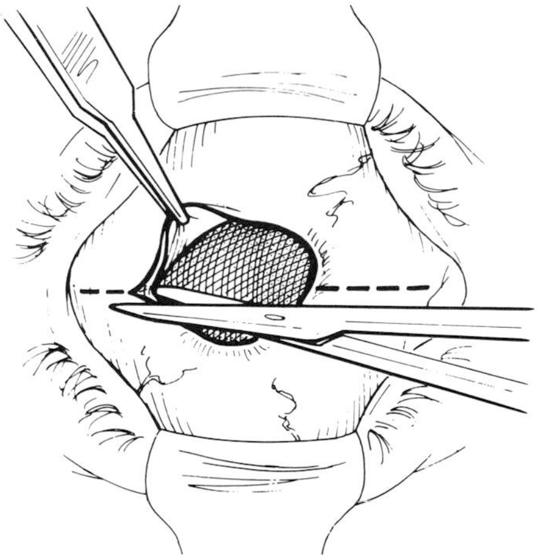

FIGURE 22–10

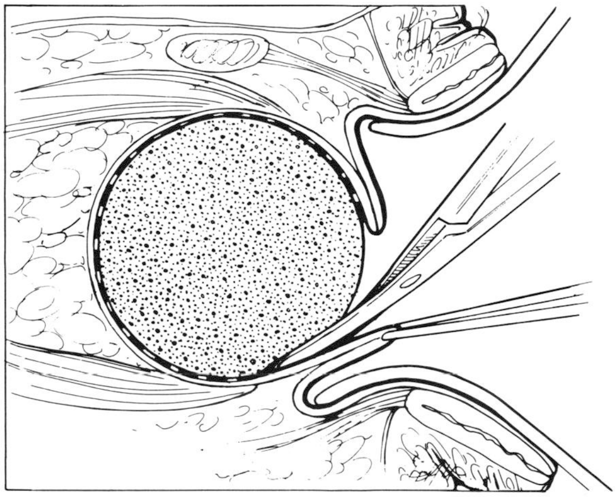

FIGURE 22–11

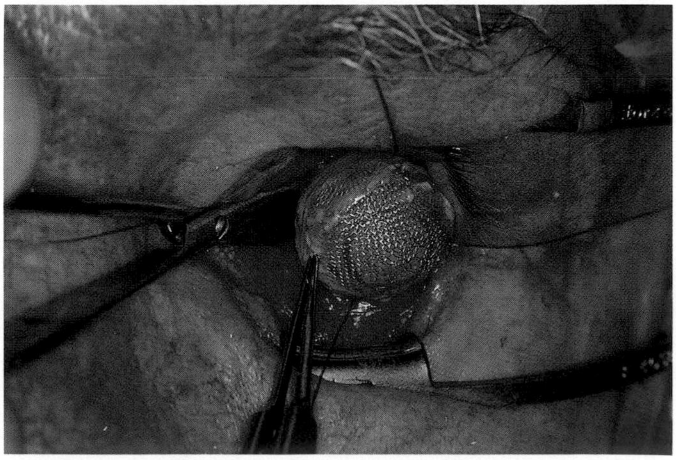

FIGURE 22–12

Figure 22–13. Sharp scissors are used to buttonhole through the fibrous Tenon's capsule posteriorly and extended into a vertical incision through the scar tissue until the intraconal orbital fat is exposed centrally and posteriorly. Hemostasis should be maintained with a bipolar cautery.

As large a spherical implant as the socket will accommodate is chosen (usually 16 mm diameter or greater) and may be wrapped in preserved sclera, polytetrafluoroethylene (Gortex), or temporalis fascia. Each of these materials can be sewn over the implant with 4–0 Vicryl sutures and provides a surface in which to secure the rectus muscles and an additional tissue barrier to prevent extrusion.

Figure 22–14. The implant is placed into the intraconal fat pad behind the pseudocapsule, and if wrapped, should be positioned with the sutured edges positioned posteriorly. If the rectus muscles can be identified, they may be attached to sides of the implant with 6–0 Vicryl sutures.

Figure 22–15. The edges of the posteriorly located Tenon's or the fibrous capsule are advanced over the implant and sutured together with interrupted 4–0 Vicryl sutures passed on a semicircle needle. If the fornices shorten while attempting to oppose these edges, they may instead be secured to the anterior surface of the implant wrapping. The anterior Tenon's capsule is closed over the implant with interrupted 5–0 Vicryl sutures followed by the conjunctival closure with a running 6–0 plain gut suture.

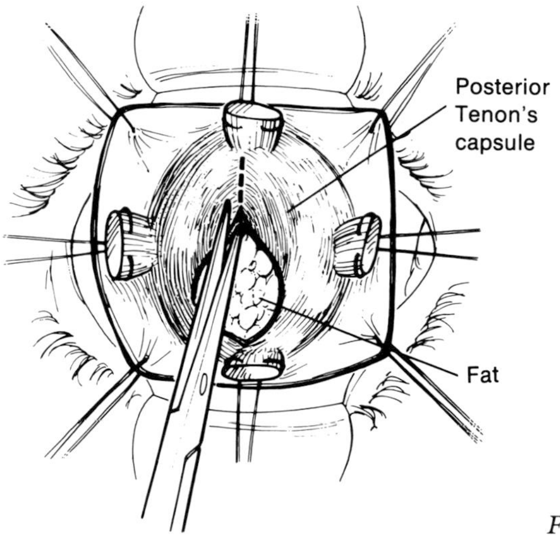

FIGURE 22–13

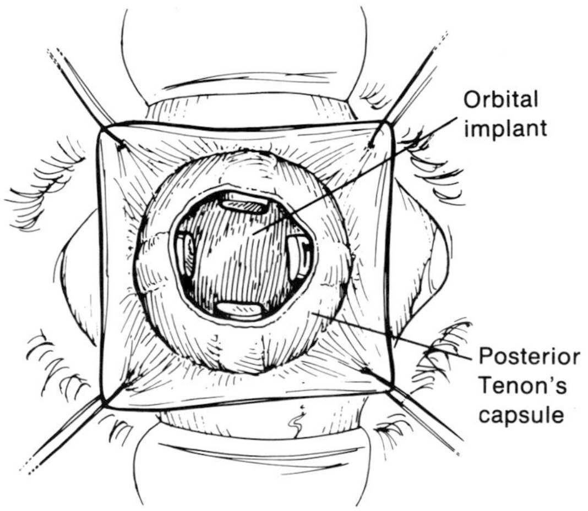

FIGURE 22–14

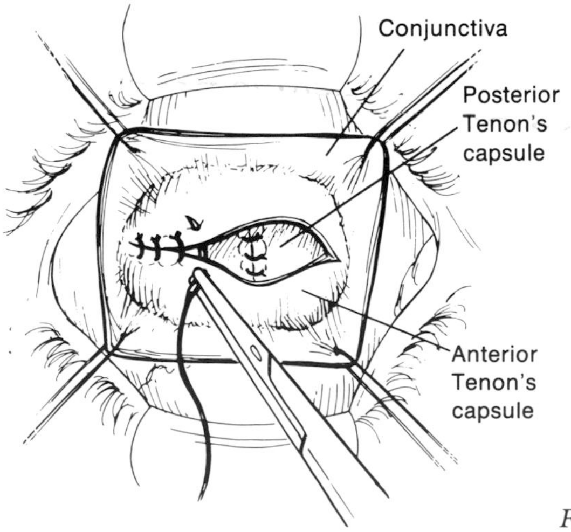

FIGURE 22–15

Figure 22–16. A cross-sectional view of the socket shows the three layers closed over the orbital implant: posterior Tenon's capsule, anterior Tenon's capsule, and conjunctiva. This technique provides three layers of tissue that act as a barrier to prevent recurrence of implant extrusion. A conformer is placed into the socket with antibiotic ointment and a pressure patch is applied as described above.

Dermis–Fat Graft Technique

Dermis–fat grafts are most useful in patients that require a secondary implant, but have a limited conjunctival socket lining or in those with recurrent extruding alloplastic implants. Other authors advocate their application as primary implants, for volume augmentation, and for expansion of foreshortened cul-de-sacs in anophthalmic sockets. The advantages for the use of dermis–fat grafts include their autogenous properties, with no risk of extrusion, physiologic volume replacement with fat, and preservation of conjunctiva. Partial absorption of the graft with loss of orbital volume is the most common complication.

When a dermis–fat graft is chosen to be placed as a secondary orbital implant, the socket is first prepared under local or general anesthesia, as described earlier under Secondary Orbital Implant Placement through the step just before inserting the implant.

Figure 22–17. The donor sites available for harvesting the graft may be either the lateral aspect of the buttocks or the left lower abdominal quadrant. Following infiltration of the surgical site with 2% lidocaine with 1:100,000 epinephrine, an ellipse, measuring approximately 25 × 30 mm, is outlined with a marker pen. A skin incision is made with a Bard–Parker size 15 blade along this mark.

Figure 22–18. The epidermis is more easily removed before harvesting the graft from the donor site. The epidermal and superficial dermal layers can be removed by sharp dissection with a blade.

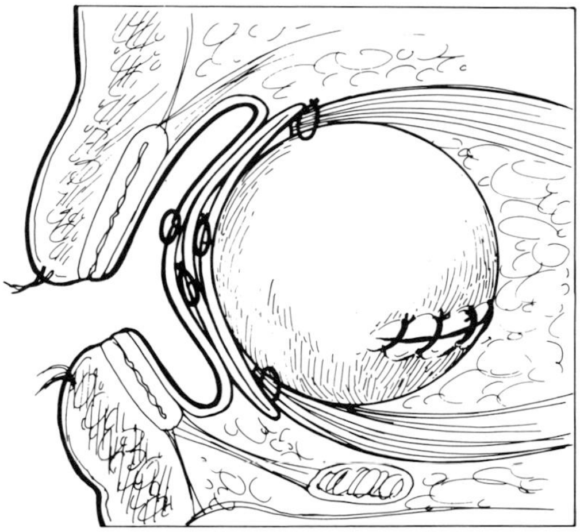

FIGURE 22–16

FIGURE 22–17

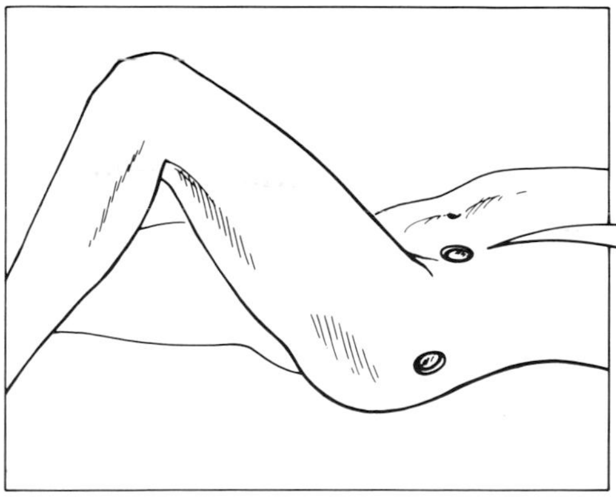

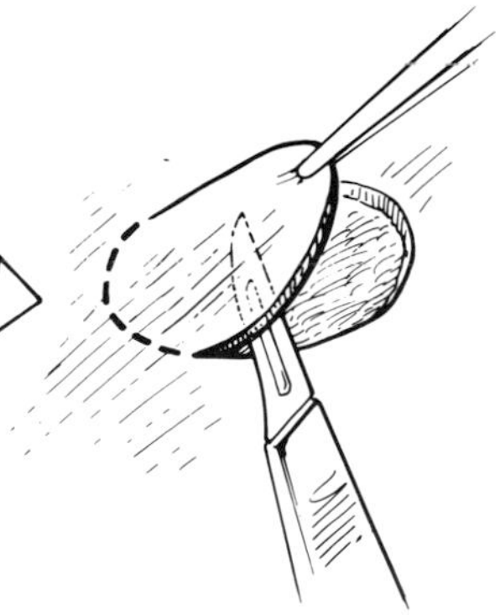

FIGURE 22–18

Figure 22–19. A dermabrader may be used to trim the epidermis. The superficial layers of skin are abraded until bleeding from the deeper dermal layers is encountered.

Figure 22–20. A cylindrical plug of dermis and fat with a depth of 25 mm is then fashioned using Steven's scissors with the blades first angled slightly away from the center of the graft to demarcate the sides and then excising it by placing the scissors along its base. If a pair of scissors or a blade is directed perpendicular or angled toward the graft's center, an insufficient volume of fat will be obtained. The harvested graft should be handled with care and may be soaked in saline until the socket is completely prepared. A bipolar cautery is utilized to control bleeding in the donor site.

The edges of deep fat at the donor site are closed with interrupted 4–0 chromic sutures. The subcutaneous tissues are apposed with 4–0 Vicryl sutures with buried knots. Skin closure is obtained with 5–0 nylon vertical mattress sutures to provide eversion of the wound edges. Surgical staples can be substituted for suture closure. Antibiotic ointment and a pressure bandage are applied.

Figure 22–21. The dermis–fat graft is transferred into the recipient bed of the intraconal space of the orbit, which can be identified by the posteriorly located fat, and excessive fat trimmed if necessary to allow a proper fit. Every effort to identify the four rectus muscles and to suture their ends to the edges of dermis of the graft in the appropriate quadrants with 6–0 Vicryl suture should be attempted. The anterior ciliary arteries accompanying these extraocular muscles theoretically contribute to the blood supply of the dermis–fat graft and the muscles will impart greater movement to the graft for improved prosthesis motility.

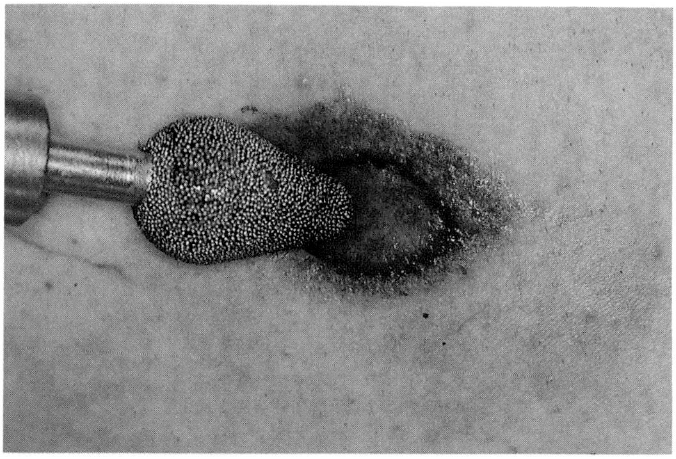

FIGURE 22–19

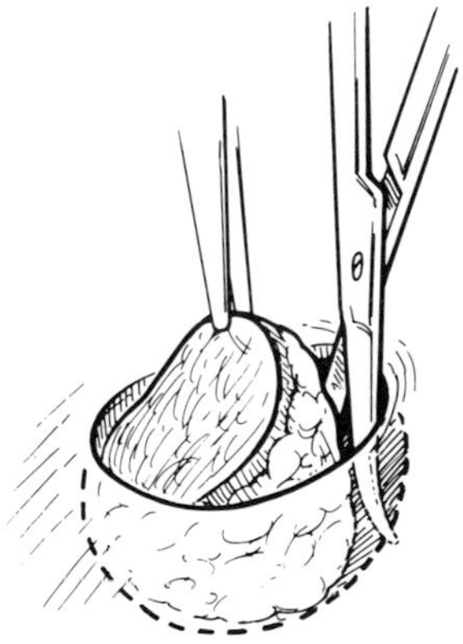

FIGURE 22–20

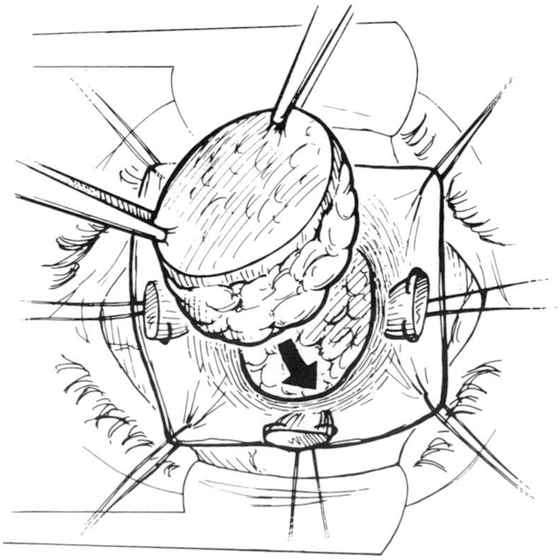

FIGURE 22–21

Figure 22–22. The anterior Tenon's capsule is secured to the peripheral edge of the dermis with interrupted 5–0 chromic or Vicryl sutures. Note the exposed horizontal rectus muscle sutured to one edge of the dermis of the graft.

Figure 22–23. The previously undermined conjunctiva is overlapped over the edge of the dermis. It is then sutured to the anterior surface of the graft with 6–0 plain or 7–0 Vicryl sutures, leaving a central zone of bare dermis measuring approximately 10 × 15 mm.

Figure 22–24. Appearance of the socket with the central portion of the dermal surface exposed and surrounding conjunctiva sutured to the periphery of the dermis.

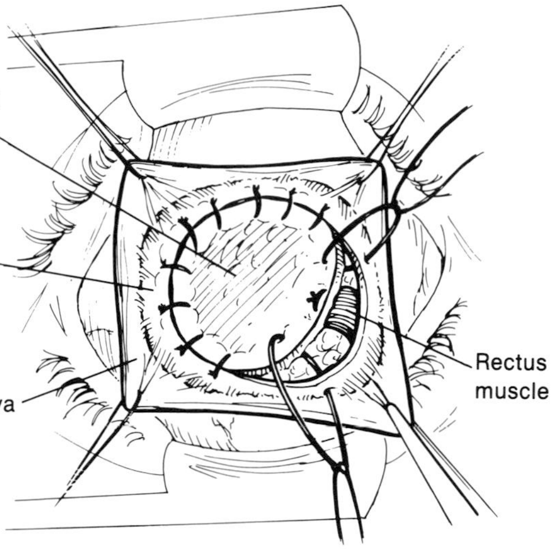

FIGURE 22–22

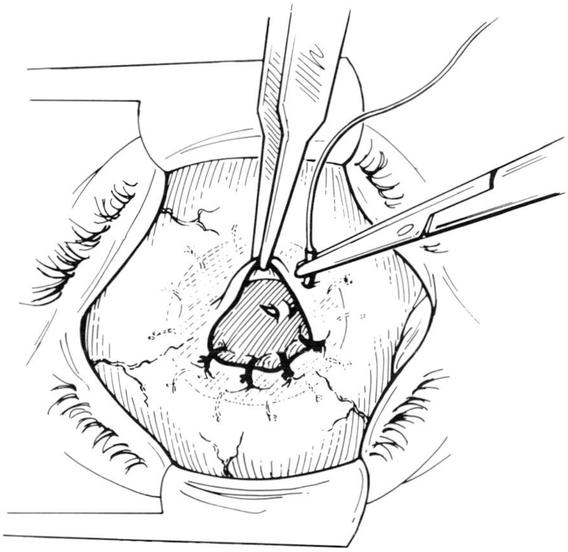

FIGURE 22–23

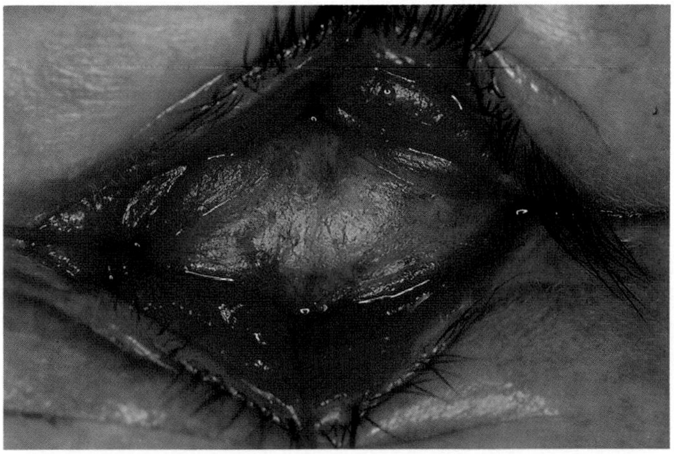

FIGURE 22–24

Figure 22–25. A cross-sectional view of the socket illustrates the fat component of the graft positioned in the intraconal space, the vertical rectus muscles and anterior Tenon's capsule sutured to the dermal borders, and conjunctiva partially advanced over the edges of dermis. A conformer is placed into the socket to maintain the fornices and prevent adhesions between the raw surface of the graft and eyelids. Antibiotic ointment and a pressure bandage should be placed as described above.

Subperiosteal Orbital Implant

Correction of enophthalmos and superior sulcus deformities can be achieved by inserting an alloplastic subperiosteal implant along the floor of the orbit. The surgical approach to the orbital floor can be transconjunctivally through the inferior fornix or transcutaneously by fashioning a lower lid myocutaneous flap. My own preference is for the infraciliary lower lid skin incision approach because surgical trauma to the conjunctiva, lower lid retractors, and orbital fat is avoided, and visualization is improved because the intact orbital septum limits the orbital tissues from herniating into the surgical site. This type of surgery can be performed under local anesthesia, but general anesthesia is preferred because of the manipulation of the deep orbital tissues and orbital bones. Hemostasis is facilitated by injecting lidocaine 2% with epinephrine 1:100,000 subcutaneously along the length of the lower lid from the margin down to the inferior orbital rim.

Two 4–0 silk sutures are placed in the medial and lateral third of the lid margin at the gray line and upward traction is applied.

Figure 22–26. An infraciliary skin incision is made with a Bard–Parker size 15 blade along the length of the eyelid, and a skin–muscle flap is dissected with scissors inferiorly down to the level of the inferior orbital rim, as shown diagrammatically in cross section. Care is taken to avoid violating the orbital septum to prevent orbital fat from prolapsing anteriorly. Bleeding points are controlled with a bipolar cautery.

With the myocutaneous flap retracted inferiorly, an incision is made with a Bard–Parker size 15 blade through the periosteum 2 mm below the edge of the inferior orbital rim. Freer periosteal elevators are used to reflect the periosteum off the orbital floor as far posteriorly as the inferior orbital fissure. Bone wax or a unipolar Bovie cautery can be used to reduce bleeding from the exposed bone. Once the floor of the orbit is adequately exposed, one of three different implants can be chosen for volume augmentation as described in the following.

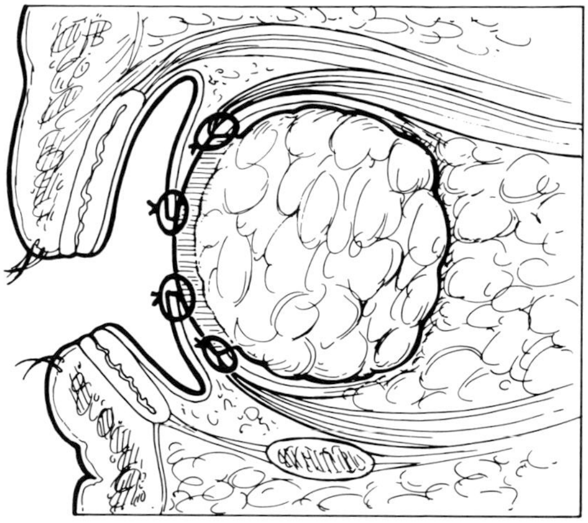

FIGURE 22–25

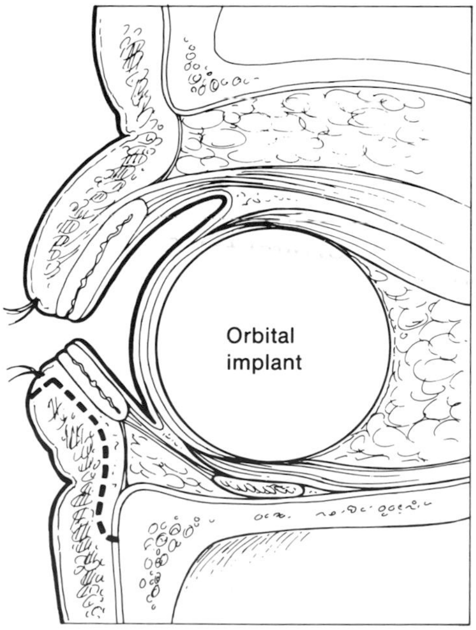

FIGURE 22–26

Technique 1: Methyl Methacrylate Resin Implants

Prefabricated subperiosteal implants are made of methyl methacrylate resin that measure 24 mm wide and 27 mm long and are available in four different heights, with their volumes ranging from 2.1 to 3.0 ml (Spivey–Allen Cosmetic Floor Implant available from Hansen Ophthalmic Lab, 2412 Towncrest Drive, Iowa City, IA). While lifting the orbital tissues from the floor with a broad malleable retractor, the largest implant that the orbit will permit is placed into the subperiosteal space along the floor with its wider and thicker end directed posteriorly. The anterior tongue-shaped extension of the implant is positioned 2 to 3 mm posterior to the orbital rim.

Figure 22–27. With the implant in proper position a few drops of cyanoacrylate tissue adhesive are applied between a dried area of the orbital bony floor and the implant to prevent implant extrusion or migration. Alternatively, the implant can be anchored into place by drilling two holes 5-mm apart in the orbital rim that exit through the orbital floor. A 3–0 Prolene or Supramid suture or 28-gauge wire is passed in a mattress fashion through the drill holes and the implant holes and tied with the knot in the orbit.

Figure 22–28. A Spivey–Allen subperiosteal implant is shown correctly positioned behind the rim and wired to the inferior orbital rim as the orbital tissues are retracted superiorly.

Technique 2: Soft Medical Grade Silicone Implant

An alternative to the hard methyl methacrylate resin implant is a soft medical grade silicone implant that can be custom fitted by contouring it to the individual socket. These implants are available in four sizes, with volumes ranging from 1.6 to 3.25 ml (Nerad-Modified Spivey–Allen Floor Implant available from Hansen Ophthalmic Lab, 2412 Towncrest Drive, Iowa City, IA). Once the proper-sized silicone implant is positioned on the orbital floor behind the orbital rim, it can be secured in place with a drop of cyanoacrylate glue.

Technique 3: Room Temperature Vulcanizing Silicone

Room temperature vulcanizing (RTV) silicone is another useful material applicable for subperiosteal orbital volume augmentation procedures.

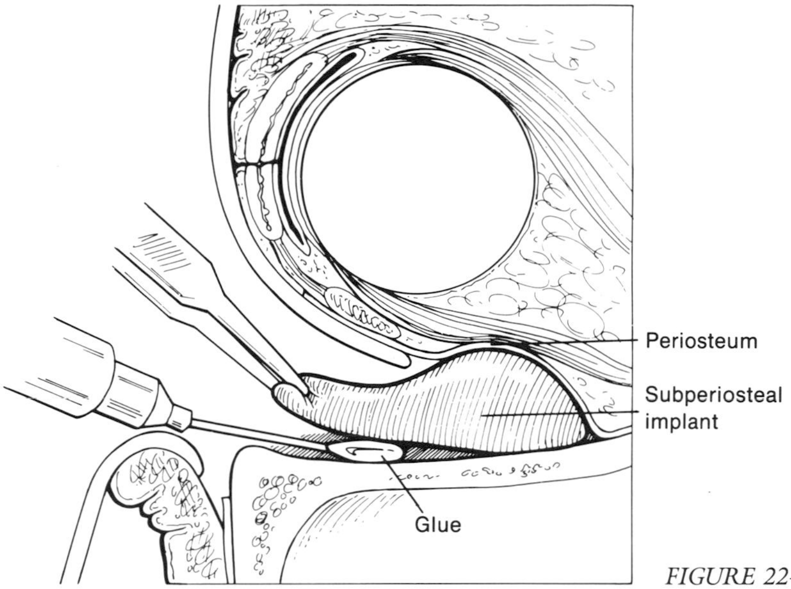

FIGURE 22–27

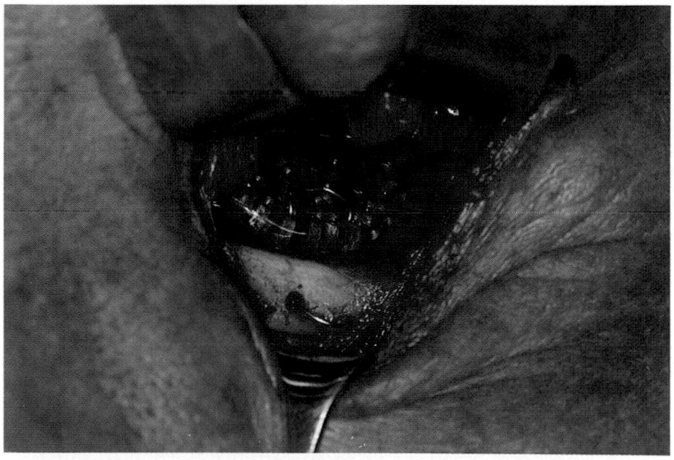

FIGURE 22–28

Figure 22–29. Once it is prepared according to Table 22–1, the RTV silicone is placed in a controlled manner onto the posterior orbital floor through tubing placed on a syringe. Approximately 1 mm of enophthalmos will be corrected with 1 ml of implant material and, therefore, the amount of silicone inserted is empirically determined and based on the degree of preoperative enophthalmos and superior sulcus deformity. Once the silicone becomes slightly firm, it can be molded or repositioned until the desired shape and position are achieved. No steps to fixate the RTV silicone to the orbital floor are necessary.

Once the selected subperiosteal implant is secured into place, the edges of periosteum are reapproximated with interrupted 4–0 Vicryl sutures using a small semicircle needle. The skin–muscle incision is closed with a running 7–0 nylon suture. A conformer is placed in the socket and the traction sutures are then secured to the forehead above the brow with Steri-strips to maintain the lower lid on upward traction postoperatively, which helps to prevent the development of lower lid retraction.

Figure 22–30. A cross-sectional view of the orbit illustrates the closure of periosteum below the inferior orbital rim and skin closure of the infraciliary incision. The subperiosteal implant adds volume to the socket and displaces the orbital implant and orbital soft tissues superiorly and anteriorly to reduce the superior sulcus deformity and enophthalmos.

Ophthalmic antibiotic ointment is applied to the socket and incision and a pressure bandage is applied.

Inferior Fornix Reconstruction

A foreshortened inferior fornix will prevent the retention of a comfortable and mobile ocular prosthesis. Preoperatively, the surgeon should assess whether the amount of forniceal conjunctiva will be sufficient to allow fornix reconstruction without a mucous membrane graft, or whether a graft will be necessary. When the socket mucous membrane is inadequate, grafting oral mucosa is required, usually in conjunction with tightening of the lower lid lateral canthal tendon.

The surgery can be performed with local anesthesia by infiltrating the lower eyelid subcutaneously and subconjunctivally with lidocaine 2% with epinephrine 1 : 100,000. With the lower lid retracted inferiorly with preplaced 4–0 silk marginal traction sutures, an incision is made with a Bard–Parker size 15 blade through the conjunctiva in the existing inferior fornix.

TABLE 22–1
Preparation of Room Temperature Vulcanizing (RTV) Silicone*

1. Place 50 ml of RTV silicone elastomer (base) in a 6-oz stainless steel mixing bowl and steam autoclave at 270°F (132.2°C) for 5 min
2. Divide the elastomer into two 25-ml portions and allow to cool to room temperature.
3. When the step of the operative procedure is reached for the use of the RTV silicone, add between 5 and 10 drops of RTV catalyst to one of the 25-ml portions of the RTV elastomer and mix thoroughly. This amount of catalyst added to the elastomer gives you 4 to 5 minutes of working time. The catalyst should not be sterilized and can be added into the elastomer directly by the circulating nurse.
4. Place the mixture into a 10-ml plastic syringe with the plunger initially removed, and then replace the plunger.
5. Add the desired amount of RTV silicone into the surgical site through the syringe outlet.
6. If the initial mixture does not vulcanize as required, use the remaining 25-ml of sterile RTV elastomer with either more or less catalyst. More catalyst will cause the RTV silicone to vulcanize more rapidly, whereas less catalyst gives you more working time.

(Adapted from Neuhaus RW, Shorr N. Moldable alloplastic material: RTV silicone #382. Presented at the Academy of Ophthalmology Scientific Meeting, Dallas, 1987.)

* *Available from Factor II, Inc., Lake Side, AZ 85929 (Item No.: Med 63-82 RTV Silicone)*

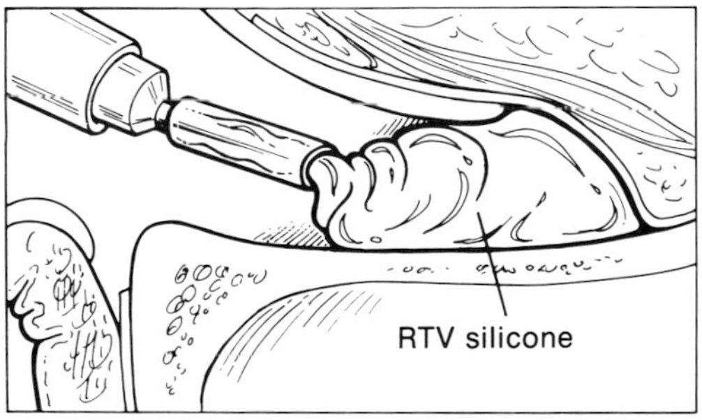

FIGURE 22–29

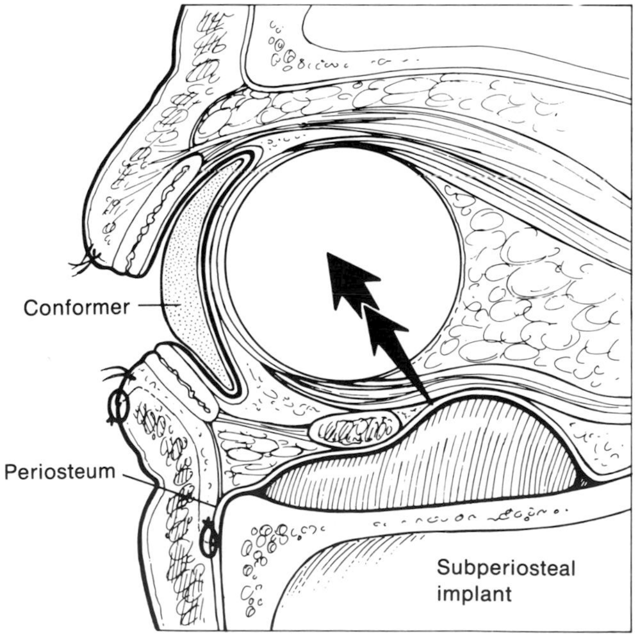

FIGURE 22–30

Figure 22–31. A cross-sectional representation of the socket shows the conjunctival incision in the inferior fornix and plane of the conjunctival undermining (*dotted line*). Dissection is then carried out inferiorly toward the inferior orbital rim (*bold line*).

Figure 22–32. The inferior forniceal conjunctiva is undermined with a blunt Wescott scissors to separate the conjunctiva from underlying scar tissue.

Figure 22–33. Sharp dissection is performed through any scar tissue and the lower lid retractors create a plane directed toward the inferior orbital rim (see Figure 22–31). Meticulous hemostasis should be achieved with a bipolar cautery. At this point, the surgeon should confirm whether there is sufficient conjunctiva or inadequate mucous membrane available for fornix re-formation.

Technique 1: Fornix Reconstruction Without a Mucous Membrane Graft

When the edges of the undermined conjunctiva can be opposed without foreshortening the fornix, re-formation of the fornix can be accomplished without a mucous membrane graft.

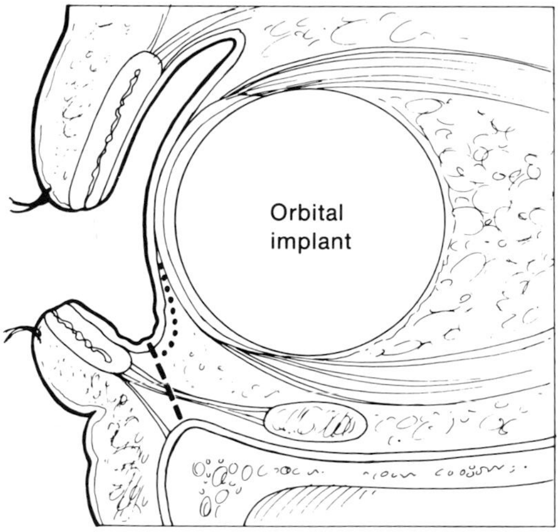

FIGURE 22–31

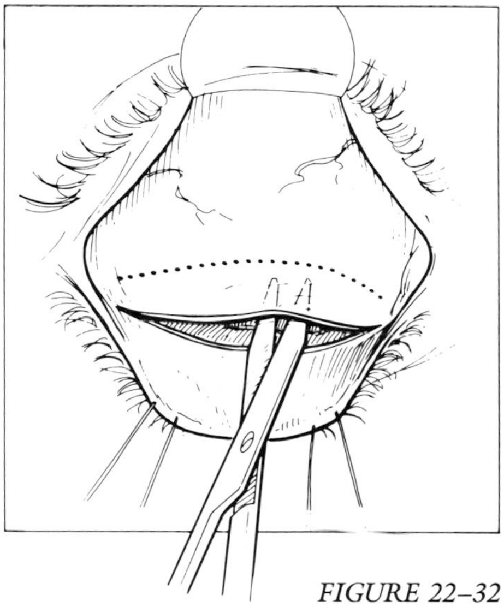

FIGURE 22–32

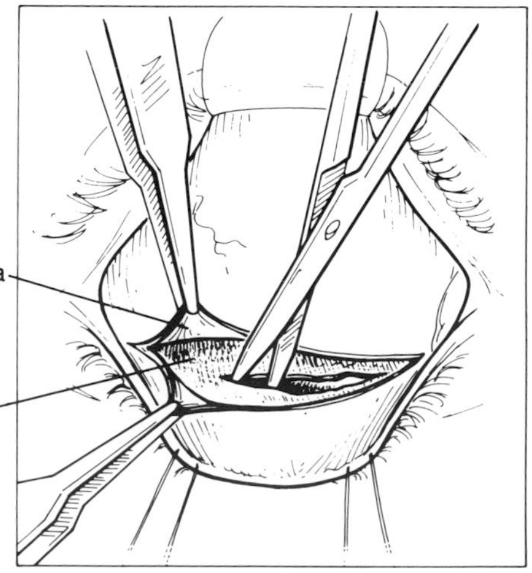

FIGURE 22–33

Figure 22–34. The conjunctival incision is closed with a running 6–0 plain suture.

Figure 22–35. A silicone retinal band (4 to 8 mm wide) is trimmed lengthwise to fit into the fornix. Three double-armed 4–0 silk or 3–0 Supramid sutures on large cutting needles are passed through the silicone stent in a horizontal mattress fashion, the conjunctiva at the proposed new fornix, the periosteum of the inferior orbital rim, and finally through the orbicularis muscle and skin anterior to the orbital rim.

Figure 22–36. The silicone stent is positioned in the deepened inferior fornix by Supramid mattress sutures.

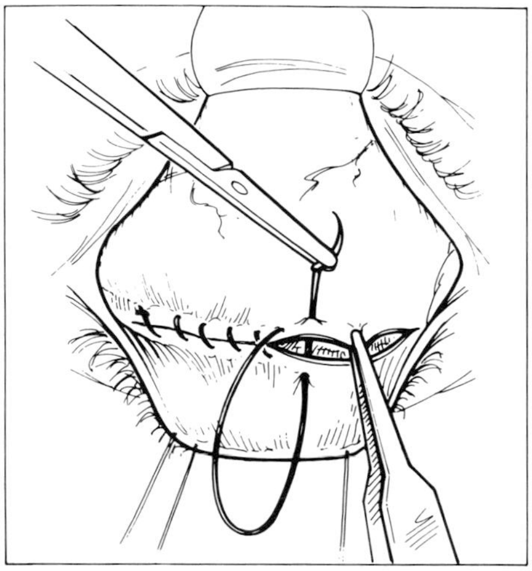

FIGURE 22–34

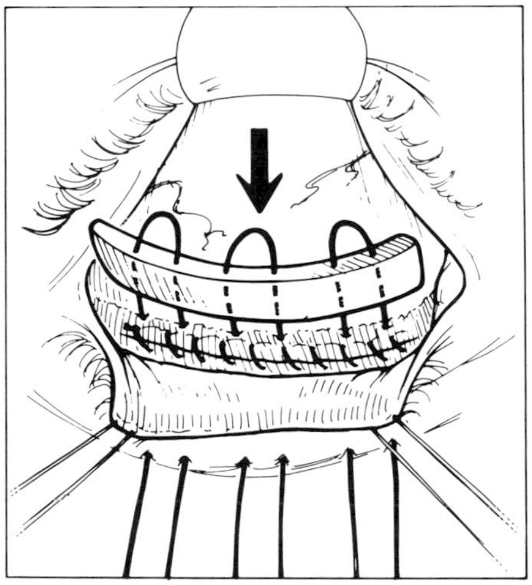

FIGURE 22–35

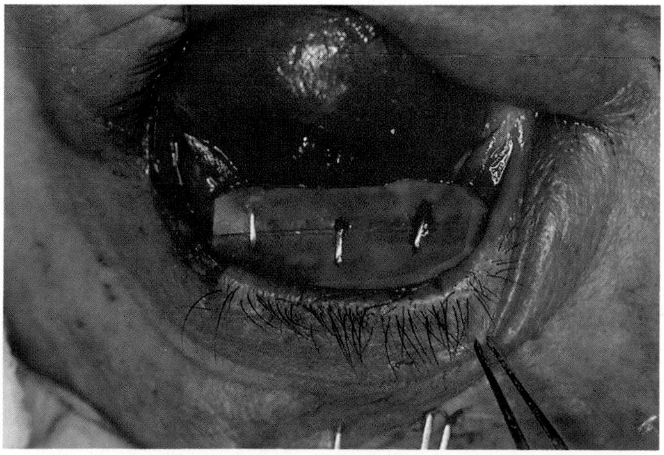

FIGURE 22–36

Figure 22–37. These mattress sutures are tied over bolsters under moderate tension, at the level of the inferior orbital rim to secure the stent and reconstructed deepened fornix toward the rim. They are left in place for 2 weeks. If sutured too tightly, necrosis of the tissues under the bolsters may result. A lateral canthal tightening procedure of the lower lid, such as a lateral tarsal strip procedure (as described elsewhere in this text), often is performed in combination with inferior fornix re-formation. Antibiotic ointment is applied to the socket and external bolsters and a conformer is inserted.

Technique 2: Fornix Reconstruction With a Mucous Membrane Graft

If when the edges of the conjunctiva are opposed the fornix is foreshortened owing to insufficient conjunctiva, a mucous membrane graft is necessary to line the re-formed fornix. A full-thickness or partial-thickness mucous membrane graft is harvested from the mouth, as described under the next section on socket reconstruction for contracted socket. The raw surface area necessary to cover with the mucous membrane graft is measured, and a graft of equal size, usually approximately 15 mm vertically by 25 mm horizontally, is laid into the recipient site.

Figure 22–38. The graft is sutured into a foreshortened inferior fornix with interrupted 7–0 Vicryl or 6–0 chromic sutures to increase the fornical depth.

Figure 22–39. Either a silicone stent as described earlier, or a methyl methacrylate conformer is inserted to immobilize the mucous membrane graft in apposition with the vascular bed in the deepened fornix. The retinal band is placed over the mucous membrane graft to immobilize it in the reconstructed inferior fornix.

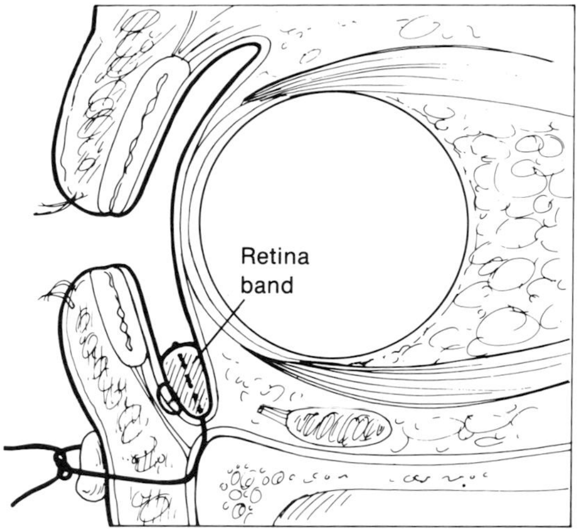

FIGURE 22–37

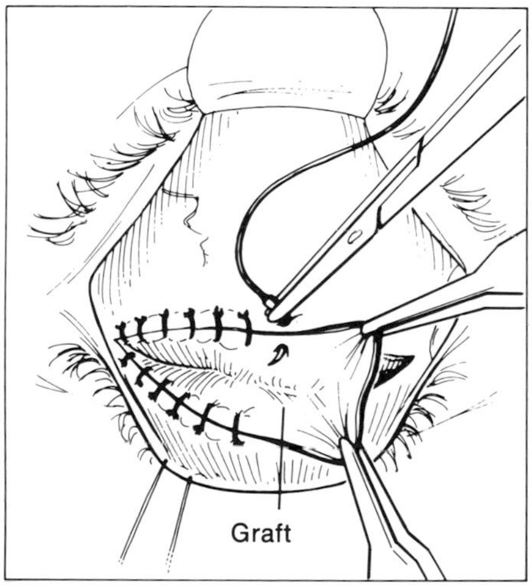

FIGURE 22–38

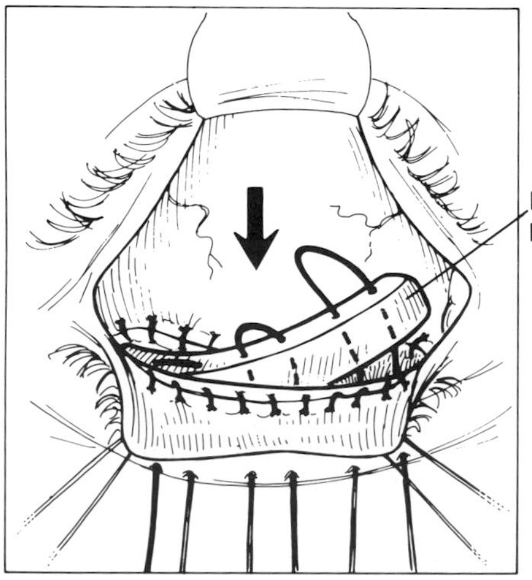

FIGURE 22–39

Figure 22–40. The graft forms the mucous membrane lining of the deepened fornix, as shown in cross section, and is secured in position by the stent.

Figure 22–41. A methyl methacrylate conformer is shown as an alternative to a silicone band to maintain the depth of the reconstructed inferior fornix. Tightening of the lateral canthal tendon with a lateral tarsal strip procedure may be performed if necessary at this point (see Chapter 10). Temporary tarsorrhaphy sutures are passed between the upper and lower eyelids utilizing two double-armed 4–0 silk sutures in a mattress fashion, which are tied over cotton bolsters (see Figure 22–41). Antibiotic ointment is placed into the socket, and a pressure patch is applied for 1 week; tarsorrhaphy sutures are removed after 2 weeks.

Socket Reconstruction for Contracted Socket

General anesthesia is usually administered for socket reconstruction because of the difficulty of anesthetizing dense scar tissue in the socket, as well as the need to obtain an oral mucosal graft. To gain adequate exposure of the contracted socket, 4–0 silk traction sutures are passed through the upper and lower eyelid margins. Lidocaine 2% with epinephrine 1:100,000 is infiltrated into the socket tissues and lids for its vasoconstrictive properties.

Figure 22–42. A horizontal incision is made through the conjunctiva across the length of the socket with a Bard–Parker size 15 blade. The conjunctiva is separated from the underlying scar tissue with scissor dissection.

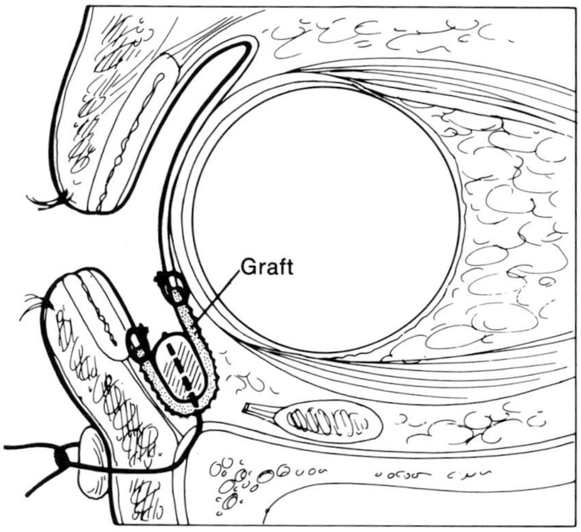

FIGURE 22–40

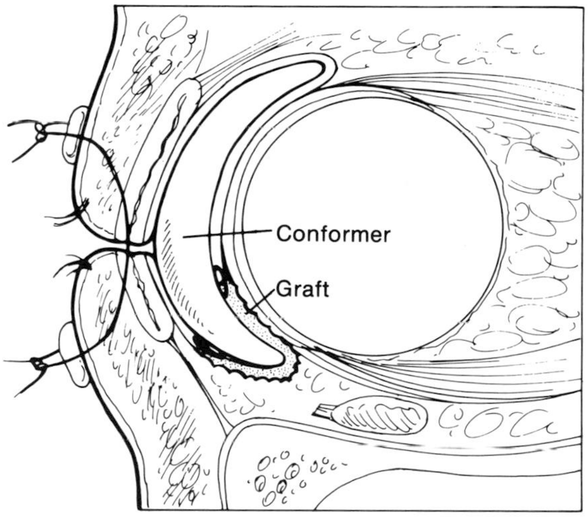

FIGURE 22–41

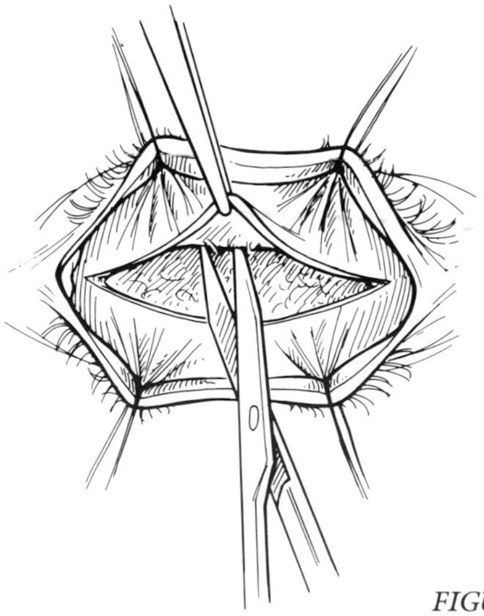

FIGURE 22–42

Figure 22–43. An attempt to spare all of the present conjunctiva is made by undermining it superiorly and inferiorly to the upper and lower tarsal borders (*dotted line*). Cauterization of bleeders with a bipolar cautery should not be excessive so as not to compromise the blood supply for the mucous membrane graft. Sharp dissection is undertaken for the excision of the scar tissue and Tenon's capsule in the central socket cavity until adequate space is created to allow formation of deep fornices.

Figure 22–44. A cross-sectional view of the socket illustrates the superior and inferior fornices of adequate depth created by dissection anterior to the scar tissue and Tenon's capsule that encapsulate the orbital implant. A mucous membrane graft must next be harvested for lining the expanded socket cavity.

Full-thickness mucous membrane is usually preferable graft material for socket reconstruction because less shrinkage will occur and it is easier to handle. On the other hand, partial-thickness mucous membrane grafts have the advantage of ease of harvesting, more rapid healing, fewer potential complications at the donor site, and the ability to reharvest a graft from the same site if additional graft material is needed at a later date.

Membrane Harvesting

Technique 1: Partial-Thickness Mucous Membrane Harvest Technique

Figure 22–45. A towel clip is placed at each end of the lower lip, and the lip is everted under tension. Lidocaine 2% with epinephrine 1:100,000 is delivered submucosally to facilitate hemostasis. Twenty to thirty milliliters of saline is injected along the length of the lip through an 18-gauge needle until the lip becomes firm and the mucosal surface is rigid. A small amount of mineral oil is applied to the mucosa for lubrication.

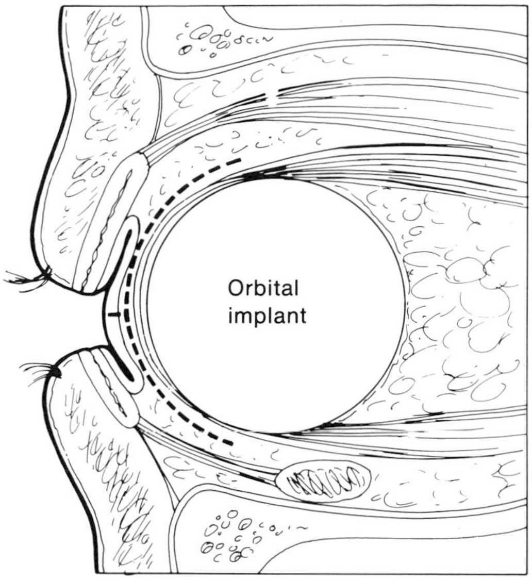

FIGURE 22–43

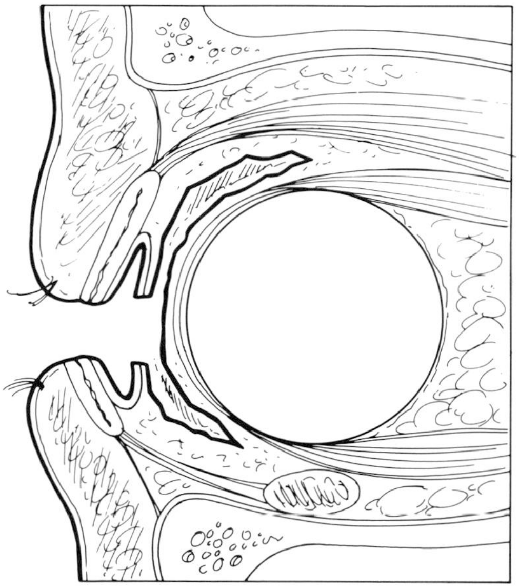

FIGURE 22–44

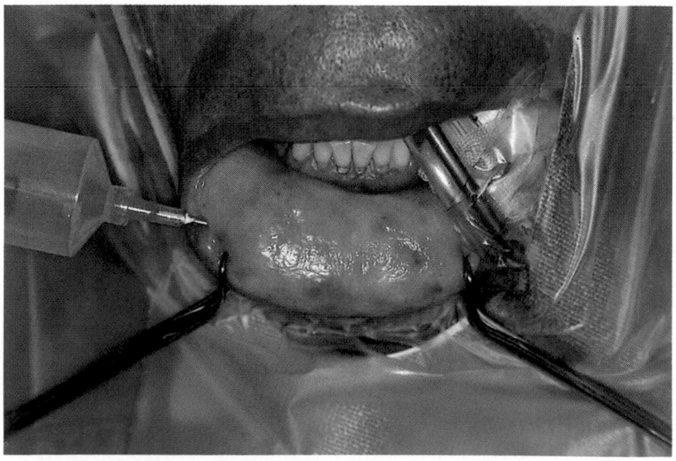

FIGURE 22–45

Figure 22–46. A Castroviejo mucotome is prepared with a 0.4-mm spacer plate (shim) and positioned at one side of the lip. With moderate pressure applied, the mucotome is advanced parallel to the lip, while toothed forceps grasp the graft as it comes through the head of the mucotome.

Figure 22–47. The mucotome is removed and the graft is cut from the attached end with Wescott scissors. The mucous membrane graft is set aside in gentamicin solution with the orientation of the mucosal surface maintained. Surgicel is applied to the graft donor site and the towel clips are removed. If more partial-thickness mucous membrane is needed for the socket reconstruction, the same technique can be used to harvest a graft from the upper lip.

Technique 2: Full-Thickness Mucous Membrane Harvest Technique

Full-thickness mucous membrane grafts can be harvested from either the lips or cheek. When the inner surface of the lips are chosen as donor sites, their preparation is similar to that described in the foregoing, including fixation with towel clips and submucosal infiltration with epinephrine-containing anesthetic solution. A marker pen outlines the graft to be obtained while avoiding the margin of the lips and frenulum, and a Bard–Parker size 15 blade is used to incise the mucosa.

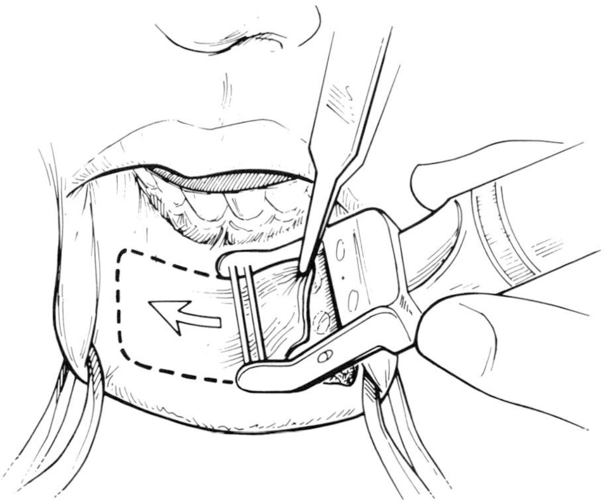

FIGURE 22–46

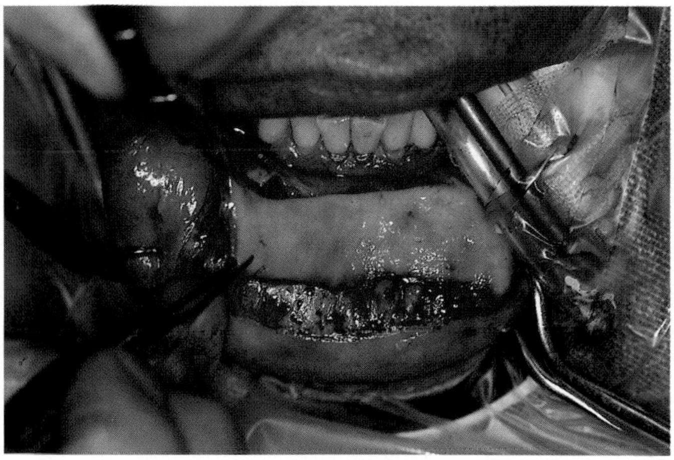

FIGURE 22–47

Figure 22–48. The full-thickness graft is excised with scissors, the attached submucosal tissue is trimmed with scissors with the graft placed over a finger, and the graft is temporarily placed into antibiotic solution. Bleeding from the donor site is controlled with a bipolar cautery, and no closure of this site is necessary. Gelfoam or Surgicel is placed over the donor site.

Figure 22–49. To obtain a full-thickness graft of the buccal mucosa, the donor site is injected with 2% lidocaine with 1:100,000 epinephrine and delineated with a marker pen. Towel clips are placed along the lateral aspect of the upper and lower lip for exposure of the cheek mucous membrane. When harvesting tissue from the cheeks, it is important to identify Stensen's duct and avoid this structure, as well as the gums. The mucosa is incised with a Bard–Parker size 15 blade and sharp and blunt scissor dissection is carried out to obtain the full-thickness mucosal graft. Closure of the donor site can be achieved with a running 5–0 chromic suture, but is usually unnecessary. Hemostasis is achieved with a bipolar cautery. The graft should be handled as described for a split-thickness graft.

Socket Conformer Insertion

Technique 1: Socket Conformer Without Orbital Fixation

Before surgery is resumed in the socket, gloves should be changed, and a different set of sterile instruments should be used because of the nonsterile field from which the oral mucous membrane was obtained.

Figure 22–50. One technique for lining the socket with the mucous membrane graft involves placing the graft directly into the socket cavity and suturing its edges to the borders of the previously undermined socket conjunctiva with 7–0 Vicryl or chromic sutures. The graft is shown partially sutured to the edge of the conjunctiva.

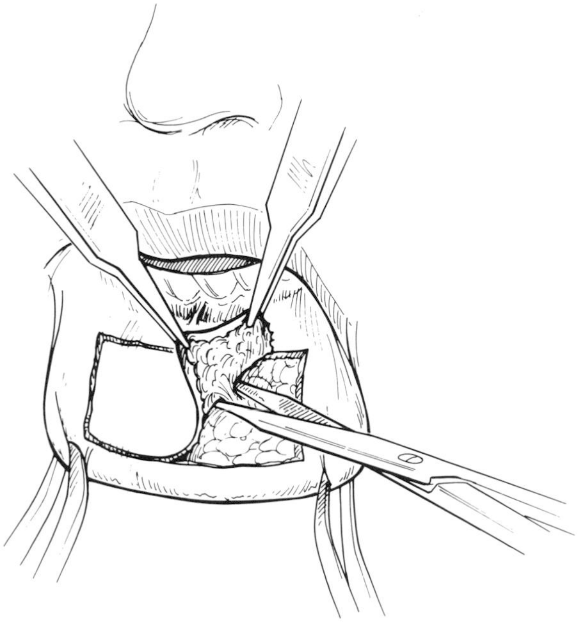

FIGURE 22–48

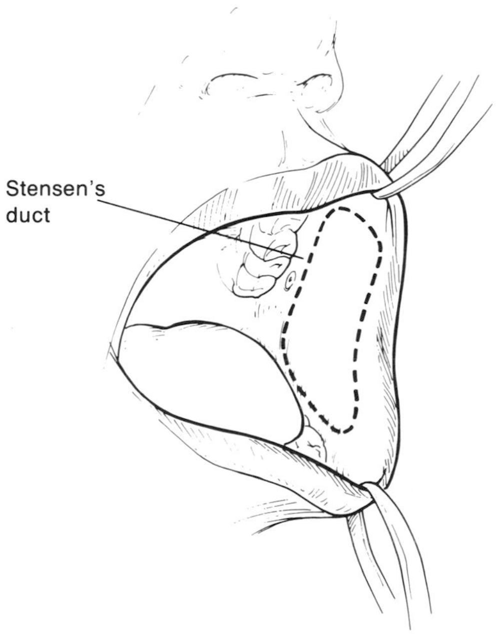

FIGURE 22–49

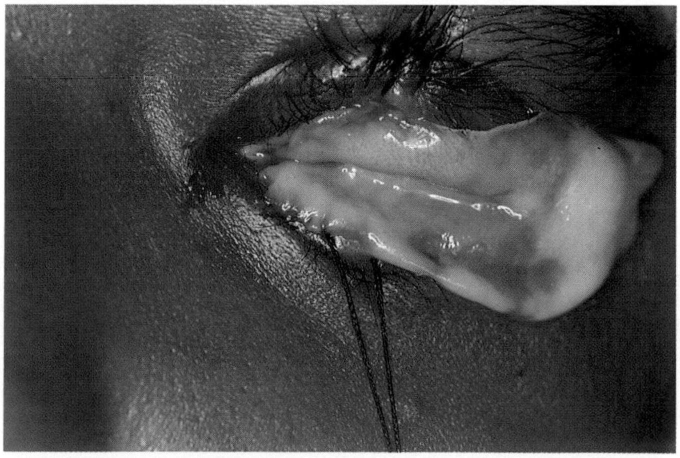

FIGURE 22–50

Figure 22–51. Enough redundancy of the graft must be allowed for re-formation of the fornices and placement of an acrylic conformer to maintain the fornices during the healing period. A conformer as large as possible, and yet still allow the eyelids to close completely without undue tension, should be placed into the socket. Antibiotic ointment is applied and the eyelids are splinted together with two 4–0 silk temporary tarsorrhaphy sutures for as long as will be tolerated, usually 3 to 6 weeks.

Technique 2: Socket Conformer With Orbital Fixation

This technique was described by Putterman (1977) and uses a prefabricated custom-designed conformer available in different sizes (available from Robert B. Scott, 111 N. Wabash Avenue, Suite 1516, Chicago, IL) that is fixated to the orbital rims to maintain the fornices and immobilize the mucous membrane graft. Gloves are changed and a new set of sterile instruments are used to continue surgery in the socket after harvesting a mucous membrane graft of adequate size that will accommodate the selected conformer. Lidocaine 2% with epinephrine 1:100,000 is injected over the central superior and inferior orbital rims.

Figure 22–52. Incisions 2-cm long are outlined (*dashed lines*) over the corresponding orbital rims, and skin and muscle are incised with a Bard–Parker size 15 blade parallel to both rims. The same blade is used to incise the periosteum, which is reflected from the orbital margin with a periosteal elevator to expose the orbital roof superiorly and floor inferiorly.

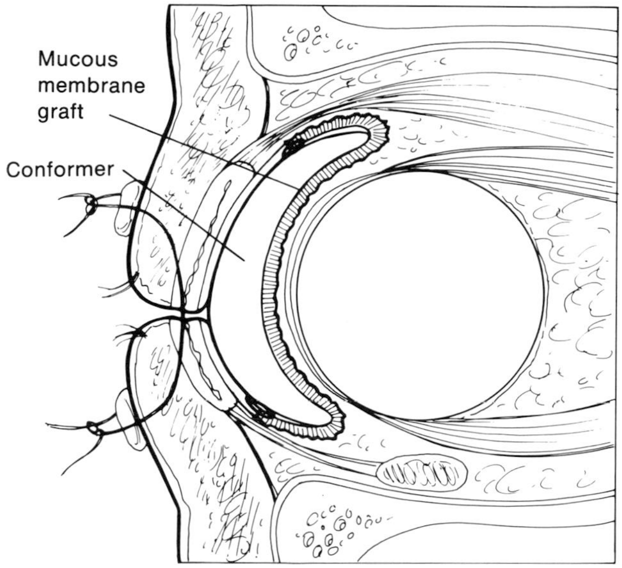

FIGURE 22–51

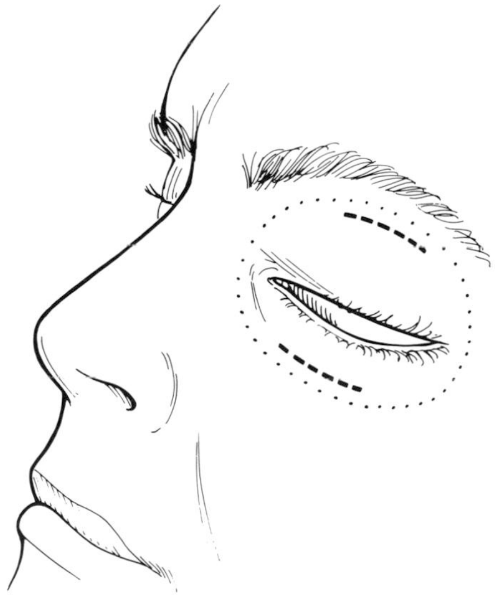

FIGURE 22–52

Figure 22–53. The orbital roof is exposed with a ribbon retractor protecting the orbital tissues, and two holes, approximately 1 cm apart, are created with a motor-driven drill in the superior orbital rim by applying the drill bit 3 mm above the margin and exiting 5 mm posterior to the rim. The cross-sectional view illustrates the course of the drill holes to which the conformer will be attached. Saline should be used to irrigate the field while drilling to minimize heat production, and a suction tip should be applied to maintain visualization. Two drill holes are created similarly in the inferior orbital rim while a ribbon retractor exposes the orbital floor.

Figure 22–54. A 2–0 Supramid suture is passed in a mattress fashion externally to internally through the drill holes. A large, loose surgical needle facilitates the passage of one arm of the suture at a time from the superior rim through the periorbita and levator muscle into the newly created superior fornix. The same needle is used to pass each arm of the Supramid suture exiting through the orbital floor into the re-formed inferior fornix. The periosteum is closed with interrupted 4–0 Vicryl sutures, the orbicularis muscle layer is reunited with 6–0 Vicryl sutures, and the skin incision is reopposed with a running 7–0 nylon suture.

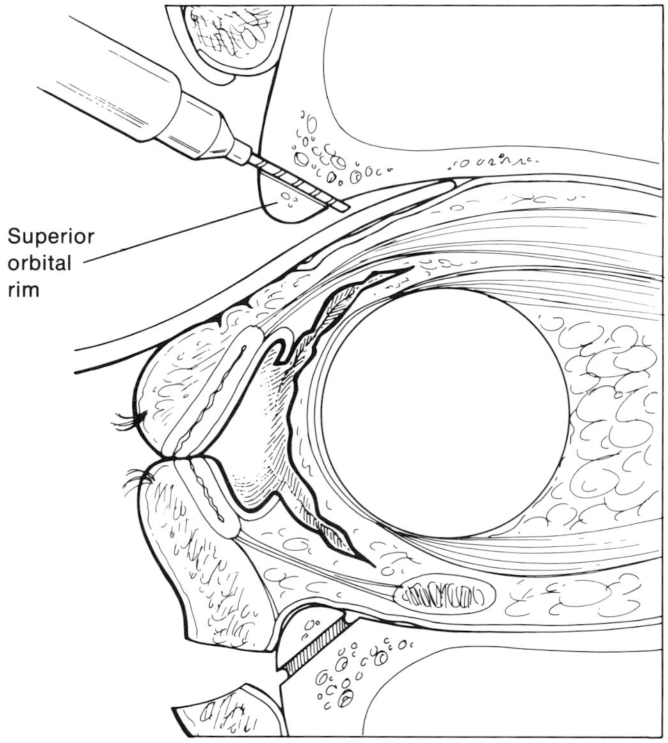

FIGURE 22–53

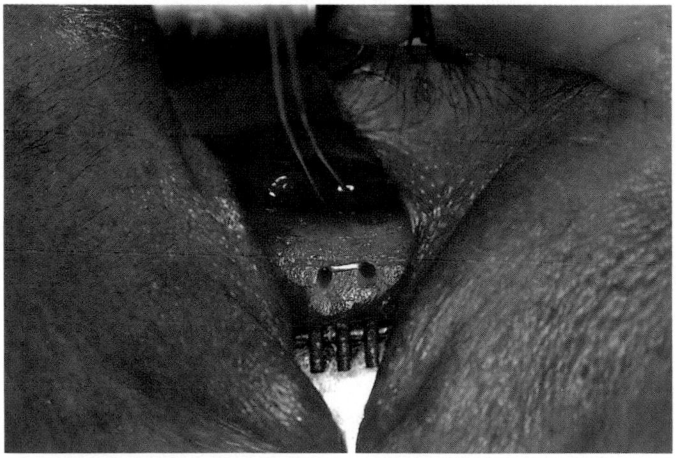

FIGURE 22–54

Figure 22–55. The mucosal graft is then wrapped around the conformer (which has a large central hole and eight smaller holes to anchor it to the orbital rim) with the raw surface outward and its edges are sutured together with 6–0 Vicryl sutures. The conformer should be entirely covered with the mucous membrane graft except for the anterior aspect of the central drainage hole.

Figure 22–56. The inferior fornix sutures are passed through the most peripheral inferior central two holes in the conformer from the external to internal surface, and then are brought through the inferior central holes exiting externally. The sutures coming through the superior fornix are passed similarly through the conformers superior central holes.

Figure 22–57. The wrapped conformer is inserted into the socket and behind the eyelids, and the sutures tied tightly so that the conformer is immobilized.

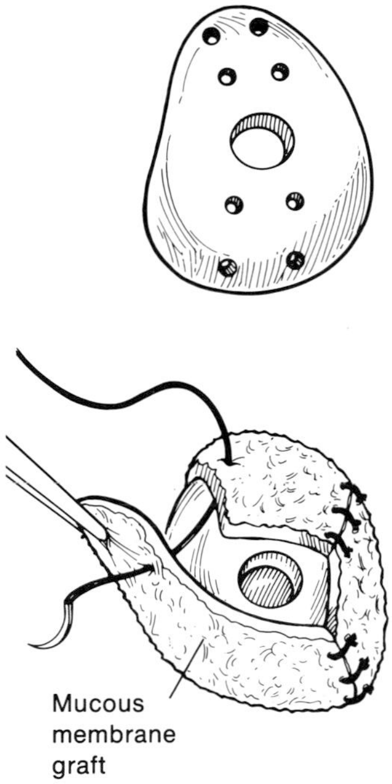

FIGURE 22–55

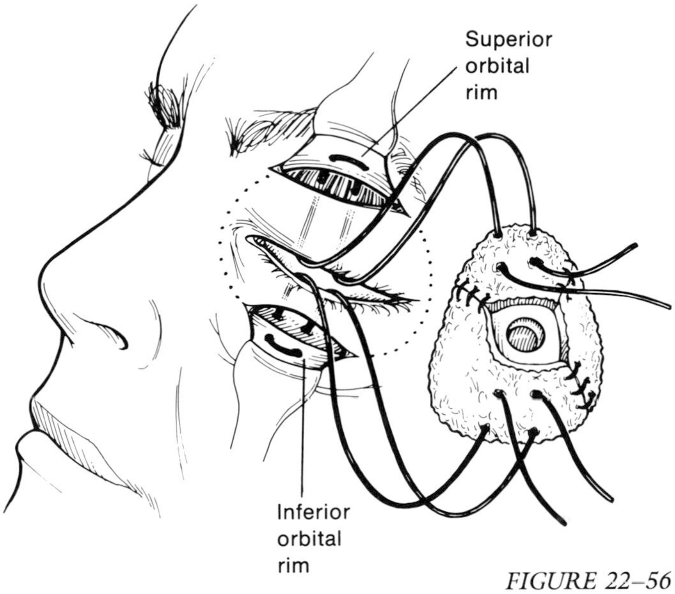

FIGURE 22–56

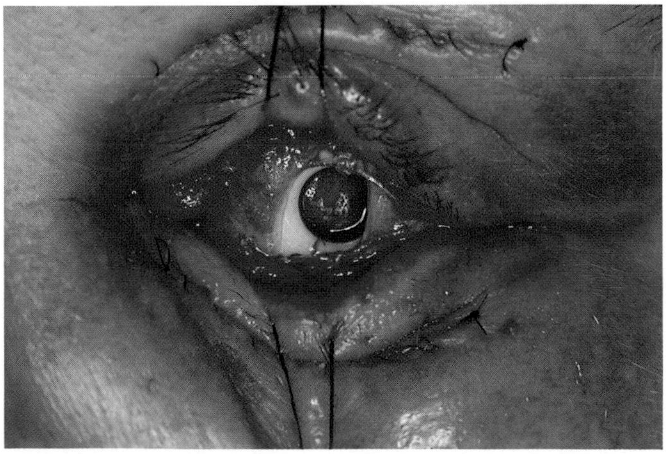

FIGURE 22–57

Figure 22–58. Two temporary 4–0 silk tarsorrhaphy sutures are tied over cotton bolsters and removed after 3 to 6 weeks. The cross-sectional diagram illustrates the reconstructed socket with a conformer wrapped with a mucous membrane graft. The pathways of the Supramid sutures are shown fixating the conformer to the orbital rims. Closure of the periosteum and skin incisions are depicted with the temporary tarsorrhaphy sutures tied over bolsters. The Supramid sutures fixating the conformer are removed after approximately 6 months, and the conformer is exchanged for an ocular prosthesis as soon as possible.

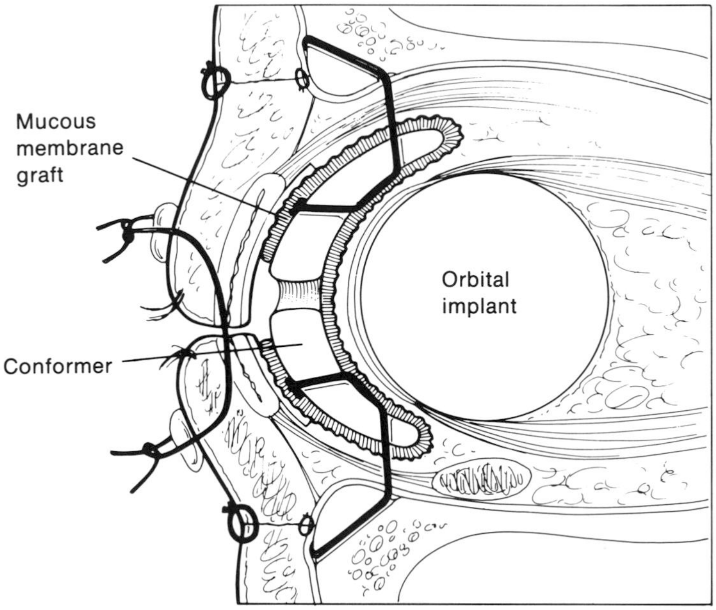

FIGURE 22–58

POSTOPERATIVE CARE

At the conclusion of all socket procedures, sterile antibiotic ophthalmic ointment should be applied followed by the placement of a polymethylmethacrylate (PMMA) conformer. Pressure bandages are always indicated to reduce postoperative bleeding and edema, fixate the conformer in the socket to maintain the eyelid position and fornices, and immobilize the socket tissues and grafts, when used. The pressure patch can be removed after 5 to 7 days, at which time the patient may start to place an antibiotic ointment into the socket three times a day for an additional 2 to 3 weeks. Broad-spectrum oral antibiotics that provide coverage for anaerobic organisms should be prescribed for all patients who undergo mucous membrane grafts. Systemic antibiotics should also be considered when socket surgery is performed in patients who are immunocompromised (e.g., diabetics), have a history of recent or chronic socket infections, or have evidence of poor socket hygiene. Once the socket is completely healed, the patient should be evaluated by an ocularist for proper prosthetic fitting.

Care of the donor site for patients in whom oral mucous membrane grafts are harvested include the use of antiseptic mouthwashes and, occasionally, lidocaine jelly. When full-thickness grafts are obtained from the cheek, the mouth should be opened widely and external pressure applied 4 to 5 times daily for 2 months to minimize contracture of the graft host site.

SURGICAL COMPLICATIONS

Early or late recurrence of orbital implant extrusion may complicate the postoperative course following the placement of a patch graft or secondary implant owing to the loss of viability of the patch graft, resorption of the material in which the implant was wrapped, contracture of the socket tissues, inadequate blood supply, too large a primary or secondary implant, or infection. Infections should be treated intensively with systemic and topical antibiotics. Once the infection clears and inflammation subsides, replacement of the implant with one that is smaller in diameter or a dermis–fat graft can be considered. Multiple extrusions, repeat surgeries, and chronic inflammation may lead to socket contracture that would require mucous membrane grafting for reconstruction. Epithelial cyst formation along the conjunctival wound may require excision.

Dermis–fat grafts have been associated with postoperative graft atrophy or necrosis, leading to insufficient volume replacement. Sloughing of the graft may be prevented by limiting the graft size to no larger than 25 mm in diameter. A secondary alloplastic implant or subperiosteal implant may be required for subsequent volume augmentation. Excessive socket volume and orbital cyst formation following dermis–

fat grafting may necessitate excision of part of the graft or cyst. Infected dermis–fat grafts should be treated with appropriate topical and systemic antibiotics. Retention of graft cilia may be only temporary, but occasionally will warrant epilation or electrolysis. Granulomas and small conjunctival cysts also may develop in the late postoperative period.

Such complications as extrusion or migration of subperiosteal orbital implants may be avoided by properly securing the implants to the orbital floor or rim; however, should these develop, the implant may need to be removed. Removal of these implants may also be indicated for such rare complications as orbital pain, facial hypesthesia, and infection. Inadequate volume augmentation of the socket with the implant can be improved by either replacing the original implant with one that is larger or placing an additional subperiosteal implant along the lateral orbital wall.

The most common complication following fornix re-formation and socket reconstruction is recurrent contracture. Sufficient dissection of the fornices and the placement of an oversized mucous membrane graft that accounts for approximately 30% natural shrinkage of the graft can help prevent this difficult problem. Also, repeat surgeries should be delayed for at least 1 year to allow resolution of active cicatricial processes. Recurrence of a foreshortened fornix that was initially re-formed with a stent alone might require a second procedure utilizing a mucous membrane graft. If a nonsecured conformer placed in the socket is expelled because of contraction of the tissues, another mucous membrane graft and use of a conformer sutured or wired to the orbital rim becomes necessary. Graft failure may result from infection, limited blood supply owing to prior irradiation or chemical burn, hemorrhage, and poor fixation to underlying tissues. The surgeon should be aware that repeat attempts of socket surgery lead to a buildup of scar tissue, and each successive procedure becomes less likely to succeed. After multiple failed reconstructive procedures, or in cases in which the eyelids are severely distorted, further surgery is not recommended; instead, an occlusive patch or orbital prosthesis may offer the patient a superior alternative. Complications at the donor site of oral mucous membrane grafts include submucosal scar formation with cicatricial bands and webs that may require reconstructive Z-plasty techniques if oral dysfunction develops.

Chapter Twenty-Three

ENUCLEATION AND TECHNIQUES OF ORBITAL IMPLANT PLACEMENT

Delyse R. Buus, Jan W. Kronish, and David T. Tse

Enucleation refers to the removal of the eye and the anterior portion of the optic nerve from the orbit. It is a complex procedure that alters the volume and normal anatomic relations of the orbit and may be complicated by eyelid malpositions, superior sulcus deformities, and implant migration or extrusion. Ideally, the technique selected should minimize the potential for development of these complications while providing for volume replacement, prosthetic motility, and maintenance of adequate fornices for prosthesis retention.

Many orbital implants have been developed in an attempt to improve the results of enucleation surgery, but most have been associated with an increase in postoperative complications. Exposed integrated implants and tantalum mesh spheres are designed to improve motility, but are now rarely used because of their high extrusion rates. The buried semi-integrated implant (Allen, Iowa, Universal) transmits movement from its irregular anterior surface to the back surface of a custom-fitted prosthesis. Excellent motility may be attained and, as the prosthesis is supported by the implant rather than the inferior fornix, lower eyelid malpositions and superior sulcus abnormalities may occur less frequently. Socket discomfort and extrusion associated with the Allen and Iowa implants have been attributed to conjunctival erosion over the surface prominences. The Universal implant was designed with lower, more rounded protrusions to reduce the incidence of these complications, and the extrusion rate appears to be comparable with that associated with spherical implants. The Universal is the only semi-integrated implant widely available.

The sphere is the most commonly used orbital implant and is positioned within the muscle cone either anterior or posterior to the posterior Tenon's capsule. The largest implant that can be accommodated within Tenon's space without undue tension at closure is generally the 18-mm sphere. Implantation behind the posterior Tenon's allows placement of a larger sphere with greater volume replacement and provides an additional tissue barrier to postoperative extrusion and migration. Motility is felt to be dependent on forniceal movement, as the smooth contour of the spherical implant cannot engage the overlying prosthesis. Attachment of the extraocular muscles to the conjunctival fornices may thus enhance prosthesis motility. Imbrication of the extraocular muscles directly in front of the implant is less efficient in transmitting movement and is associated with postoperative sphere migration.

Recently, a fully integrated orbital implant composed of porous durapatite (hydroxyapatite), an inorganic substrate of bone, has been introduced. Fibrovascular ingrowth into this porous spherical implant reduces the potential of implant migration and extrusion, and allows the implant to be coupled directly to the prosthesis, thereby providing superior prosthetic motility. The implants are wrapped in preserved sclera to provide a surface onto which the extraocular muscles are attached. Thorough screening and appropriate precautions must be taken when implanting donor material, such as preserved sclera, to reduce the risk of transmission of infectious disease. Once the implant is incorporated in the orbital tissues (approximately 6 months after implantation), a peg that inserts into the implant integrates with the ocular prosthesis to transmit the full range of implant motility.

INDICATIONS

The choice between enucleation and evisceration is often controversial. However, in the surgical management of a suspected intraocular malignancy, enucleation is the procedure of choice. Evisceration risks incomplete tumor removal, and precludes an intact specimen for pathologic examination. In the presence of an inadequate scleral shell, such as may occur with severe trauma, phthisis bulbi, or following scleral buckling procedures, enucleation is also preferable to optimize volume replacement. Enucleation removes uveal tissues more effectively than evisceration, and is indicated when the slight risk of sympathetic ophthalmia following evisceration is unacceptable.

Enucleation may be considered in the treatment of any painful or unsightly blind eye for pain control or cosmetic rehabilitation. However, superior cosmesis and motility are usually achieved if the natural globe can be preserved and fitted with a scleral shell or cosmetic contact lens. A Gunderson flap may improve tolerance of a scleral shell if corneal sensation is problematic. It is often possible to restore comfort to a blind painful eye nonsurgically with topical medications, cyclocryotherapy, or retrobulbar alcohol injections. In children particularly, the globe should be preserved whenever possible to provide a stimulus for orbital growth and development.

PATIENT PREPARATION

The procedure is explained, including the temporary use of a conformer and the plan for prosthesis fitting at 5 to 6 weeks following surgery. The patient is prepared for the loss of full motility and the possibility of an asymmetric appearance. The potential complications of infection and extrusion should also be discussed.

ENUCLEATION

Enucleation may bc pcrformed under local retrobulbar or general anesthesia. If the eye to be removed is not readily apparent by external examination, the operative side should be reconfirmed by reviewing clinic notes, the operative consent, and by performing an indirect ophthalmoscopy in the operating room. The unoperated fellow eye is protected with a metal Fox shield under the drape throughout the procedure.

A speculum is placed between the eyelids and a 360° conjunctival peritomy is performed adjacent to the corneal limbus with Westcott scissors.

Tenon's capsule is separated from the underlying sclera to the level of the rectus muscle insertions. A Stevens tenotomy scissors is passed into each quadrant and is gently spread to separate Tenon's capsule from the sclera between the rectus muscles. A muscle hook is passed behind a rectus muscle insertion.

Figure 23–1. A locking suture of double-armed 5–0 Vicryl is placed in the muscle tendon near the insertion, and the muscle is then disinserted. The ends of the suture are clamped to the surrounding drape with a hemostat. This procedure is repeated with the remaining rectus muscles. A 1- to 2-mm stump of medial and lateral rectus tendon left adherent to the sclera is useful for traction later in the procedure.

Figure 23–2. The superior oblique muscle is identified with a small muscle hook and detached from the globe. The inferior oblique muscle is also isolated with a small muscle hook, and cross-clamped with a hemostat before transection. Any remaining adherent tissues should be separated from the globe with Stevens scissors as far posteriorly as possible.

A horizontal rectus muscle insertion is grasped with a hemostat, and the globe is gently elevated. A large curved hemostat is passed behind the globe from the temporal side. The optic nerve position is determined by strumming the nerve with the closed instrument. The tips are then opened and placed on either side of the optic nerve as far posteriorly as possible. The nerve is clamped for 5 minutes. The hemostat is removed and a curved enucleation scissors is passed behind the globe in a similar fashion. The nerve is then transected, taking care to avoid trauma to the rectus muscles, and the globe is removed.

Figure 23–3. Alternatively, the globe can be removed with the enucleation snare. With gentle upward traction on the globe, the wire is slowly tightened as the snare is advanced posteriorly. For hemostasis, the wire is allowed to constrict the nerve for 5 minutes before transection.

Once the globe is removed, the socket is packed with a moistened gauze pad and pressure is applied for several minutes. When the gauze is removed, the socket is inspected and any residual bleeding points are cauterized with a bipolar cautery. Three different techniques to insert an orbital implant are discussed below.

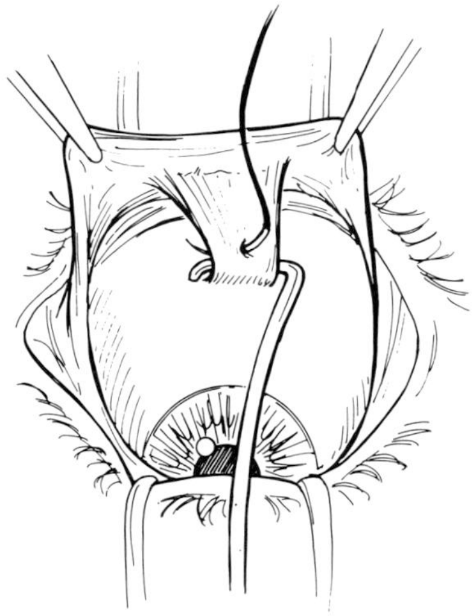

FIGURE 23–1

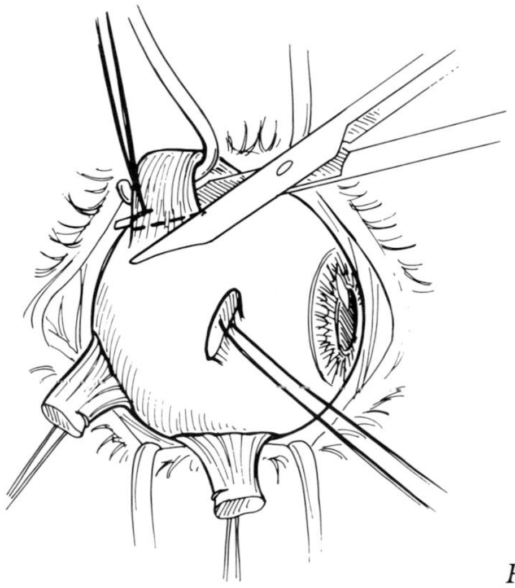

FIGURE 23–2

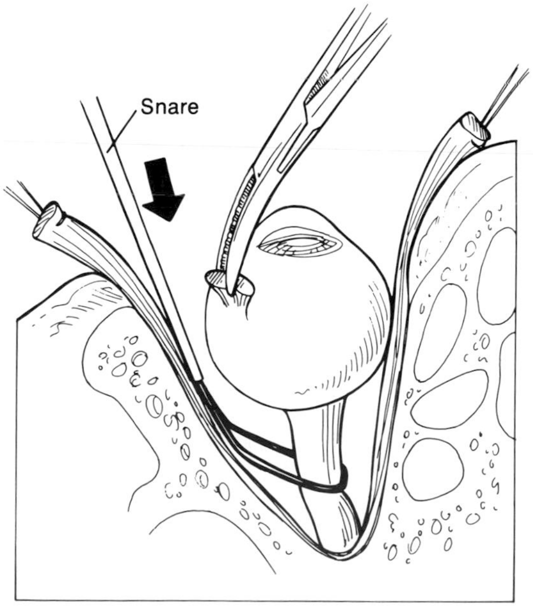

FIGURE 23–3

TECHNIQUES OF ORBITAL IMPLANT PLACEMENT

Universal Implant

The Universal implant is a quasi-integrated, completely buried motility implant made of compression-molded methyl methacrylate resin. The implant comes in small, medium, and large sizes. It has a convex, hemispheric posterior surface. On the anterior surface, there are four smooth mounds, with a horizontal and a vertical groove between them. Holes and tunnels are placed on various parts of the implant for suture passage and fibrous tissue ingrowth. The largest implant that can be accommodated without undue tension at closure of the muscles and Tenon's capsule should be selected.

Figure 23–4. The implant is placed within Tenon's capsule with the assistance of the Ferguson clips placed at the corner of each mound. The implant is oriented so that the rectus muscles will lie in the grooves between the mounds. A double-arm 4–0 chromic suture on a large needle is passed through each of the tunnels on the anterior surface of the implant. The vertical rectus muscles are united first, followed by the horizontal rectus muscles.

Figure 23–5. Each arm of the vertically preplaced suture is used to engage the cut end of the vertical rectus muscle tendon from its undersurface. The needle should engage the muscle about 2 mm from the severed edge to prevent the suture cheese-wiring through the tissue.

Figure 23–6. The ends of the chromic suture are then tied, thus joining the vertical muscles. To reinforce this union, both arms of the locking 5–0 Vicryl suture left at the stump of the inferior rectus muscle are passed through the cut edge of the superior rectus muscle. The sutures are then tied. Similarly, the arms of the superior rectus locking suture are brought around the edges of the inferior rectus and passed through the inferior rectus tendon from the underside.

Figure 23–7A, B. The procedure is repeated with the horizontal rectus muscles. An additional suture may be used to secure the vertical rectus stump to the horizontal rectus muscle stump. The Ferguson clips are then removed.

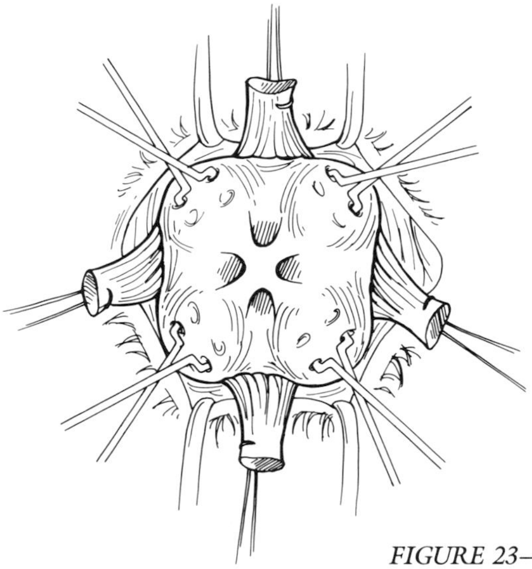

FIGURE 23–4

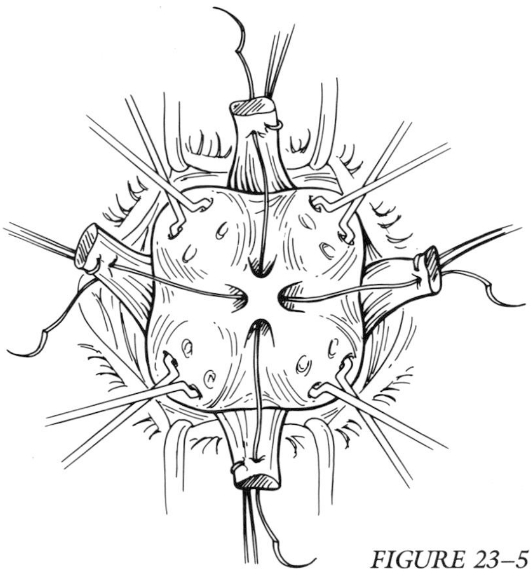

FIGURE 23–5

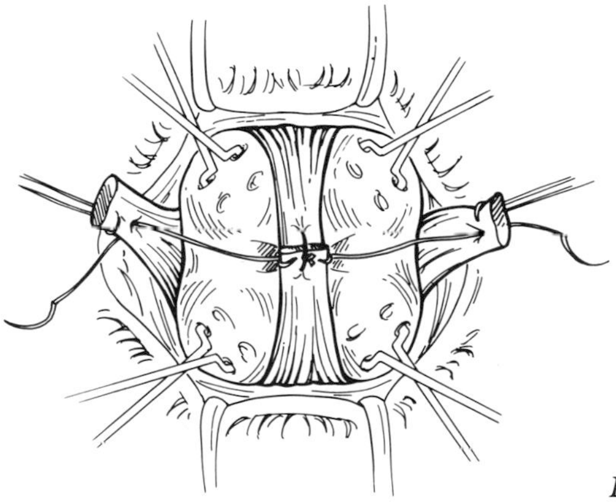

FIGURE 23–6

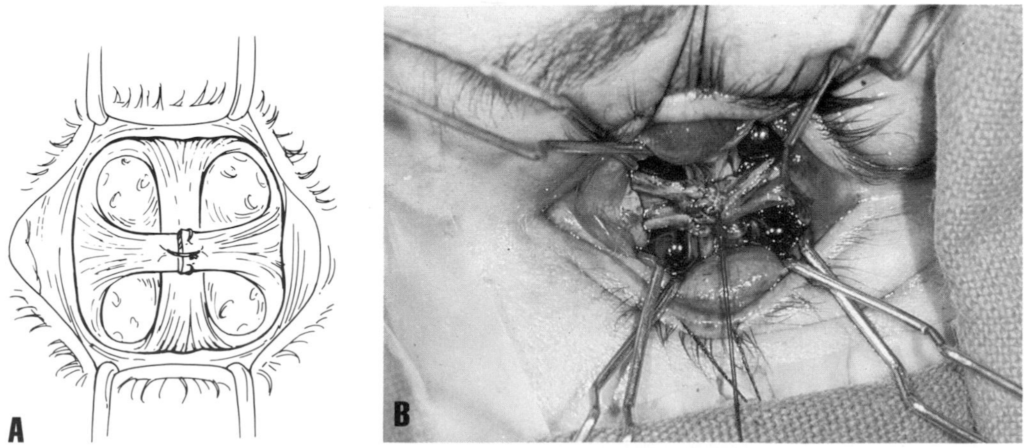

FIGURE 23–7

Figure 23–8. The anterior Tenon's capsule is closed horizontally with multiple interrupted 5–0 Vicryl sutures. Proper closure of this layer is important to prevent conjunctival dehiscence over the mounds.

Figure 23–9. The conjunctiva is closed with a running 5–0 or 6–0 chromic suture. Antibiotic ointment is applied to the fornix and a conformer is placed. A pressure dressing is applied to minimize postoperative edema.

Sphere Implant

When a silicone or acrylic sphere orbital implant is chosen, one additional step during the isolation and disinsertion of the extraocular muscles during enucleation is to suture the end of the inferior oblique muscle to the inferior border of the lateral rectus muscle to enhance the support of the implant. Also, some surgeons prefer to pass the locking sutures through the cut ends of the medial and lateral rectus muscles and do not engage the vertical rectus muscles, thereby allowing them to retract. Care is taken throughout these steps to avoid disturbing the intermuscular septum that provides a barrier to implant migration.

Figure 23–10. Once the globe is removed and all bleeding points are cauterized, the largest sphere implant that the orbit will accommodate (usually 20 or 22 mm diameter) is placed into the intraconal fat pad. The intraconal fat can be visualized through the vent created in the posterior Tenon's capsule after cutting the edges of the optic nerve.

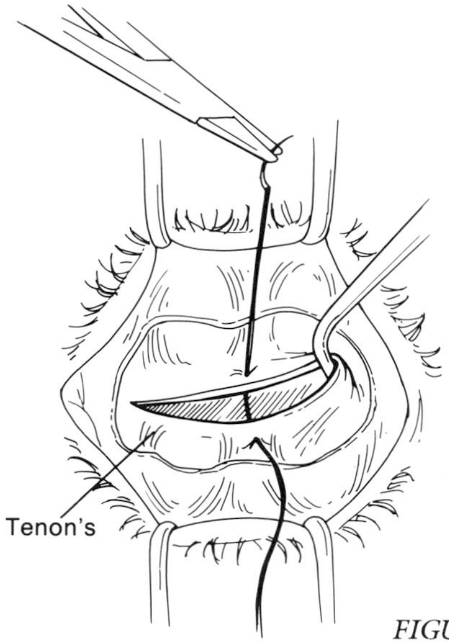

FIGURE 23–8

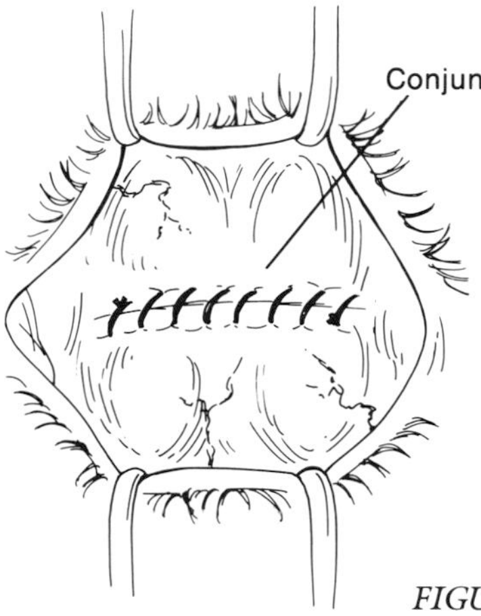

FIGURE 23–9

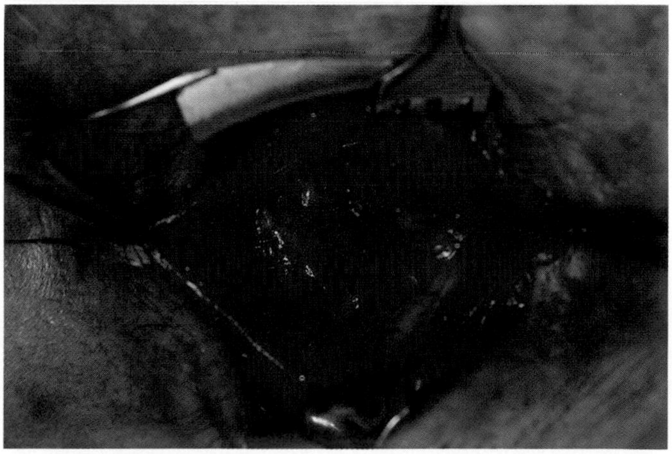

FIGURE 23–10

Figure 23–11. The implant is placed through the opening in the posterior layer of Tenon's capsule. Although rarely necessary, scissors may be used to enlarge the rent in posterior portion of Tenon's capsule to accommodate the implant. It is unnecessary to wrap the sphere implant in donor sclera or fascia lata when placed behind posterior Tenon's capsule, which represents an additional tissue barrier to prevent extrusion. The edges of posterior Tenon's capsule should be approximated without tension in a vertical orientation with interrupted 4–0 Vicryl sutures (see Figure 23–11).

Figure 23–12. The double-armed Vicryl sutures secured to the ends of the rectus muscles are passed through the anterior layer of Tenon's capsule and conjunctiva into the corresponding conjunctival fornices to transmit greater mobility to the prosthesis.

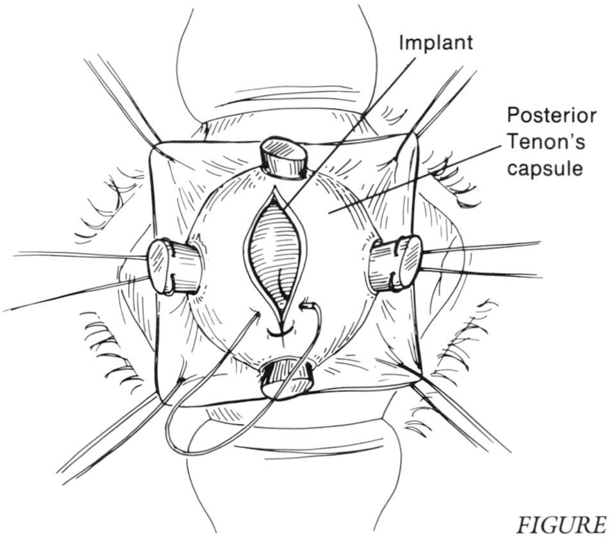

FIGURE 23–11

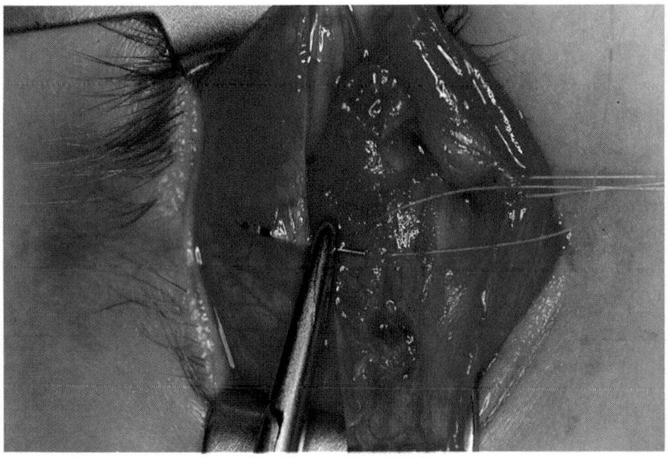

FIGURE 23–12

Figure 23–13. The anterior Tenon's capsule is closed horizontally with interrupted 5–0 Vicryl sutures with the knots buried. The edges of conjunctiva are united with a running 6–0 plain gut suture.

Figure 23–14. A cross-sectional view of the orbit illustrates the sphere positioned posteriorly to the posterior Tenon's capsule, the anterior Tenon's capsule, and the conjunctiva. Antibiotic ointment and an acrylic conformer are placed into the socket and a firm pressure bandage applied.

Hydroxyapatite Integrated Orbital Implant

From a selection of 16, 18, 20, and 22 mm diameter hydroxyapatite implants (Integrated Orbital Implants, 12526 High Bluff Drive, Suite 300, San Diego, CA), the largest one that will fit into Tenon's capsule without undue tension at closure of the anterior Tenon's capsule and conjunctiva is chosen. Wrapping the implant in preserved sclera obtained from a whole cadaver eye facilitated the introduction of the rough-surfaced hydroxyapatite sphere and a covering on which to suture the extraocular muscles is provided. Relaxing incisions must be made in the donor tissue, where the cornea was excised from the sclera to accommodate the implant, and these incisions are reunited with interrupted 4–0 Vicryl sutures.

Figure 23–15. A hydroxyapatite spherical implant is shown wrapped in sclera. The exposed area of hydroxyapatite will be positioned posteriorly in the orbit. Four perforating "windows," each measuring approximately 3 × 6 mm, are made in the sclera a few millimeters anterior to the equator of the sclera-wrapped implant with Stevens scissors or a blade at the proposed 12:00, 3:00, 6:00, and 9:00 o'clock meridians. The wrapped hydroxyapatite implant is placed within Tenon's capsule with the exposed portion of the implant oriented posteriorly to promote fibrovascular ingrowth from the orbit.

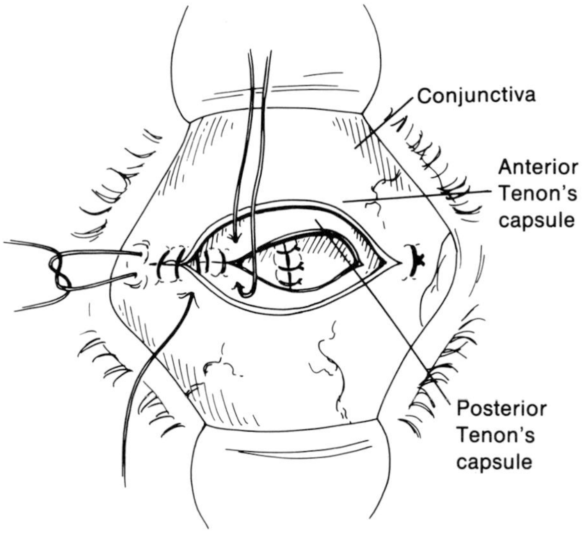

FIGURE 23–13

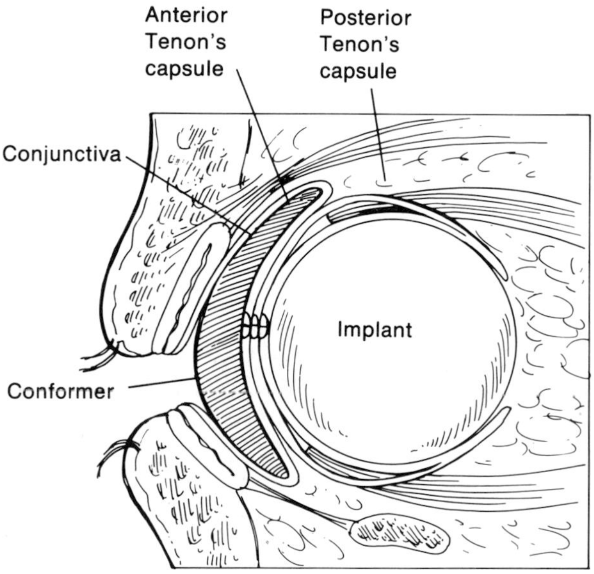

FIGURE 23–14

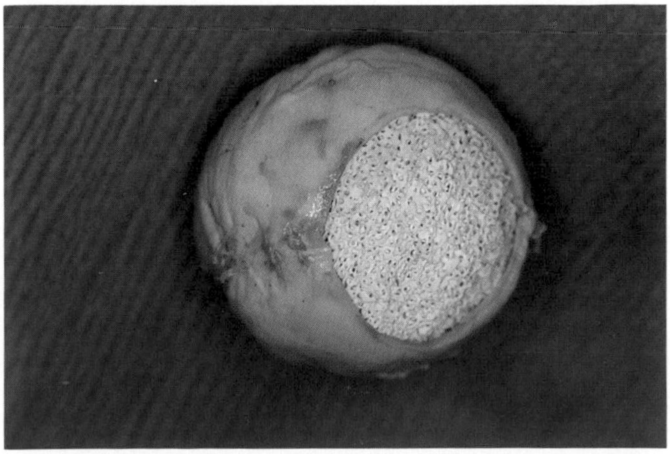

FIGURE 23–15

Figure 23–16. A cross-sectional view of the orbit shows the implant inserted within Tenon's capsule.

Figure 23–17. The rectus muscles are sutured to the anterior lip of the corresponding scleral windows with the double-armed Vicryl sutures in a mattress fashion. One of the rectus muscles is shown sutured to the scleral wrapping. This step approximates the cut edge of the rectus muscle with the exposed portion of the hydroxyapatite material to promote fibrovascular ingrowth. The anterior layer of Tenon's capsule is closed over the implant with interrupted 5–0 Vicryl sutures. The conjunctival edges are reapproximated with a running 6–0 plain gut suture. Sterile ophthalmic antibiotic ointment is placed in the socket, an acrylic conformer is inserted, and a pressure dressing is applied.

Six weeks after surgery, the patient is fitted with a standard customized ocular prosthesis. If one chooses to integrate the prosthesis with the implant, it is necessary to wait at least 4 to 6 months to insert a motility peg into the implant. This period is allotted to permit the implant to become fully integrated and vascularized with the surrounding orbital tissues. Vascularization within the hydroxyapatite implant can sometimes be verified with a bone scan.

The method to insert the peg first involves administering a standard retrobulbar anesthetic block. A 3-mm incision through conjunctiva, Tenon's capsule, and the scleral wrapping is made with a size 15 Bard–Parker blade in the central portion of the socket to expose the hydroxyapatite implant.

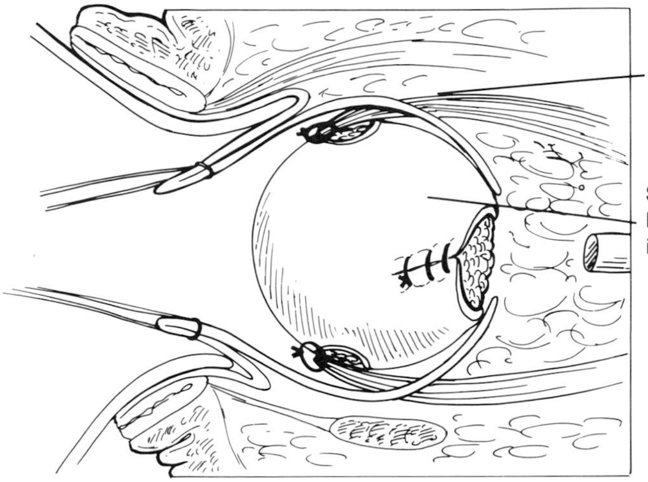

FIGURE 23–16

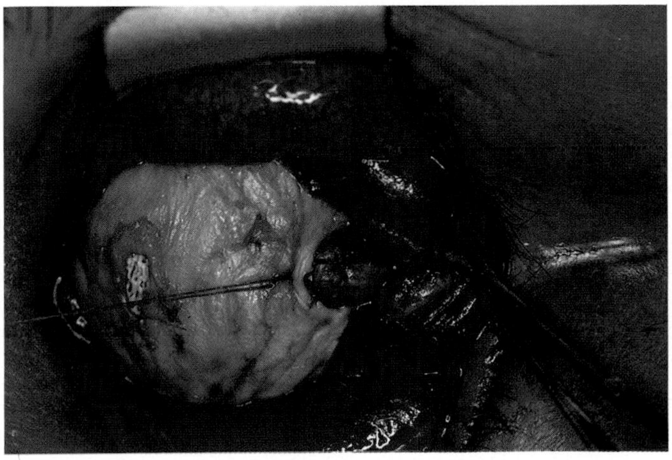

FIGURE 23–17

Figure 23–18. An air-powered drill, with a 3-mm–diameter cutting burr, is held perpendicular to the implant surface, and a hole is drilled into the implant to a depth of 11 to 13 mm. The debris is rinsed out and a temporary 2.5 × 10-mm acrylic flat-headed peg is inserted into this hole. This hole becomes lined with conjunctival epithelium after approximately 6 weeks, at which time the flat-headed peg is exchanged for a peg with a rounded cap.

Figure 23–19. The ocular prosthesis can be modified to couple with the round head of the peg in a ball-and-socket fashion to transmit the movement of the implant directly to the prosthesis.

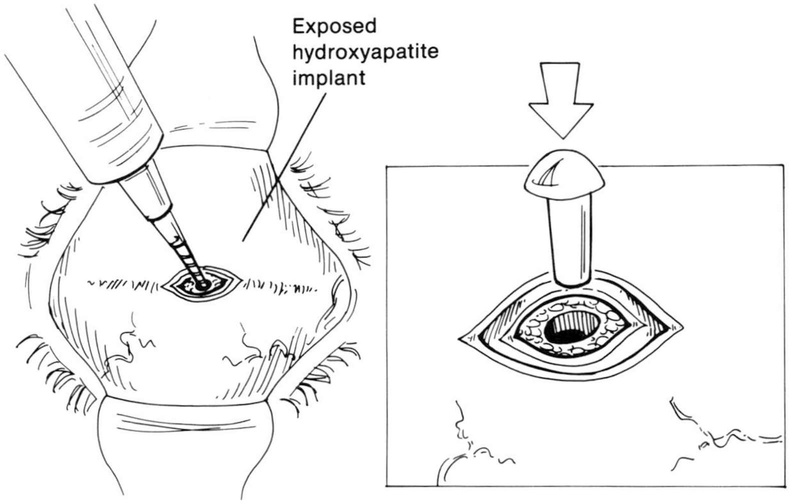

FIGURE 23–18

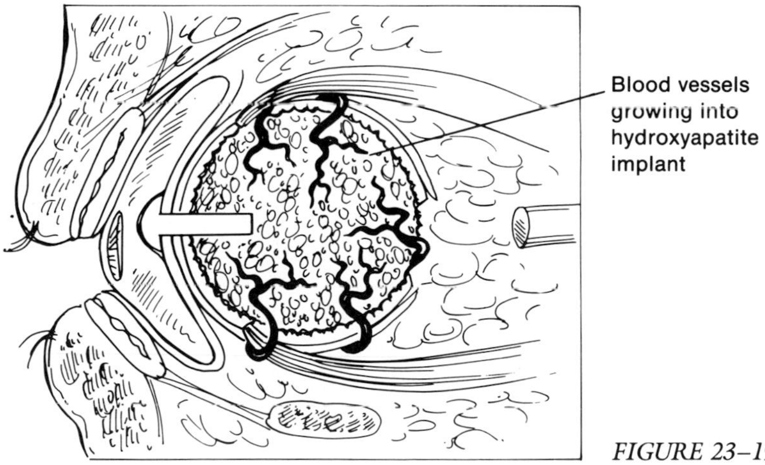

FIGURE 23–19

POSTOPERATIVE CARE

Systemic antibiotics are usually prescribed for 7 to 10 days after surgery. The pressure dressing is removed 5 days postoperatively, and antibiotic ointment is continued for 2 to 3 weeks. The socket should be sufficiently well healed to allow fabrication of a custom prosthesis within 6 to 8 weeks. In the interim, the conformer is left in place to maintain the fornices and prevent socket contraction. Polycarbonate glasses are recommended to protect the remaining eye.

POSTOPERATIVE COMPLICATIONS

Postoperative implant extrusion is most commonly due to improper wound closure, placement of an oversized implant, or infection. Early extrusion without infection can be corrected by placement of an appropriately sized implant and careful closure of all tissue layers, particularly the Tenon's capsule. Late extrusion has been associated with conjunctival epithelial ingrowth into the implant cavity and requires obliteration of the epithelial lining or relocation of the implant behind posterior Tenon's capsule.

Infections should be treated promptly with topical and systemic antibiotics. Removal of the implant becomes necessary if the infection is refractory or extrusion appears likely. A secondary implant can be placed once the infection has resolved completely.

Implant migration is most commonly associated with imbrication of the muscles in front of a spherical implant. Modification of the prosthesis is often sufficient to compensate for an implant malposition. In some cases, replacement of the orbital implant behind posterior Tenon's capsule may be needed to improve prosthesis fit and appearance.

A volume deficit may be manifested by enophthalmos, superior sulcus deformity, or lower eyelid malpositions caused by a heavy, oversized prosthesis. If these deformities persist, despite prosthesis modification, volume augmentation may be provided by placement of a larger orbital implant, placement of a subperiosteal orbital floor implant, or a dermis–fat graft.

Chapter Twenty-Four

EVISCERATION

Delyse R. Buus
David T. Tse

Evisceration is a surgical procedure in which the entire intraocular contents are removed and the scleral shell is left in situ. Evisceration can be performed with or without keratectomy. Since the sclera, Tenon's capsule, extraocular muscle attachments, and orbital suspensory structures are virtually undisturbed, evisceration is associated with better postoperative cosmesis and motility than with enucleation. There is less tendency for postoperative enophthalmos, superior sulcus deformity, or ptosis. Additionally, evisceration is simpler and quicker to perform than enucleation, which permits performance of this procedure on even the most debilitated patient.

INDICATIONS

The relative indications for enucleation versus evisceration are controversial. Sympathetic ophthalmia, although rare, is the most feared complication associated with this technique. In contrast with enucleation, in which uveal tissue is completely removed, pigmented melanocytes remain within the perineural region and emissary channels of the sclera following evisceration and may potentially incite an inflammatory response in the fellow eye. The benefits of improved cosmesis must be weighed against the risk of sympathetic ophthalmia, and the decision made depending on the particular clinical situation, the philosophy of the surgeon, and the informed preference of the patient.

Evisceration is particularly suited for the treatment of medically uncontrolled endophthalmitis or corneal ulceration in which vision and the structural integrity of the globe cannot be preserved. In this clinical setting, the intraocular abscess is evacuated, with minimal orbital tissue disruption. The intact scleral shell serves as a barrier for the spread of infection into the orbit and the potential subarachnoid space of the optic nerve, thereby minimizing the risk of orbital cellulitis or meningitis. Additionally, excessive bleeding from inflamed orbital tissues is avoided. In the presence of a localized anterior infectious scleritis, evisceration remains an option if adequate sclera will be available following excision of the infected tissues. However, if there is extensive scleritis or an extrascleral abscess has developed, enucleation is necessary for optimal removal and drainage of the infected tissues.

CONTRAINDICATIONS

Evisceration is contraindicated for patients in whom an intraocular tumor is suspected or cannot be assured by clinical, computed tomography scan, or ultrasound examinations. This procedure should not be considered if a complete histopathologic examination of the globe is needed. Evisceration should also be avoided if the scleral shell is thinned or inadequate, such as in a posterior staphyloma, posterior segment trauma, or phthisis bulbi. In cases of fungal endophthalmitis, the tendency for early invasion of the scleral wall may also argue for enucleation, rather than evisceration.

SURGICAL PROCEDURE

Evisceration is performed under general or local retrobulbar anesthesia. Retention of the cornea has been advocated to allow for a larger implant and greater volume replacement. However, because of the potential for persistent sensation, thinning, and perforation of the cornea, we prefer the evisceration technique that includes keratectomy.

A speculum is placed between the eyelids. A 360° limbal peritomy is performed. The Tenon's capsule and conjunctiva are separated from the underlying sclera anterior to the tendinous insertions of the rectus muscles.

The anterior chamber is entered at the posterior surgical limbus with a size 11 blade. Care is taken to avoid penetrating the iris, lens, or the ciliary body. A cataract scissors is used to perform the keratectomy.

Figure 24–1. Once the corneal button is removed and the anterior chamber exposed, bacterial culture specimen may be collected.

Figure 24–2. While grasping the scleral rim with a forceps, a small evisceration spatula is inserted into the suprachoroidal space at the scleral spur. The ciliary body should be detached circumferentially from the sclera first, before proceeding with any posterior dissection. Care is taken to keep the spatula held with pressure against the scleral wall while separating the uveal tissue off the inner surface of the globe.

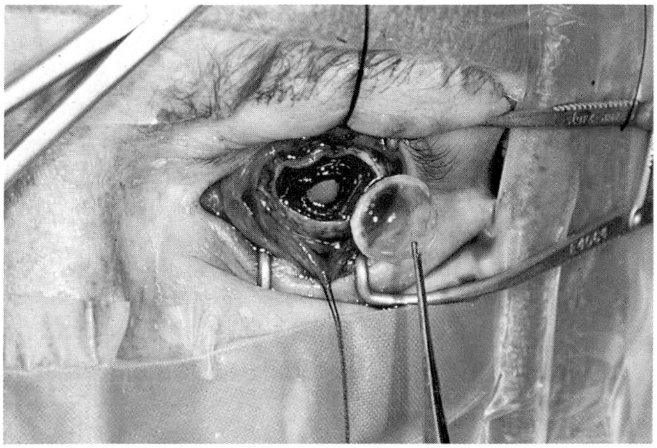

FIGURE 24–1

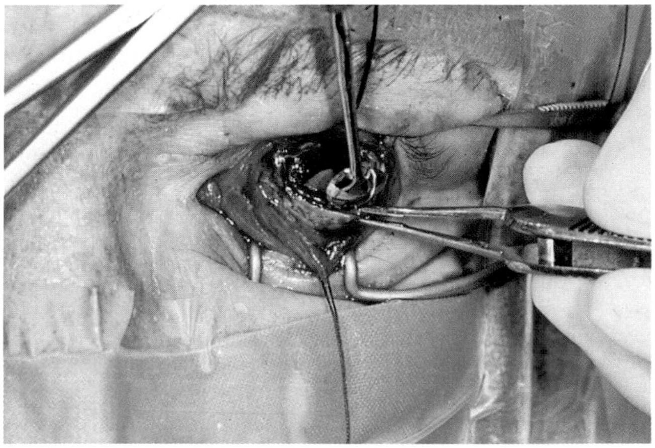

FIGURE 24–2

Figure 24–3. The spatula is swept 360° in a posteriorly directed spiral fashion to remove the intraocular contents. Bleeding is encountered when the choroid is separated from the attachments at the vortex veins. Once dissection reaches the optic nerve head, a larger evisceration spatula is used to sever the final uveal attachment at the lamina cribosa. The contents of the globe are then totally removed with the spatula.

The scleral cavity is irrigated with balanced salt solution, and bleeding from the optic nerve head and vortex veins can be controlled with bipolar cauterization. Unipolar cautery should be avoided, as current may be preferentially conducted along the optic nerve and cause chiasmal damage. The scleral cavity is carefully inspected for any remnants of uveal tissue.

Figure 24–4. The inner surface of the scleral shell is then scrubbed with cotton-tipped applicators moistened with 70% ethanol to denature and remove any residual uveal pigment. In cases of endophthalmitis, cotton applicators soaked in povidone–iodine (Betadine) are also used to scrub the scleral surface. This is followed by irrigation with copious amounts of normal saline and an antibiotic solution.

The scleral aperture is enlarged to a horizontal ellipse by excising triangular wedges of sclera at the 3:00 and 9:00 o'clock positions.

A size 14- or 16-mm spherical alloplastic implant is then placed within the scleral cavity. When eviscerating for endophthalmitis, some surgeons prefer to omit placement of the implant at this stage and to delay wound closure for 3 to 4 days. The scleral cavity is packed with iodoform-impregnated gauze; the dressing is changed twice daily. The rationale is to permit inflammation to subside and granulation to commence, which tends to help minimize the risk of implant extrusion. It has been our experience however, that most of these implants are retained, even in the presence of preexisting infection. If the implant does extrude, the patient will be no worse than had the procedure been done without an implant.

Figure 24–5A, B. Since the scleral shell tends to shrink with time, the largest implant that will allow closure without undue tension should be selected.

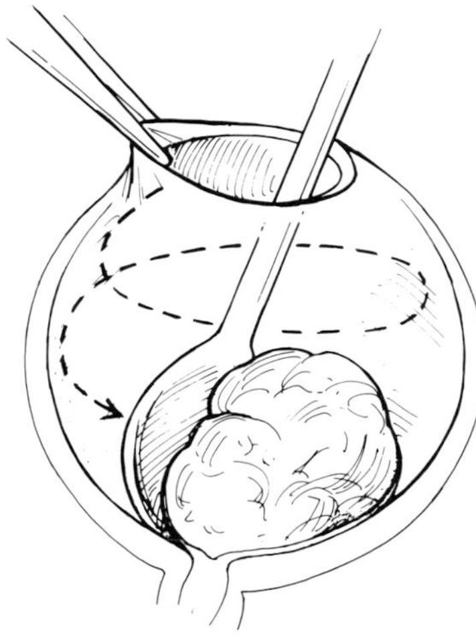

FIGURE 24–3

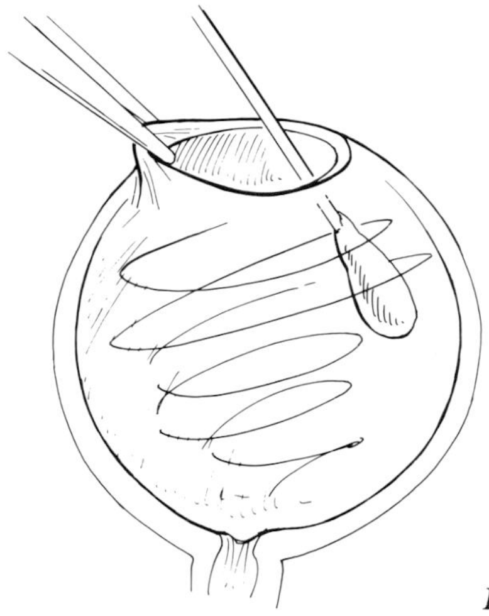

FIGURE 24–4

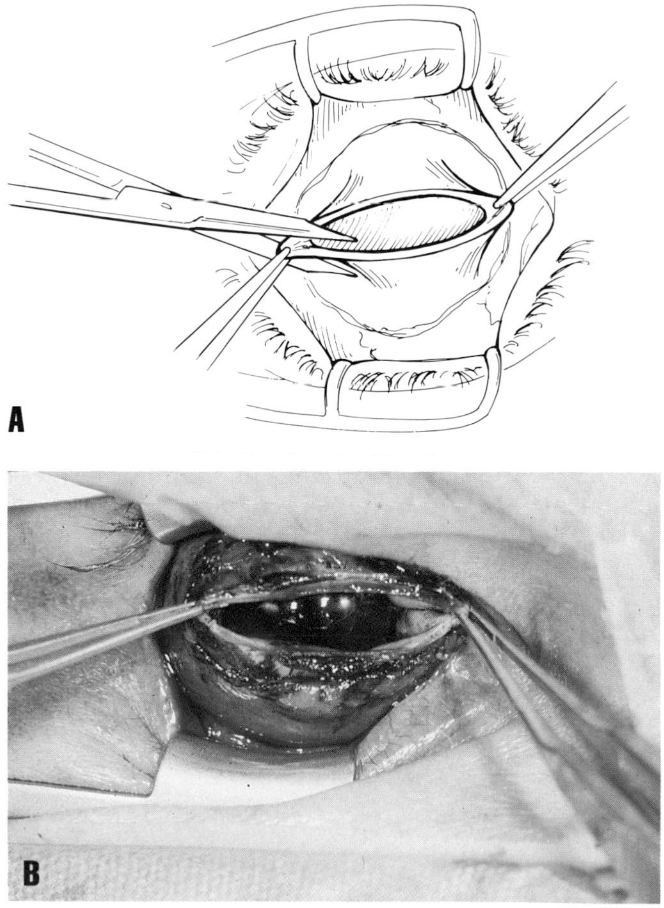

FIGURE 24–5

Figure 24–6. The scleral edges are united with interrupted 5–0 Vicryl sutures.

Figure 24–7. The Tenon's capsule is reapproximated with interrupted 5–0 Vicryl sutures.

Figure 24–8. The conjunctiva is closed with a running 5–0 chromic suture. Antibiotic ointment is applied to the socket and a conformer is positioned. A pressure dressing is applied over the operative site.

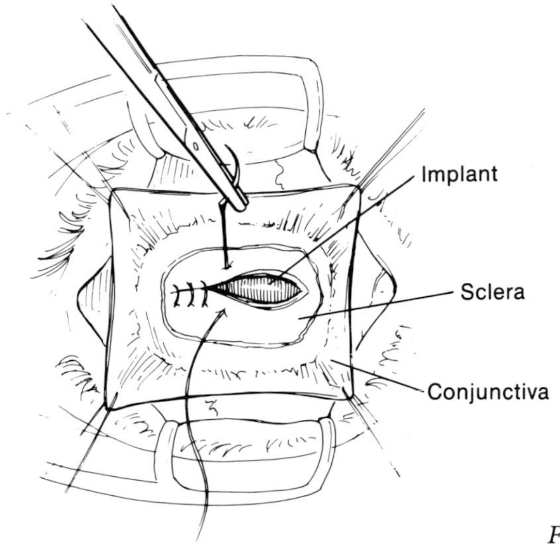

FIGURE 24–6

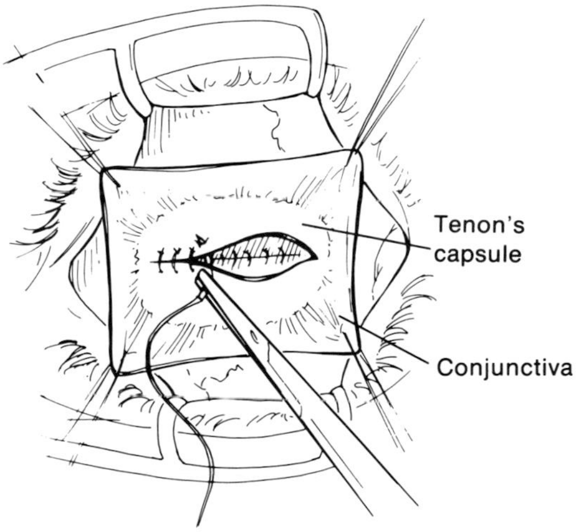

FIGURE 24–7

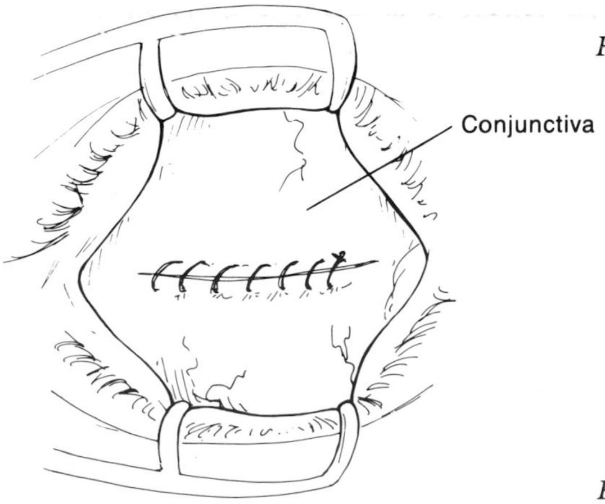

FIGURE 24–8

POSTOPERATIVE CARE

The pressure dressing is removed 5 days after surgery. It may be removed earlier for inspection if there is concern for postoperative infection; the dressing is then reapplied. Antibiotic ointment is continued for 2 weeks. Systemic antibiotic therapy, guided by culture and sensitivity results, is usually administered for an additional 7 to 10 days postoperatively. The temporary conformer is left in the fornix until the patient is fitted with a prosthesis by the impression technique 6 to 8 weeks following surgery.

POSTOPERATIVE COMPLICATIONS

Infection may occur following evisceration. It is possible to eradicate the infection with antibiotic therapy first, without removing the implant. However, if the infection does not respond to optimal medical therapy, the implant should be removed, and a secondary implant should be inserted at a later date, after complete resolution of the infection.

Proper selection of implant size and careful wound closure are important prerequisites in preventing implant extrusion. However, if implant extrusion occurs shortly after surgery, an attempt should be made to replace it immediately and scleral edges reapproximated carefully. If scleral shrinkage precludes proper wound closure, an implant encased in a donor sclera is inserted into the cavity; the edges of the host sclera are then sutured onto the surface of the donor sclera. The Tenon's capsule and conjunctiva are closed over the scleral wound in separate layers.

Chapter Twenty-Five

EXENTERATION

Delyse R. Buus
David T. Tse

Exenteration involves the removal of the soft-tissue contents of the orbit including the eye, extraocular muscles, periorbita, and part or all of the eyelids.

Exenteration is most commonly performed in the treatment of malignant tumors of the eye and ocular adnexa. This includes primary orbital tumors, ocular and eyelid neoplasms with orbital invasion, lacrimal gland malignancies, and tumors extending into the orbit from the adjacent cranial or nasal cavities or from paranasal sinuses. Recent studies suggest that exenteration may offer no benefit over enucleation with local excision in the management of choroidal melanomas with extrascleral extension. In the management of certain neoplasms, such as orbital lymphoma and rhabdomyosarcoma, radiation and chemotherapy have supplanted exenteration as primary therapeutic modalities. In each case, a review of recent treatment advances for the tumor in question is advised. In some cases of orbital metastases or advanced orbital disease, palliative exenteration may be warranted for tumor debulking or pain control. On rare occasions, exenteration may be indicated in the treatment of nonmalignant conditions such as severe trauma, mucormycosis, meningioma, orbital contracture caused by sclerosing pseudotumor, and congenital deformities.

PREOPERATIVE EVALUATION

A definitive pathologic diagnosis based on permanent histologic sections must be established before proceeding with orbital exenteration. Under no circumstances should exenteration be performed based on frozen-section interpretation of a biopsy. Preoperatively, the extent of the lesion should be evaluated by physical examination, computed tomography, magnetic resonance imaging, and ultrasound, as indicated. The surgical procedure may then be modified, depending on the biologic activity, extent, and location of the disease process. For tumors involving the posterior aspect of the orbit, the eyelid skin may be preserved to partially line the exenterated socket. In contrast, partial or complete excision of the eyelids is usually required for lesions arising from the eyelids, conjunctiva, or the anterior segment. If the extent of skin involvement cannot be determined clinically, Mohs microscopically controlled excision may be helpful in clearing the epithelial margins and allowing maximal preservation of the uninvolved eyelid skin. In some cases, bone removal may be required if tumor invasion into the bony orbit has occurred. Malignancies arising from the nose, paranasal sinuses, or cranial cavity often require collaboration with a neurosurgeon or otolaryngologist for optimal management.

Following removal of the orbital soft tissues, the socket may be lined with a split-thickness skin graft, or it may be allowed to granulate by secondary intention. The placement of a skin graft prolongs the surgical procedure slightly and involves a second operative site. However, it shortens the socket healing process and provides a smooth, clean socket surface. Healing by granulation results in a thicker, irregular socket surface, which may obscure detection of early tumor recurrence.

Transposition of the temporalis muscle and fascia has been advocated to minimize the depth of the socket postoperatively. The disadvantages of this technique include a cosmetic depression in the temporal area and masking of tumor recurrences by the resultant thick apical lining. However, in some cases of exenteration involving extensive tissue loss or compromised vascularity following radiation therapy, local tissue flaps including the temporalis and median forehead flaps may be used.

PATIENT PREPARATION

The patient must be prepared for the loss of the eye and for the cosmetic deformity that results from orbital exenteration. Hypesthesia of the forehead and cheek owing to removal of branches of the fifth nerve during exenteration should be anticipated. Also, the patient should be aware of the possibility of tumor recurrence or metastatic spread, despite surgical intervention. Discussing the options for cosmetic rehabilitation preoperatively, with the use of photographs to demonstrate the postsurgical appearance with an orbital prosthesis, may be beneficial in gaining acceptance of the planned procedure.

SURGICAL PROCEDURE

Exenteration is performed under general anesthesia.

Figure 25–1. The planned incision is marked and the periocular region infiltrated with lidocaine (Xylocaine) with epinephrine for hemostasis. If eyelid skin cannot be preserved, the incision is made directly over the orbital rim. A 4–0 silk traction suture is passed through the upper and lower eyelid margins and tied together.

Figure 25–2. The incision is made over the orbital rim and is continued through the underlying orbicularis until the periosteum of the orbital rim is exposed.

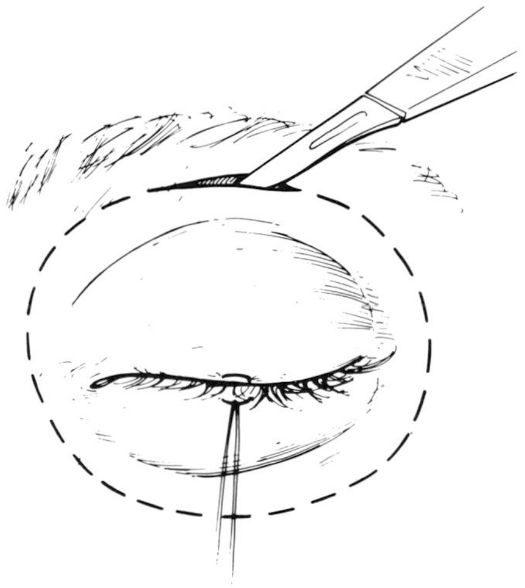

FIGURE 25–1

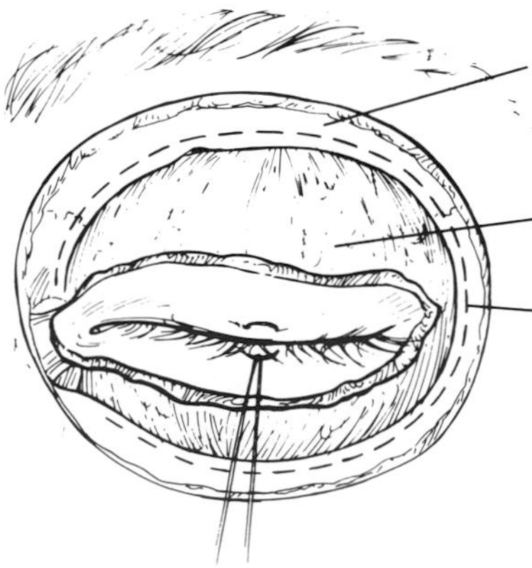

FIGURE 25–2

Figure 25–3. If the eyelid skin is to be preserved, the initial incision is made adjacent to the lashes, a myocutaneous flap is elevated anterior to the orbital septum until the orbital rim is reached.

The orbital rim is further exposed by separating the periosteum from the overlying orbicularis with a periosteal elevator.

Figure 25–4. An incision is then made in the periosteum with a size 15 blade, 2 to 3 mm outside the orbital rim. This incision is continued around the circumference of the orbital aperture.

Figure 25–5. The periosteum is elevated off the orbital rim with a periosteal elevator. Bleeding from the bone may be controlled with the Bovie cautery or bone wax.

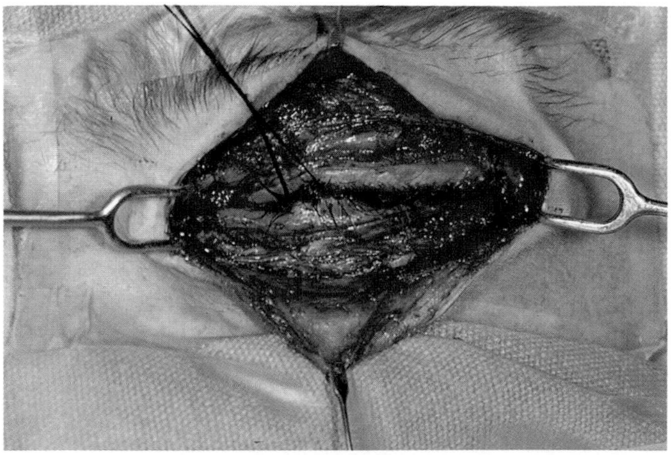

FIGURE 25–3

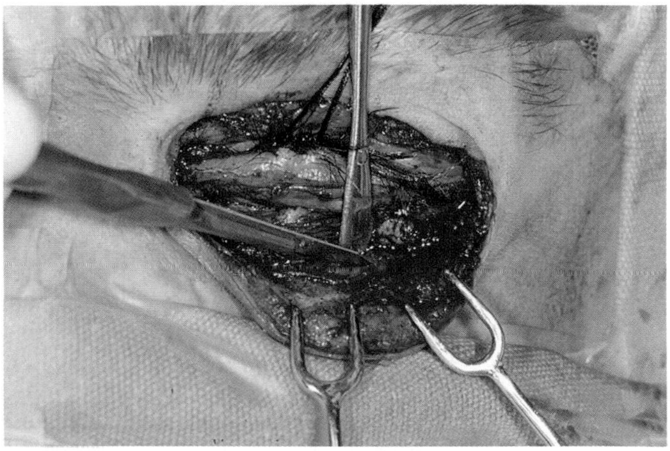

FIGURE 25–4

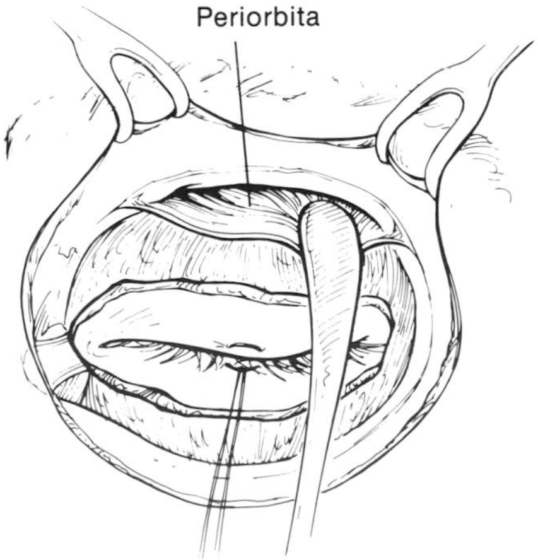

FIGURE 25–5

Figure 25–6. The periorbita is then gently separated from the orbital walls. Care should be taken to avoid inadvertent perforation of the bony walls, particularly the thin medial wall. The perforating vessels, including the anterior and posterior ethmoid arteries, are cauterized and transected as they are isolated. Tight adhesions of the periorbita to the bone will be encountered at the insertion of the trochlea, and the medial and lateral canthal attachments. Sharp dissection may facilitate separation in these areas.

Figure 25–7. The lacrimal sac is identified within the lacrimal fossa. The surrounding periorbita is separated from the orbital wall until the sac is isolated. It is then transected with the Bovie knife.

Figure 25–8A, B, C. The raw edges of the lacrimal sac (**A**) are turned inward and sutured with 5–0 Vicryl sutures (**B**). (**C**) This is a mucosal turnover flap which effectively closes off the nasolacrimal duct, thereby minimizing the chance of fistula formation.

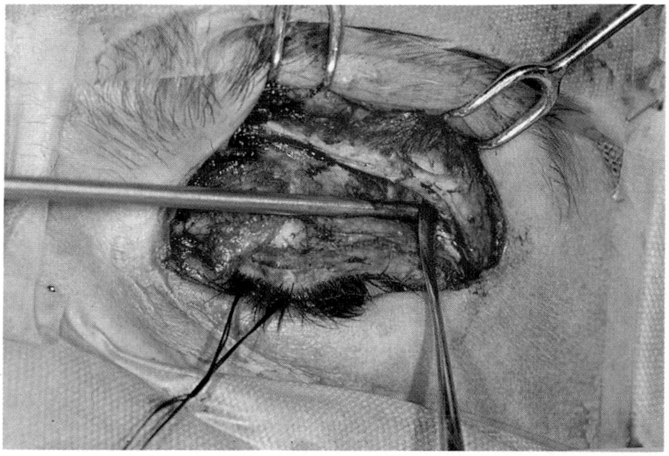

FIGURE 25–6

FIGURE 25–7

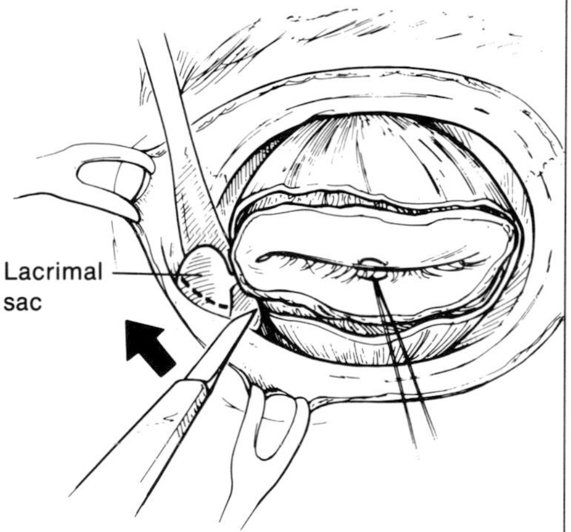

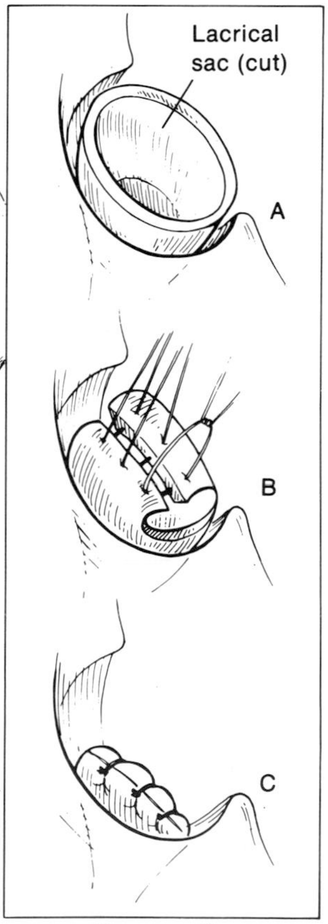

FIGURE 25–8

Turnover flap

Figure 25–9. The inferior orbital fissure is isolated and partially transected with the Bovie knife.

Figure 25–10A. Once dissection has reached the orbital apex, an enucleation snare is passed around the orbital contents from the temporal side, to avoid injury to the lamina papyracea.

Figure 25–10B. With upward traction on the silk sutures, the snare is slowly constricted as it is passed posteriorly. The snare is then tightened until it is compressing the apical tissues. It is left in this position for 5 minutes to provide hemostasis.

Figure 25–11. The snare is then tightened until the tissues are transected. Alternatively, the apical tissues may be cross-clamped with a curved hemostat, and then transected with curved enucleation scissors. Any oozing from the apical stump is controlled by direct pressure with a 4 × 4 gauze or cautery. The bony socket is then inspected for evidence of tumor invasion, and bone is removed if required. If apical extension is suspected, additional biopsies of the stump may be taken and sent for frozen-section examination. The orbit is then loosely packed with a moistened 4 × 4 gauze while harvesting the skin graft.

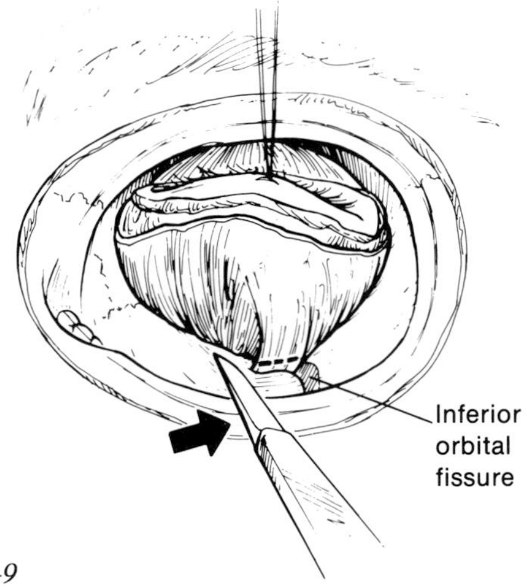

FIGURE 25–9

FIGURE 25–10

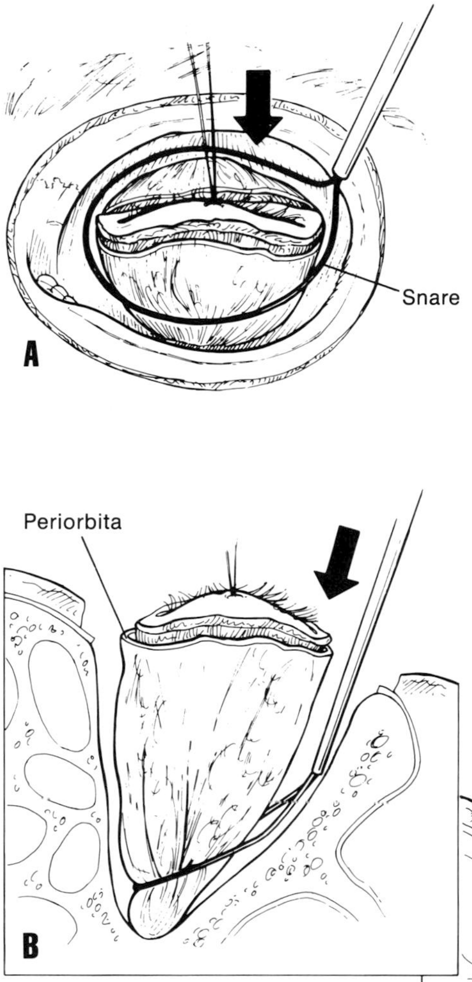

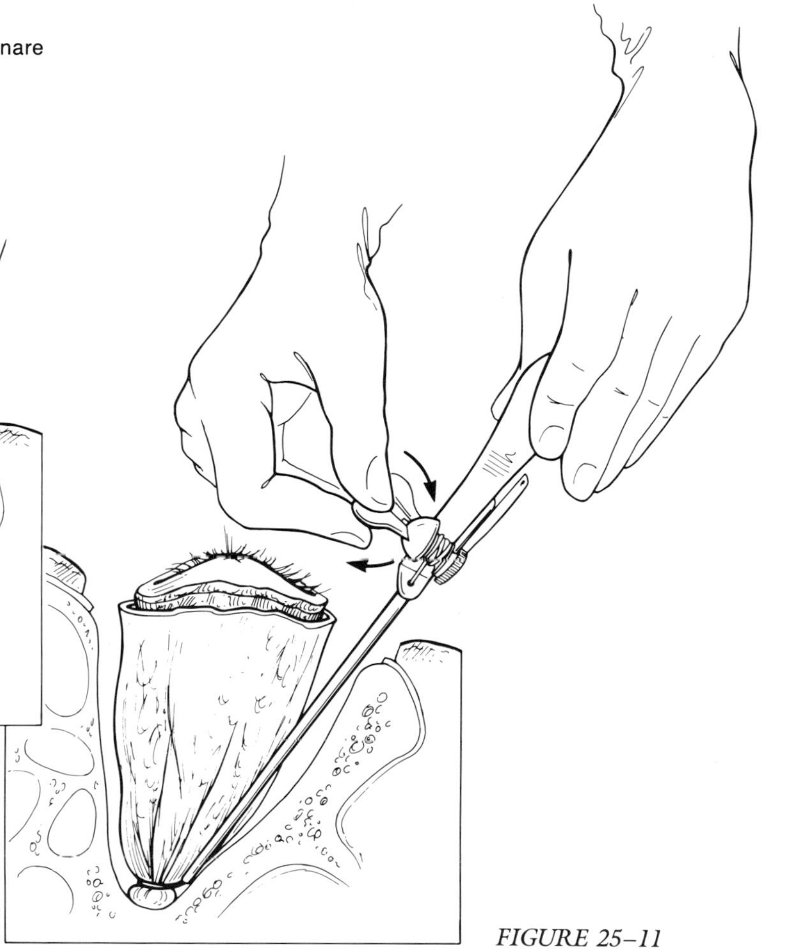

FIGURE 25–11

Figure 25–12. The skin graft is harvested from the non–hair-bearing anterior or inner surface of the upper thigh. The skin is coated with a thin layer of mineral oil, and a 0.3-mm (0.012-in.) split-thickness graft is harvested with a dermatome. The skin surface should be flattened with a tongue blade during the harvesting procedure to ensure a graft of uniform thickness. A graft of 2 × 3 in. (5 × 7.5 cm) is adequate in most cases.

Figure 25–13. As the skin graft emerges from the dermatome, the graft should be grasped with a pair of forceps and gently guided away from the cutting edge. A 5 × 7 in. (12.5 × 17.5 mm) Xeroform gauze is then applied onto the donor site. Direct pressure is applied until bleeding has stopped. The Xeroform is left in place, and the area is dressed with a Curlex wrap.

Figure 25–14. The skin graft is passed through a 1:1 ratio mesher. Meshing the graft allows it to cover a greater surface area to conform to the concavity of the exenterated socket, and facilitates drainage of serosanguinous fluid from under the graft.

Figure 25–15. The graft is then sutured to the skin edges with 5–0 Vicryl interrupted sutures. It is not necessary to trim the graft to fit, as it will conform to the contour of the orbit. A Tefla pad, with its cotton layer removed, is placed over the skin graft in the socket.

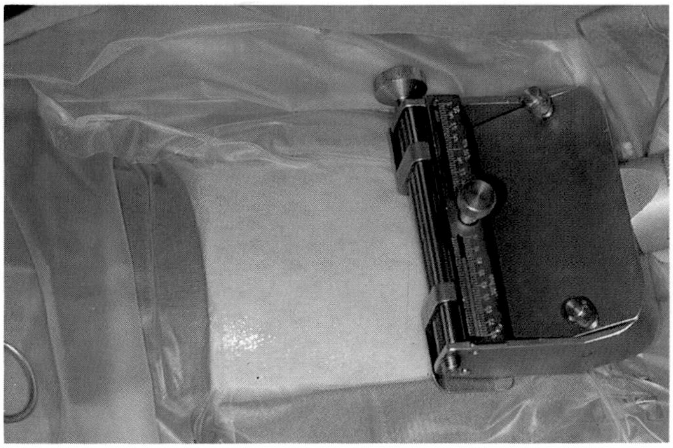

FIGURE 25–12

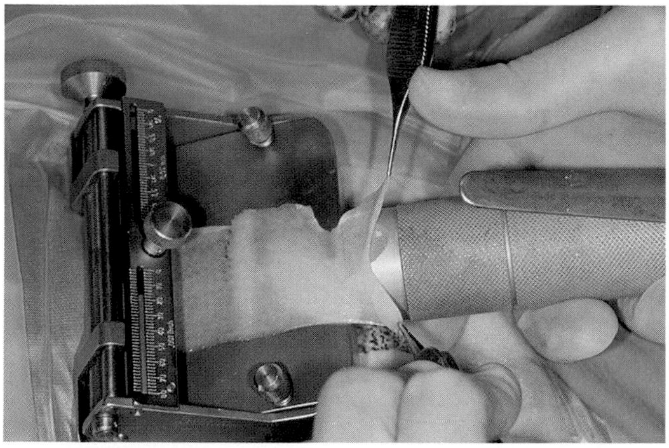

FIGURE 25–13

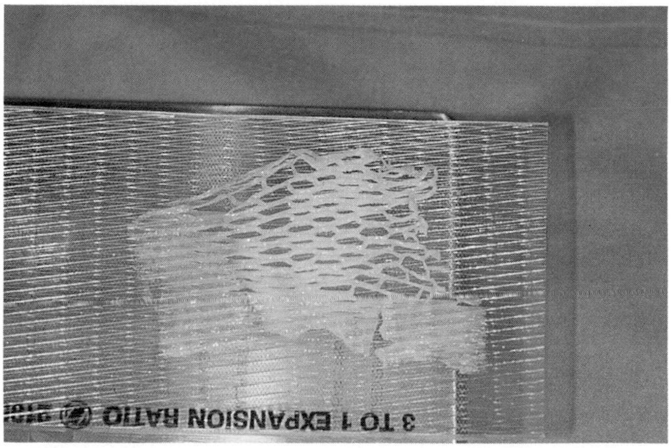

FIGURE 25–14

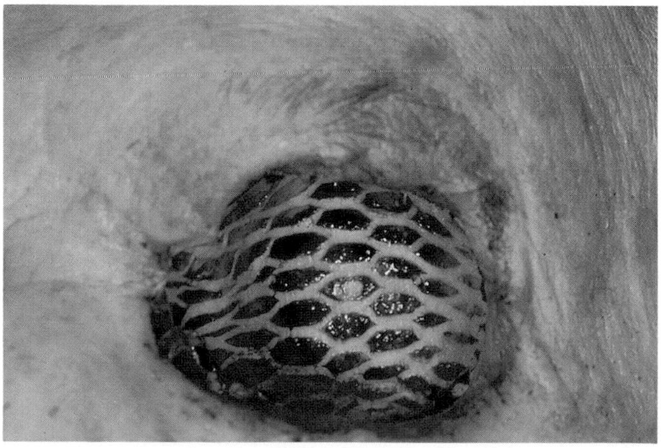

FIGURE 25–15

Figure 25–16A, B. Three sterile surgical scrub sponges (without the detergent) are moistened with gentamicin solution and packed into the socket.

Figure 25–17. The packing is held within the socket by three interrupted 4–0 silk sutures passed through the intact skin overlying the orbital rim. A pressure dressing is applied over the sponges. If the socket is to heal by granulation, it is packed loosely with ½-in. iodoform gauze coated with antibiotic ointment before applying a pressure dressing.

POSTOPERATIVE CARE

The patient is placed on a regimen of broad-spectrum oral antibiotics postoperatively. In 5 days, the pressure dressing is removed, and wet to dry dressing changes begun. With use of clean technique, 4 × 4 gauze pads are moistened in a solution of equal parts hydrogen peroxide and povidone–iodine (Betadine). The gauze is wrung out well, unfolded, and loosely packed into the socket. All areas of the socket should be in contact with the gauze, which will serve to debride the socket of old blood and keratin when removed. Initially, the dressings are changed twice a day for a month, decreasing to once a day, and then every other day as healing progresses. The patient is seen weekly for the first month to remove any crusts formed within the socket. The orbit is usually well epithelialized within 3 to 4 months. Dressing changes for the granulating socket consist of changing the antibiotic-coated Xeroform gauze daily until epithelialized. The patient is then referred to an ocularist for a custom-fitted orbital prosthesis. The Xeroform gauze is left in place over the donor site on the thigh until it falls off spontaneously.

COMPLICATIONS

The most common complication encountered in an orbital exenteration procedure is intraoperative bleeding. To minimize this problem, aspirin and other anticoagulants should be discontinued before surgery, if possible. The most important factor in avoiding intraoperative hemorrhage is careful attention to hemostasis during the procedure. Cerebrospinal fluid leak is an uncommon, but potentially serious, complication of exenteration, because of the risk of meningitis in untreated or persistent cases. This complication results from inadvertent penetration of the dura, most commonly at the superior orbital fissure. A small leak may close spontaneously, but larger leaks require treatment. Autogenous fat graft, temporalis muscle pedicle flap, or repair of the

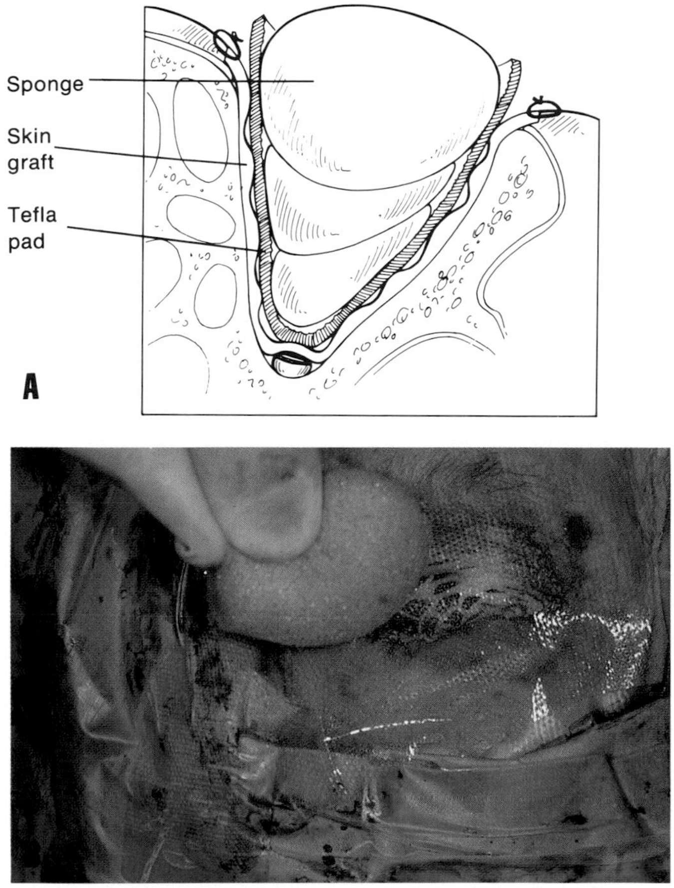

FIGURE 25–16

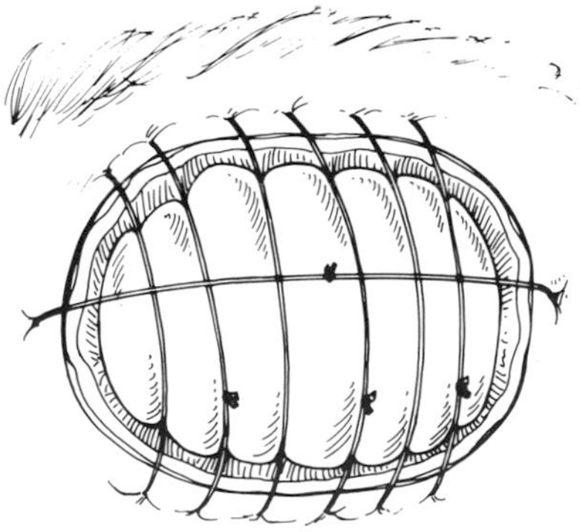

FIGURE 25–17

dural tear by direct closure or a lyophilized dural graft are treatment options. A simple, effective technique is the application of tissue adhesive (Histoacryl blue) to the area of leakage.

Postoperative infection is uncommon, and it is usually the result of improper dressing changes and poor socket hygiene. Debridement of the socket at postoperative visits, and temporary increases in the frequency of dressing changes, will usually suffice to control low-grade infections or discharge. Topical and systemic antibiotics may be needed if the infection is more severe. Fistulas into the ethmoid and maxillary sinuses may result from bony defects in the floor or medial wall of the orbit. Small, asymptomatic sinoorbital fistulas usually do not require treatment. Larger fistulas may cause chronic discharge and interference with prosthesis wear, if not repaired.

Chapter Twenty-Six

MANAGEMENT OF THYROID-RELATED EYELID RETRACTION

David T. Tse

Retraction of the eyelids is one of the most common ophthalmic manifestations of Graves' disease. This malposition may occur with or without exophthalmos and is responsible for functional and cosmetic problems in many patients with thyroid-related eye disease. The etiology of eyelid retraction in Graves' disease is not clearly understood, but several factors seem to be contributory. In the upper lid, these factors include (1) Mueller's muscle overaction from sympathetic stimulation, (2) levator contraction from degeneration and thickening of the levator muscle or the aponeurosis, (3) levator adhesions to the orbicularis muscle and orbital septum, and (4) overaction of the levator–superior rectus complex in response to a hypophoria produced by fibrosis and retraction of the inferior rectus.

In the lower eyelid, adrenergic stimulation of the Mueller's muscle plays a smaller role, but fibrosis of the inferior rectus exerting a retraction action on the lower eyelid through its capsulopalpebral head appears to be more influential.

SURGICAL INDICATIONS

Surgical treatment of eyelid retraction is usually reserved for patients whose endocrine status and eyelid height have been stable for at least 6 months to 1 year, and in whom retraction causes significant exposure keratopathy, lagophthalmos, chronic conjunctival injection, and cosmetic imperfection.

Several surgical procedures have been described to bring the retracted upper eyelid downward. These included levator tenotomy or recession, Mueller's muscle resection or myectomy, and combined levator tenotomy and mullerectomy. However, I prefer the aponeurotic approach described by Harvey and Anderson (1981) because it is anatomically, surgically, and physiologically sound. In this technique, the Mueller's muscle is completely extirpated, the lateral horn of the levator severed, and the aponeurosis recessed. Additionally, this anatomic approach is similar to that used in aponeurotic ptosis surgery.

SURGICAL TECHNIQUE

Upper Eyelid

Local anesthesia is preferable whenever feasible. This permits lid height, contour, and symmetry to be adjusted intraoperatively. A full-face preparation is given, and the head is draped with 3-M 1000 surgical drape. The use of an open-face adhesive drape allows the patient to sit up in the middle of the surgery for lid height adjustment, without having to constantly adjust any loose head drape during this maneuver.

The normal skin crease is marked with a fine-tipped marking pen. For unilateral retraction cases, the skin crease is marked to correspond with the natural crease contour of the contralateral upper eyelid. Topical tetracaine may be instilled into the upper cul-de-sac intermittently throughout the procedure. Subcutaneous infiltration of lidocaine 2% with 1 : 100,000 epinephrine is given along the preplaced marking with a 30-gauge needle. The anesthetic solution should be delivered slowly to minimize patient discomfort, and no more than 1.5 ml is needed. A swollen lid will render fine lid height and contour adjustments suboptimal later on in the procedure.

A 4–0 double-armed silk traction suture is placed in the central margin of the upper lid and anchored to the surgical drape inferiorly with a hemostat. The needle is passed through the tarsal plate in a lamellar fashion, avoiding the marginal arcade and preventing unnecessary bleeding. When secured inferiorly, this traction suture puts all lid structures posterior to the orbicularis on stretch, while allowing the overlying skin and orbicularis to be mobilized. The skin is incised along the preplaced lid crease marking with a scalpel. All bleeding points are cauterized with a bipolar cautery.

The skin and orbicularis are grasped with a forceps on both sides of the incision centrally.

Figure 26–1. The orbicularis is tented anteriorly as far as possible from the posterior structures and a full-thickness vertical incision of the muscle is made with a Westcott scissors.

Figure 26–2. A full-thickness incision through the orbicularis muscle places one at the avascular postorbicular fascial plane, where the shiny surface of the orbital septum can be seen. Bleeding from the muscle layer should be cauterized immediately so that this important tissue plane is not obscured.

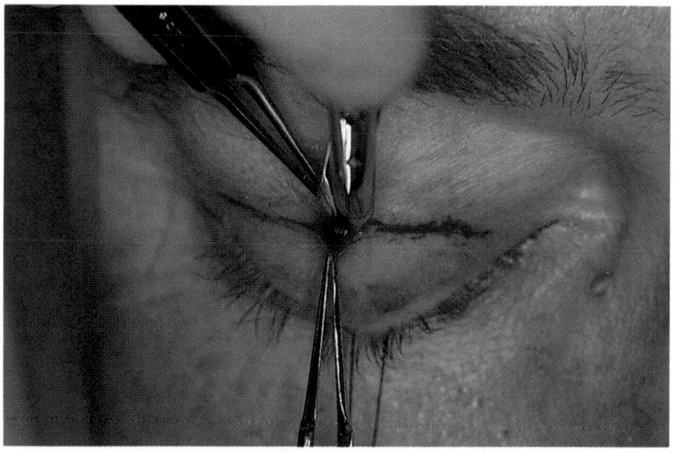

FIGURE 26–1

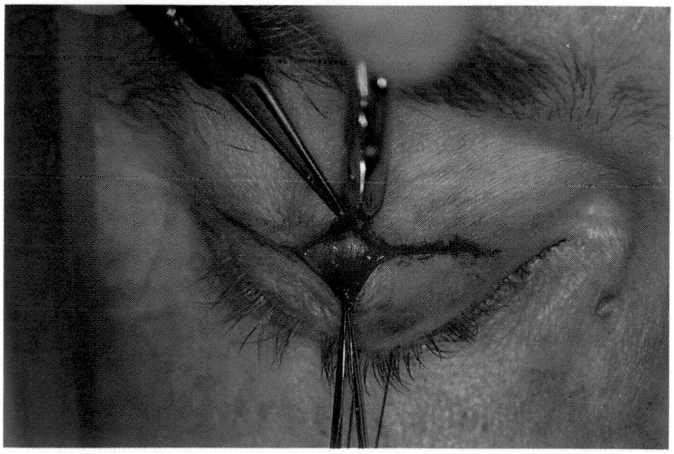

FIGURE 26–2

Figure 26–3. One blade of a scissors is passed bluntly in this plane medially and laterally to open the full length of the incision.

With the edges of the incision retracted apart, the underlying levator aponeurosis and the orbital septal attachment to the aponeurosis can be identified.

Figure 26–4A, B. The lid margin suture is then released and gentle retrograde digital pressure is applied onto the globe to prolapse the preaponeurotic fat pad. The yellowish fat pad can be seen bulging forward and distending the overlying thin, translucent orbital septum. The tip of the instrument is pointing at an intact orbital septum, with its attachment to the aponeurosis. A horizontal snip with scissors directed perpendicularly is used to buttonhole the orbital septum above its fusion with the aponeurosis.

Figure 26–5. This allows the yellow preaponeurotic fat with its intact capsule to herniate through the buttonhole. The preaponeurotic fat pad is a key anatomic landmark to identify in this procedure. The entire orbital septum is opened by placing one blade of a Westcott scissors behind the septum and extending the incision medially and laterally. Incision of the septum should always be made over a bulging fat pad, using it to insulate the scissors from making iatrogenic defects in the aponeurosis.

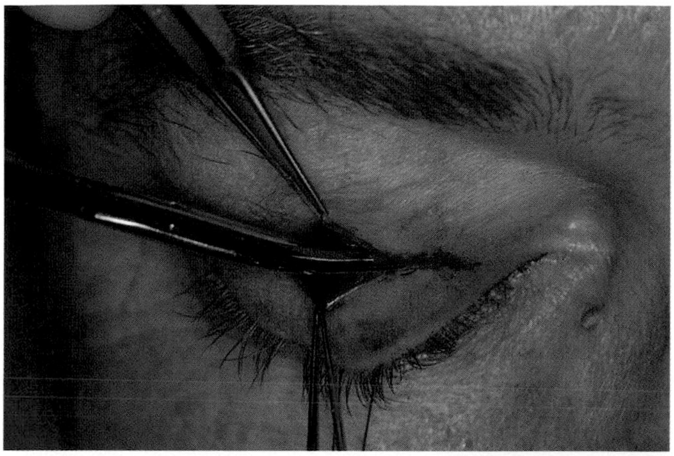

FIGURE 26–3

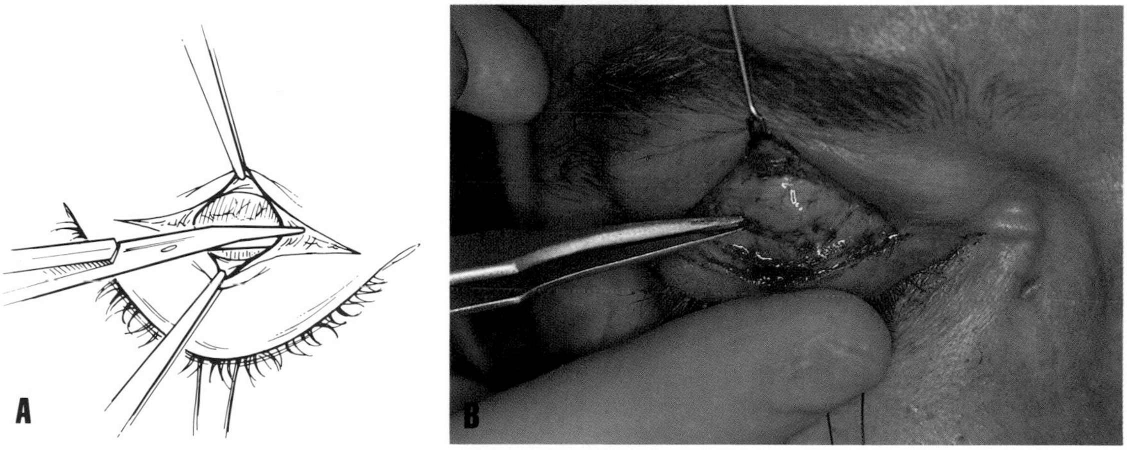

FIGURE 26–4

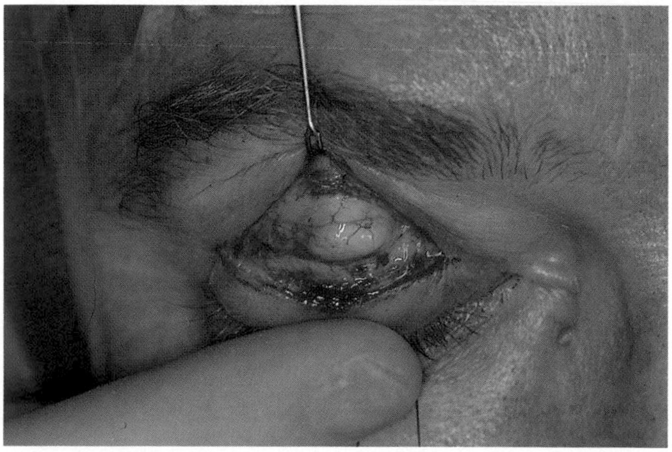

FIGURE 26–5

Figure 26–6. With the skin edge retracted superiorly, the full expanse of the preaponeurotic fat is displayed.

Figure 26–7. The preaponeurotic fat is gently teased away from the underlying white glistening structure with a cotton tip applicator. This structure, located immediately beneath the fat pad, is the levator aponeurosis. The forceps is grasping this structure. While grasping the glistening tissue with a forceps and asking the patient to look down and up, this structure can be easily confirmed as the mobile, force-generating levator aponeurosis. The Whitnall's ligament can be identified at the superior limit of the aponeurosis. Once the entire fat pad has been dissected free from the aponeurosis, it is retracted superiorly with a self-retaining Jaffe retractor to expose the shiny anterior surface of the levator aponeurosis.

Figure 26–8. A metal lid plate is inserted into the superior fornix to protect the globe, while local anesthetic is injected under the levator aponeurosis with a 30-gauge needle to hydraulically separate the aponeurosis from Mueller's muscle. One should avoid infiltrating the anesthetic too close to Whitnall's ligament or into the levator muscle, as paresis of the levator will affect the outcome of lid height adjustment later on.

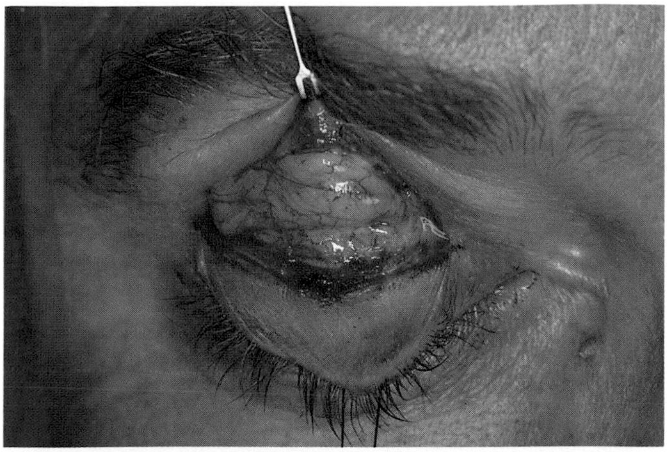

FIGURE 26–6

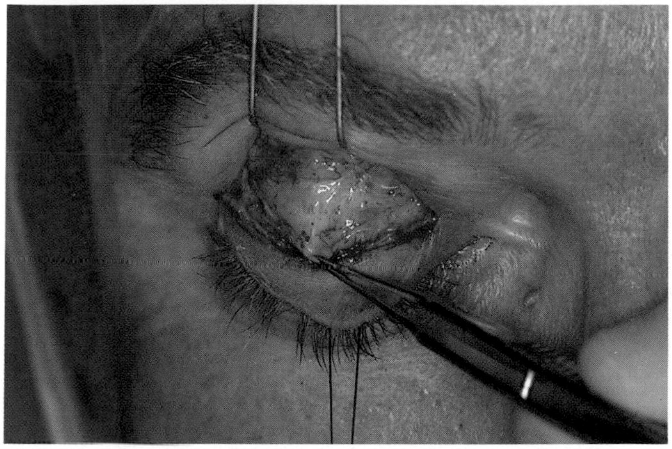

FIGURE 26–7

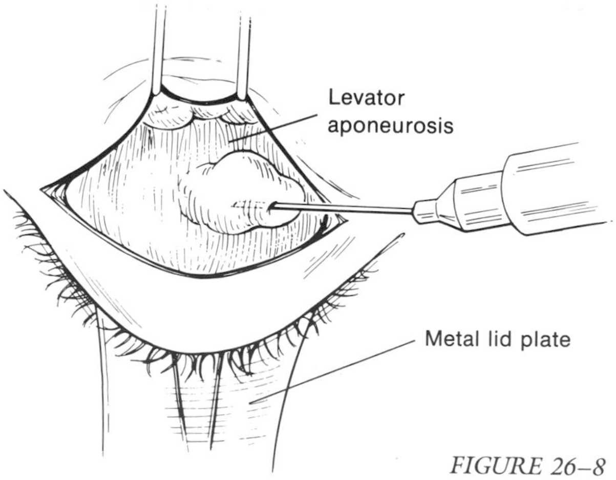

FIGURE 26–8

Figure 26–9A, B. A snip incision of the aponeurosis is made at the superior margin of the tarsal plate to expose a distinct tissue plane between the aponeurosis and the anterior surface of Mueller's muscle. One blade of a Westcott scissors is passed bluntly in this plane medially and laterally to sever the attachment of the aponeurosis from the tarsal plate. Sharp dissection is used to fully detach the undersurface of the aponeurosis from Mueller's muscle. Care is taken not to buttonhole the aponeurosis. Blunt dissection within this tissue plane is discouraged, since it may cause dehiscence of the aponeurosis.

Figure 26–10A, B. With forceps lifting up the aponeurosis, the peripheral arcade of vessels is seen in Mueller's muscle just above the tarsal border. Mueller's muscle can be seen as a thin vascular structure with vertically oriented muscle fibers inserting onto the superior border of the tarsal plate. Frequently, fatty infiltration and fibrosis of the muscle are seen in patients with Graves' disease. Bleeding from Mueller's muscle is usually moderate because of the highly vascular nature of the tissue. It should be stopped immediately, with pinpoint cautery, before proceeding with further dissection. Meticulous hemostasis is critical at this juncture of the procedure, as uncontrolled bleeding will obscure this tissue plane and make further dissection more difficult. To avoid thermal damage to the cornea, one must lift the tissue off the globe with the bipolar tip, before cauterizing.

Figure 26–11. Dissection is carried superiorly to the level of the Whitnall's ligament. Laterally, care is taken to carefully dissect out the lateral horn (shown retracted by a skin hook) of the aponeurosis as it bisects the lacrimal gland. Up to this point, the procedure is identical with the technique of aponeurotic ptosis surgery. The only difference is that one does not need to inject anesthetic under the aponeurosis in ptosis surgery. Instead of recessing the aponeurosis and extirpating Mueller's muscle, the aponeurosis is advanced onto the tarsal plate and Mueller's muscle is preserved in ptosis repair.

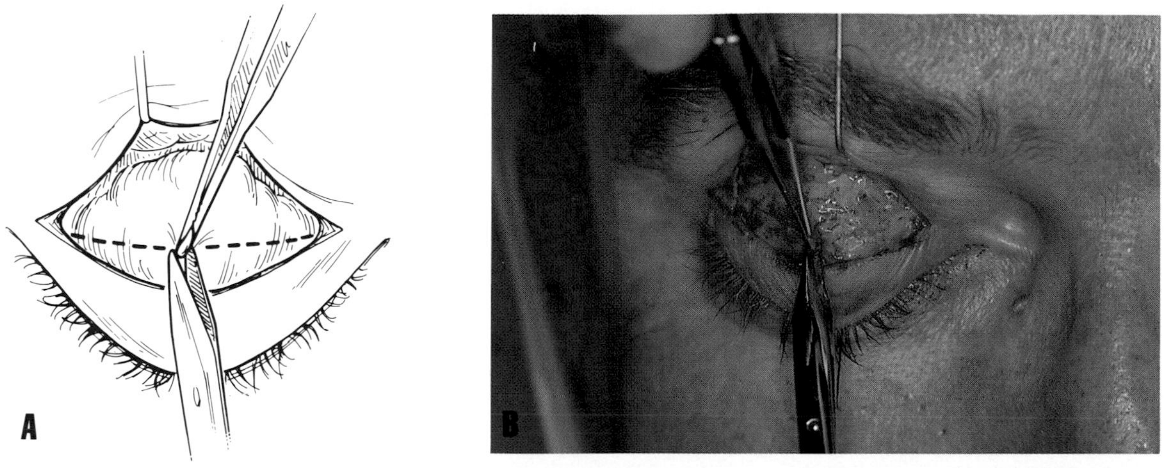

FIGURE 26–9

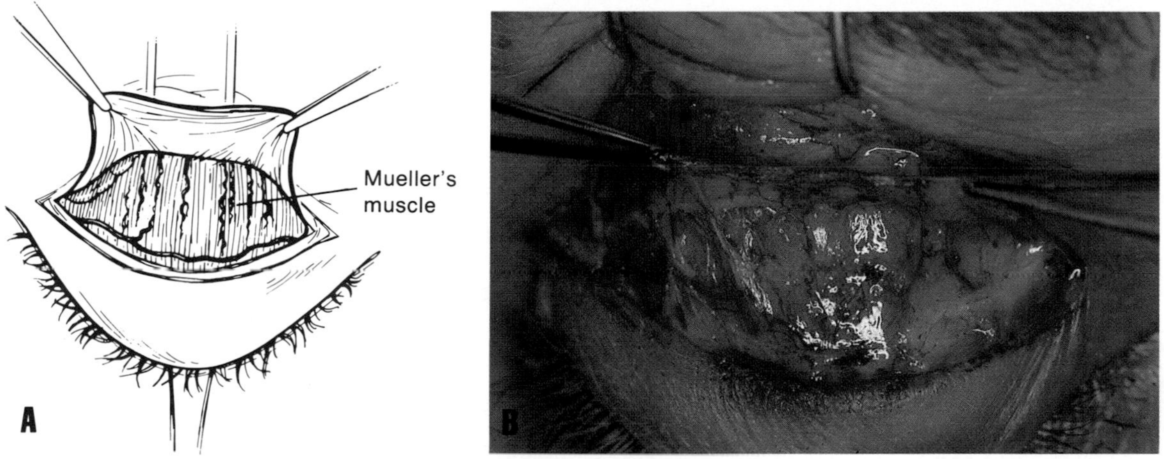

FIGURE 26–10

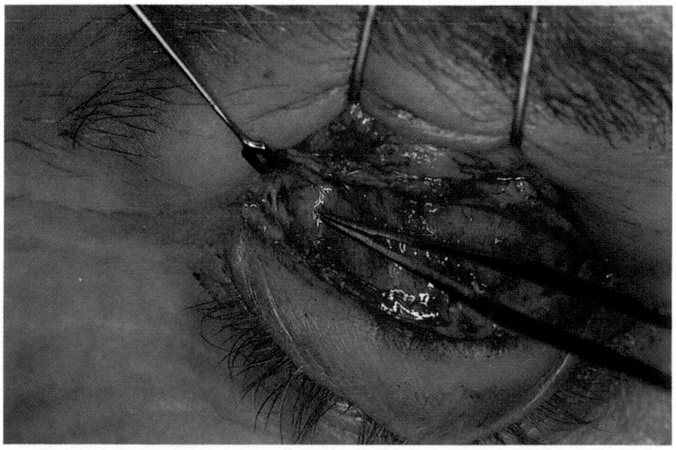

FIGURE 26–11

Figure 26–12A, B. With the freely mobilized levator aponeurosis retracted superiorly, lidocaine 2% with epinephrine is injected under Mueller's muscle to balloon it away from the underlying conjunctiva. A metal lid plate is placed in the superior fornix to protect the globe.

Figure 26–13. Starting at the midtarsal border, Mueller's muscle is tented upward with a forceps and opened with a Westcott scissors. A dissection plane beneath Mueller's muscle could be achieved in most cases. Once within this plane, the conjunctiva is put on stretch over a lid plate and sharp dissection will easily separate the sympathetic muscle from the conjunctiva. Small conjunctival buttonholes can be repaired with 7–0 chromic sutures.

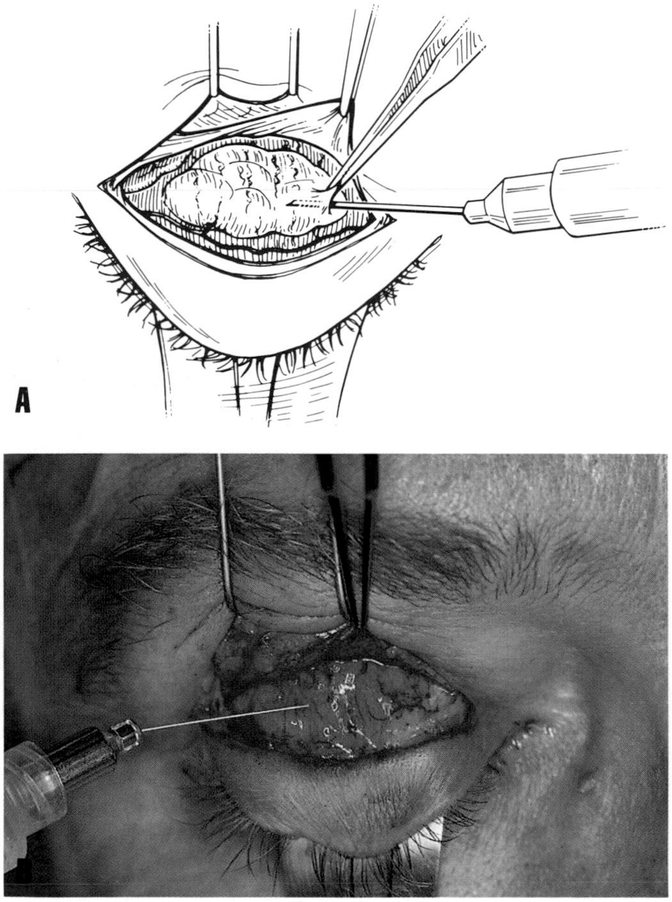

FIGURE 26–12

Figure 26–14. Stripping of the Mueller's muscle is continued superiorly to the fornix. Laterally, one must be certain to extirpate all of Mueller's muscle and scar tissue, since it is here that the eyelid retraction is most prominent and most difficult to recess. Temporally, meticulous dissection is mandatory to avoid injury to the palpebral lobe of the lacrimal gland. Bleeding usually ceases when Mueller's muscle is completely separated from the conjunctiva.

Figure 26–15. The Mueller's muscle is then extirpated en bloc with a scissors.

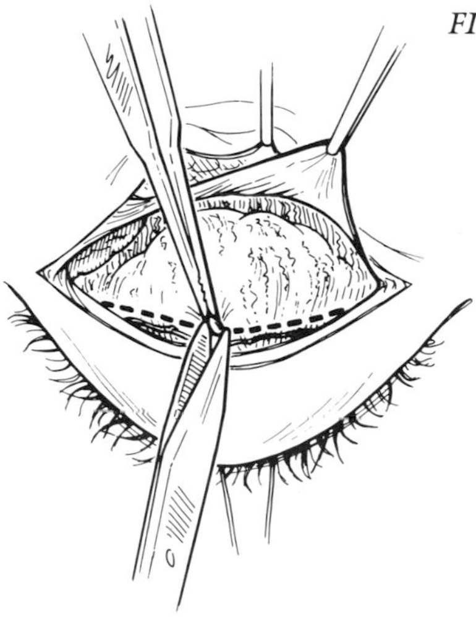

FIGURE 26–13

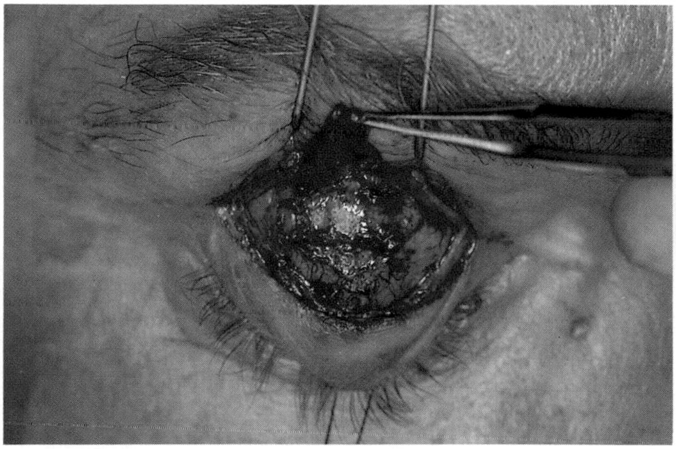

FIGURE 26–14

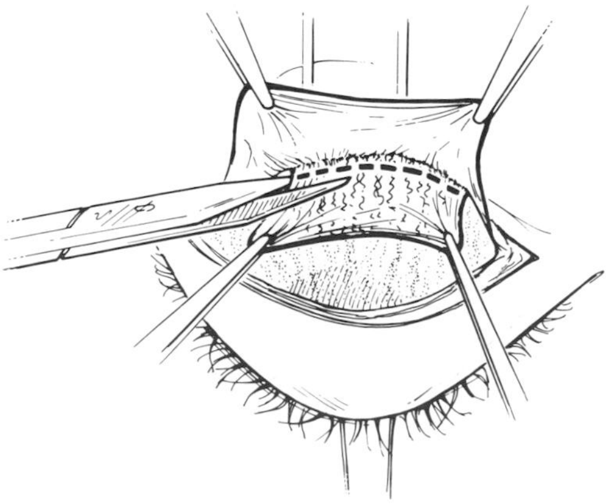

FIGURE 26–15

Figure 26–16A, B. The lateral horn of the levator aponeurosis is grasped with a forceps and severed from its lateral wall attachment with a blunt Westcott scissors. One blade of the scissors is inserted under the aponeurosis and directed superotemporally. The lacrimal gland and any surrounding vessels must be carefully insulated before the lateral horn is cut. As it is cut, one can feel the "give" and the lateral aponeurosis becomes fully mobile.

The upper two-thirds of the pretarsal orbicularis is undermined, thereby baring the anterior surface of the tarsal plate. A strip of pretarsal orbicularis is excised along the length of the eyelid to minimize a thickened appearance at the incision site.

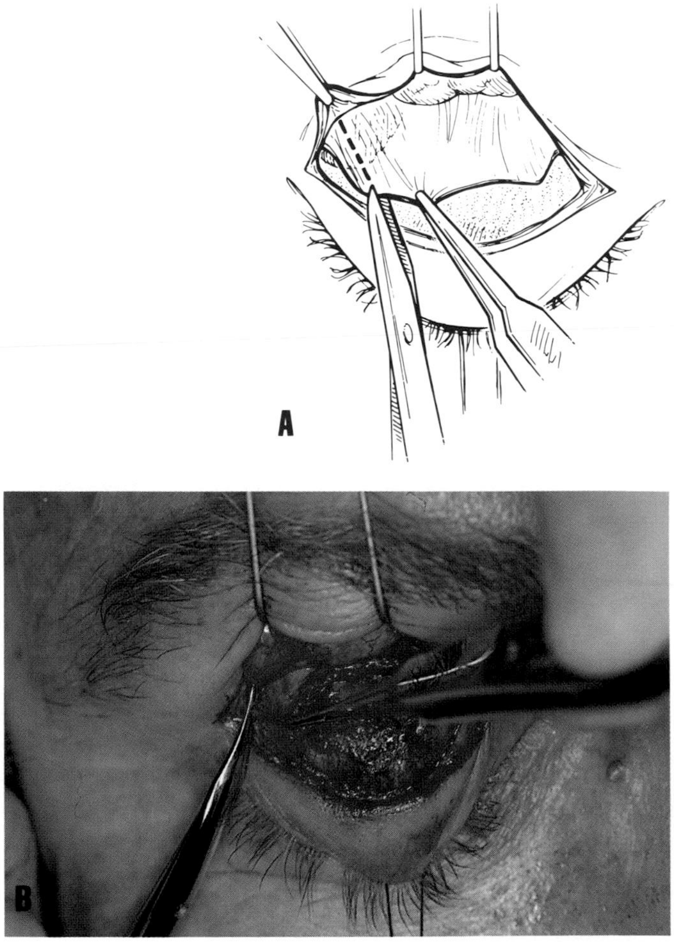

FIGURE 26–16

Figure 26–17A, B. The levator aponeurosis is then sutured either onto the conjunctiva or the upper edge of the tarsal plate, with 6–0 chromic sutures. Two to three interrupted sutures are placed over the central portion of the eyelid. A spatula needle facilitates a lamellar tarsal pass. Full-thickness tarsal sutures should be avoided to prevent corneal abrasion.

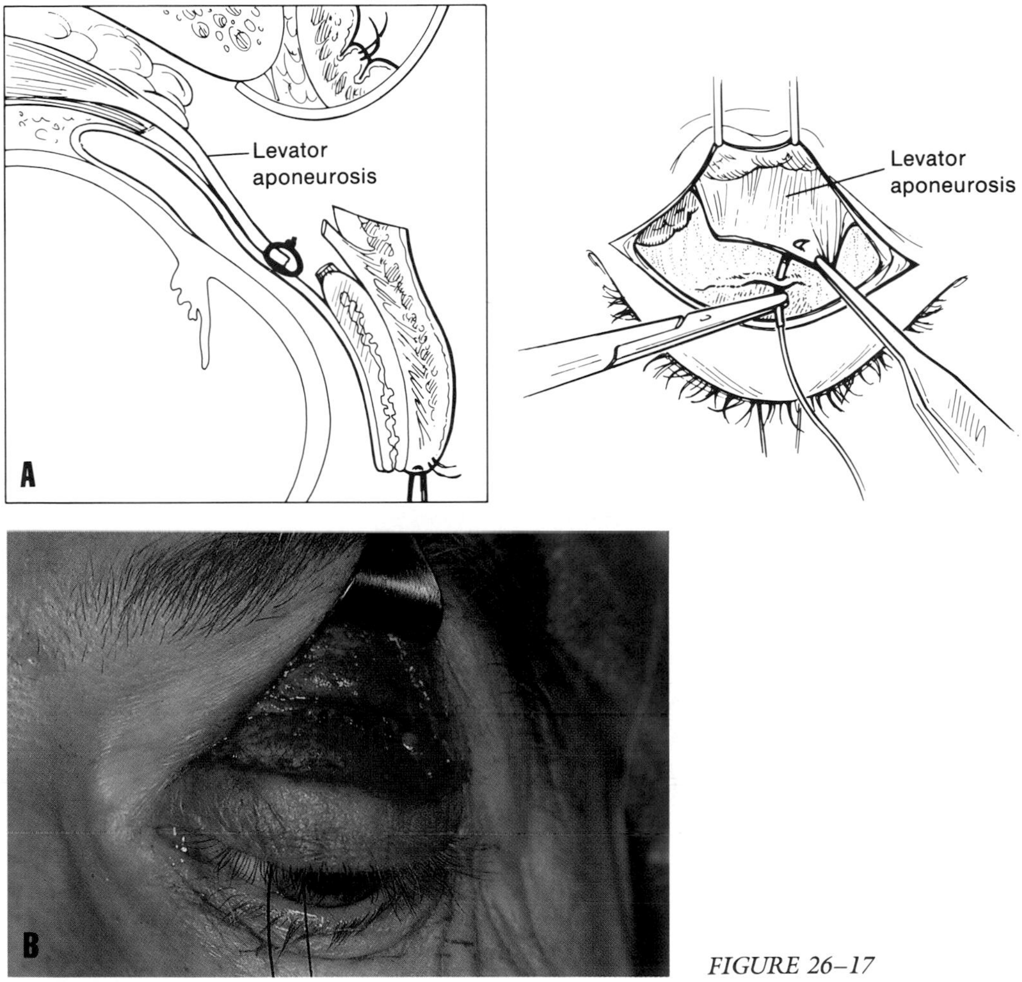

FIGURE 26–17

Figure 26–18. The patient is brought to a sitting position, and lid height and contour are assessed. Adjustments are made to place the eyelid at the desired level and contour. It may be necessary to recess the aponeurosis 5 to 10 mm from the superior tarsal margin to effect a suitable eyelid lowering. There is no need to overcorrect lid height, as one would in a ptosis correction, to compensate for anesthetic paralysis of the protractors. In an aponeurosis recession procedure, the lid height determined intraoperatively should be the postoperative height. Additional reinforcing sutures are placed to fixate the aponeurosis to the new position. Care should be taken not to alter the contour of the eyelid while placing these additional sutures. The prolapsing preaponeurotic fat pad, if prominent, can be clamped and excised as in a blepharoplasty. The severed stump must be cauterized before allowing it to retract into the orbit. Excess skin is marked and excised from the superior margin of the incision. The skin incision is closed with a running 7–0 nylon suture.

Figure 26–19A, B. The patient's appearance before surgery (**A**) can be contrasted with that immediately after surgery (**B**).

Postoperative Management

Bacitracin ophthalmic ointment is applied onto the incision three times daily for a week. An ice pack is placed over the lid to reduce postoperative edema. The suture is removed in 5 to 7 days. Any lid height or contour asymmetry should be corrected within the first week.

Lower Eyelid

In patients with 2 mm or less of lower eyelid retraction, a conjunctival approach with complete extirpation of the retractors (capsulopalpebral fascia and sympathetic muscle) is performed. For patients with 3 mm or more of lower eyelid retraction, the conjunctiva and retractors are recessed and a hard palate mucosal graft is used as a "spacer" to lengthen the posterior lamella.

Lidocaine 2% with 1:100,000 dilution of epinephrine is injected subconjunctivally with a 30-gauge needle. Two 4–0 silk sutures are placed along the lid margin for traction during surgery and left as modified Frost sutures to suspend the lower eyelid at the end of the procedure. One suture is positioned along the medial third of the lid, and the other is at the lateral third. The needle is passed through the tarsal plate in a lamellar fashion, avoiding the marginal arcade vessels.

The lid is everted over a metal lid plate and an infratarsal snip incision is made with a blunt-tipped Westcott scissors. The incision is through both conjunctiva and retractors, until the postorbicular fascial plane is identified. Through this opening, the horizontally oriented preseptal orbicularis muscle fibers can be seen. Meticulous hemostasis should be obtained to prevent bleeding from obscuring this tissue plane.

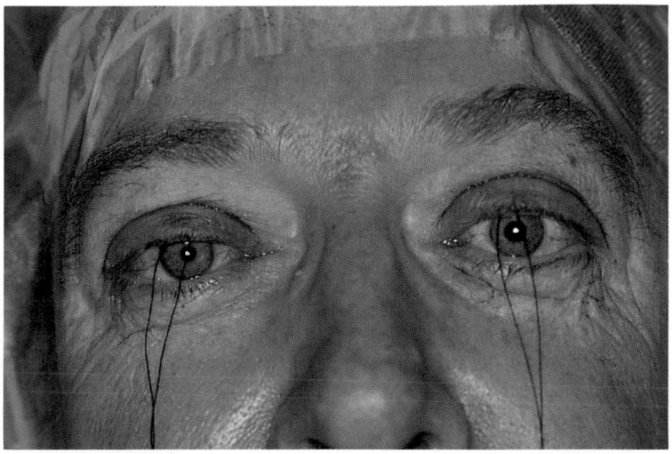

FIGURE 26–18

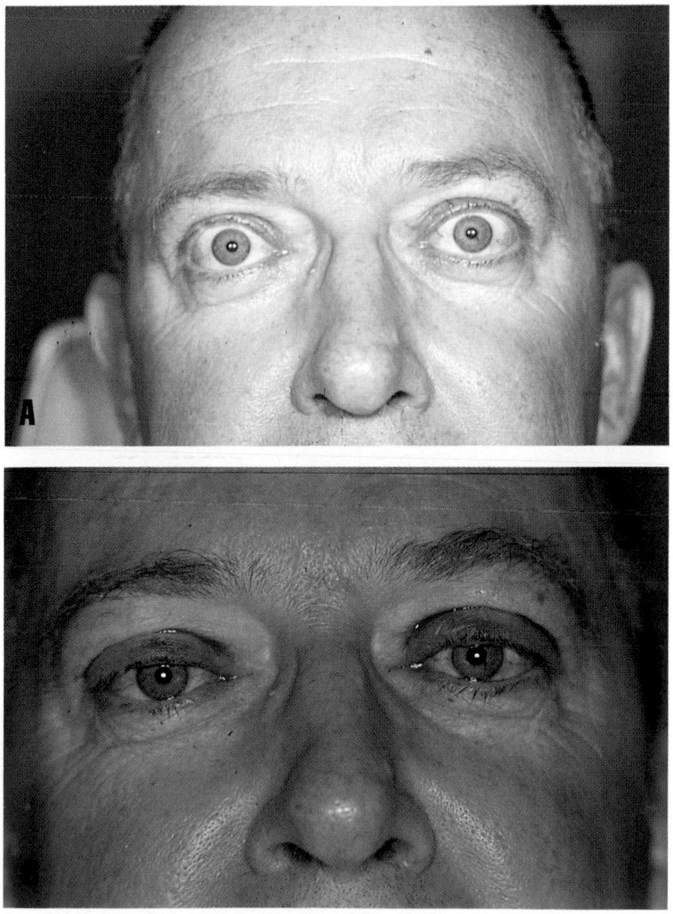

FIGURE 26–19

Figure 26–20A, B. A surgeons view while operating on the left lower lid is shown. With one blade of the scissors inserted into this tissue plane, the infratarsal incision is completed with cuts medially and laterally. A foreceps is grasping both the conjunctiva and the retractors. This incision extends from below the punctum to the lateral canthus. Using sharp dissection, the anterior surface of the lower eyelid retractors is separated from orbital septum and the preaponeurotic fat pad. Anatomically, the retractors of the lower eyelid lie immediately posterior to the fat pads. Prolapsing orbital fat can be removed in the same manner as in a lower eyelid blepharoplasty. To verify that the lower eyelid retractors have been dissected free from the anterior lamella, the patient is asked to look down while the surgeon gently lifts up the eyelid with the traction sutures. If separation within this plane is complete, one should see the disinserted edges of the conjunctiva and retractors pulled deep into the fornix, without tugging on the anterior lamella.

Figure 26–21. The retractors are then ballooned away from the underlying conjunctiva with local anesthetic.

Figure 26–22. The capsulopalpebral fascia or aponeurosis, together with the sympathetic muscle are carefully dissected off the conjunctiva. The dissection is carried inferiorly to Lockwood's ligament. Lockwood's ligament, a whitish transverse suspensory ligament located anterior to the inferior oblique muscle, is formed by fusion of fascial fibers from several structures (see Chapter 1 for review of lower eyelid anatomy). Inferior dissection of the retractors should stop at this landmark. Dissection beyond this structure will invariably encounter the inferior oblique muscle or the insertion of the inferior rectus.

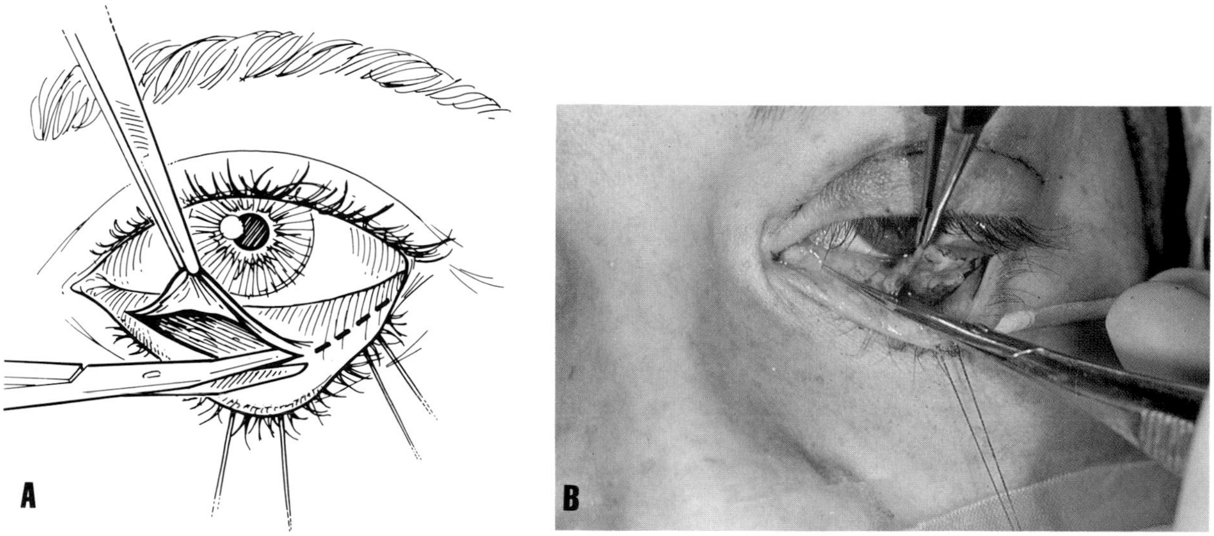

FIGURE 26–20

FIGURE 26–21

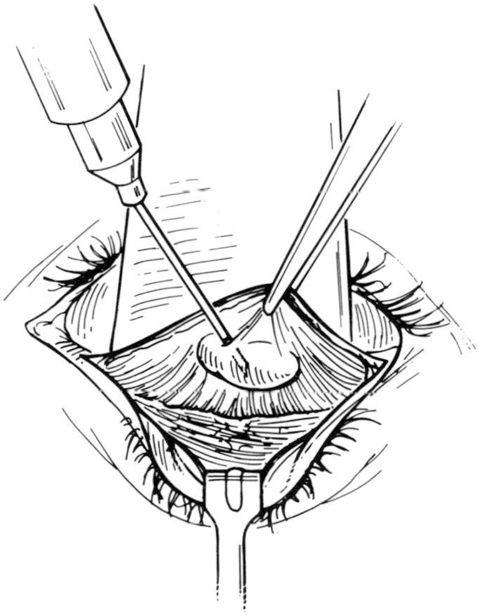

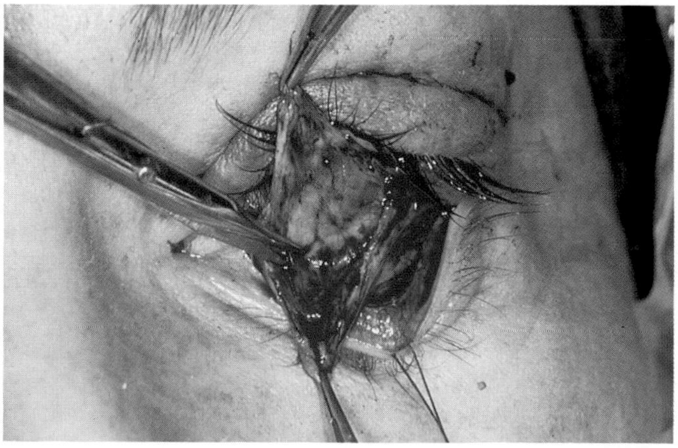

FIGURE 26–22

Figure 26–23A, B. The retractors are then amputated above the Lockwood's ligament with a scissors. The severed stump of the retractors should be cauterized before allowing it to retract into the orbit.

Figure 26–24. The conjunctiva is sutured to the inferior margin of the tarsal plate with a 7–0 chromic suture in a running horizontal mattress fashion. One should be careful not to expose the suture or the knots.

Antibiotic ointment is instilled into the fornix and the two 4–0 silk sutures are taped to the forehead to put the lower lid on stretch. The modified Frost sutures are removed in 4 to 5 days.

For patients with more than 3 mm of lower eyelid retraction, extirpation of the retractors alone will not be sufficient to effect the desired lid elevation. In this group of patients, the conjunctiva and retractors are recessed en bloc, and an autogenous hard palate mucosa is used as an interpositional graft to lengthen the posterior lamella. When inserted under the inferior margin of the tarsal plate, it also serves as a scaffold to provide support for the anterior lamella. Hard palate mucosa closely approximates lower eyelid tarsus in terms of contour, thickness, and rigidity. The mucosal surface is lined by keratinizing, stratified squamous epithelium, and it is well tolerate when grafted into the lower lid. Hard palate mucosa is abundant and easily obtained with minimal donor site morbidity. As an autograft it is not at risk for rejection, and it has shown only minimal shrinkage following grafting.

Harvesting of Hard Palate Mucosa

The surgery is usually performed under local anesthesia using a side mouth gag. The graft is taken from the hard palate between the alveolar ridge and the midline, extending posteriorly to within 1 to 2 mm of the soft palate. The graft is harvested lateral to the midline as the mucosa located centrally is too thin to be used as a posterior lamella splint. A graft twice the height of the measured amount of lid retraction is obtained. A mixture of equal amounts of lidocaine 2% with 1:100,000 epinephrine and bupivocaine 0.75% is injected into mucosa and mucoperiosteum.

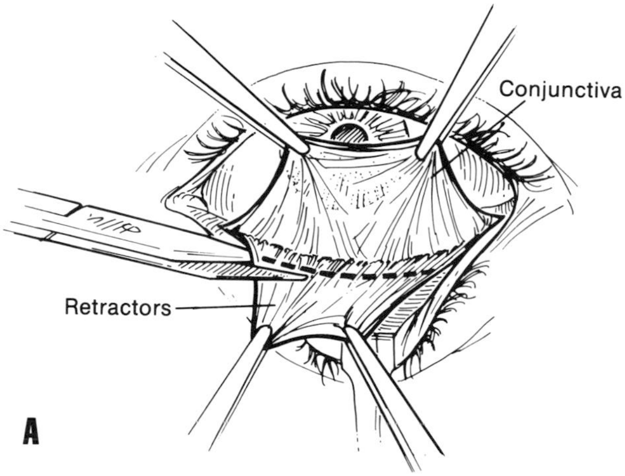

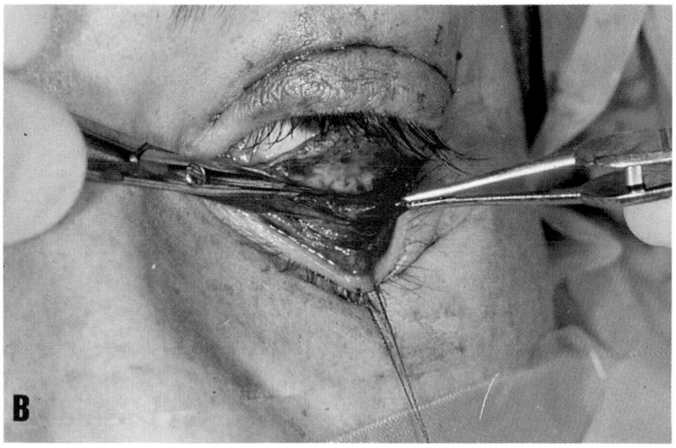

FIGURE 26–23

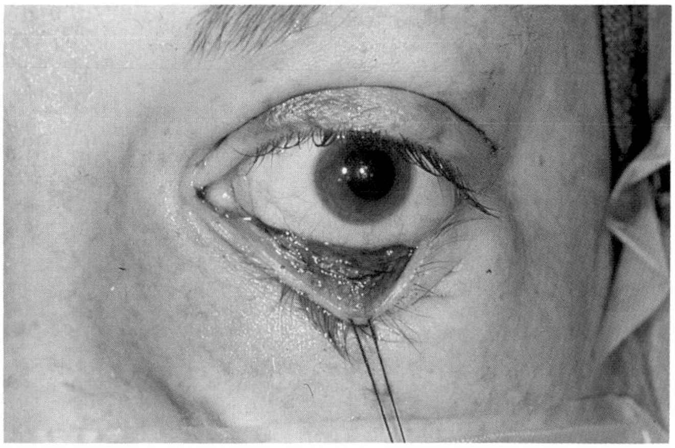

FIGURE 26–24

Figure 26–25. The dimensions of the graft are outlined on the donor site with a marking pen. Note the location of the greater palatine artery and nerve. The posterior limit of the incision should not go beyond the second molar, to avoid damage to the lesser palatine artery, which courses through the deep submucosal tissue at the junction of hard and soft palate. The greater palatine artery which courses within the mucoperiosteum adjacent the alveolar ridge can be damaged if the incisions are made too deep. If the vessel is inadvertently cut, brisk bleeding may be encountered, but can be stopped with a bipolar cautery. A damp 4 × 4 gauze may be loosely packed in the buccal recess to catch any blood runoff. Two parallel incisions the desired length of the graft are made through mucosa with a size 15 Bard–Parker blade. Care should be taken to avoid incising the underlying mucoperiosteum. As the incision is made, a suction tip is placed next to the incision to continuously evacuate any mucosal ooze, before allowing the blood to run toward the oropharynx. This is particularly important in avoiding gagging when harvesting the graft in an awake patient.

Figure 26–26. The hard palate mucosa is elevated off the mucoperiosteum with a right-angled Beaver size 66 blade. The graft is incised at each end to complete its removal.

Figure 26–27. The donor sight is shown after removal of the graft. Hemostasis is obtained by bipolar cautery and the mucosal defect is covered with collagen and periodontal paste. An upper denture or prefitted acrylic plate may be applied at the conclusion of the procedure to provide patient comfort.

Figure 26–28. Typically, the size of the graft ranges between 30 and 35 mm long and 10 to 13 mm wide when harvested. Note the rugae at right lateral portion of the specimen. The adherent mucous glands and submucosa are trimmed from the undersurface of the graft with a scissors. The graft is wrapped in a moist soak. For surgeons who do not wish to harvest their hard palate grafts, the graft can be obtained by an oral surgeon at the time of lid surgery.

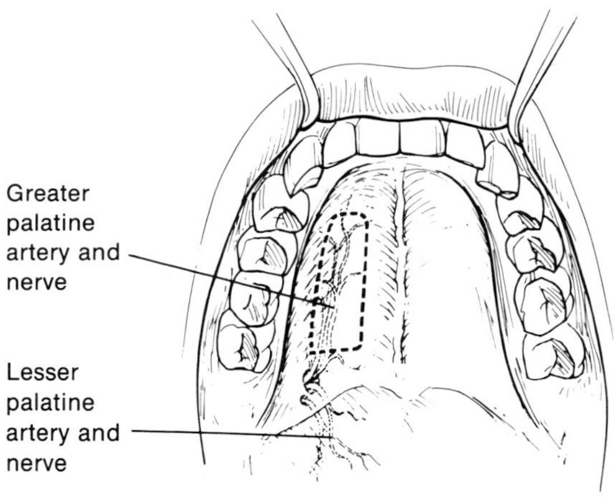

FIGURE 26–25

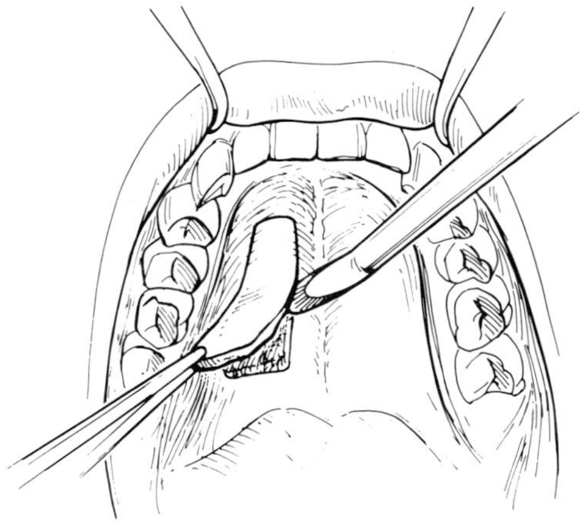

FIGURE 26–26

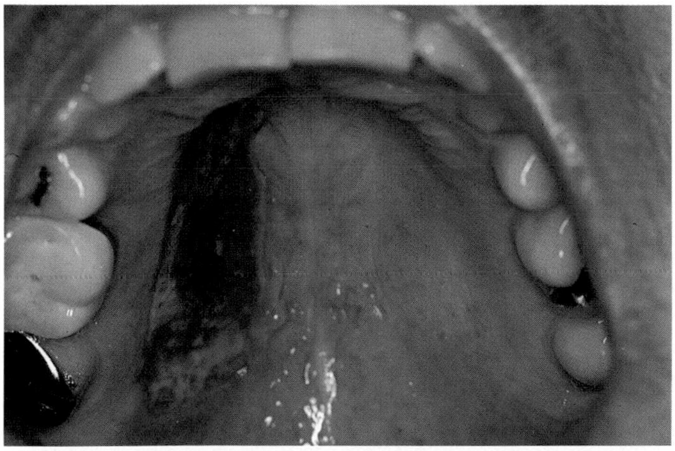

FIGURE 26–27

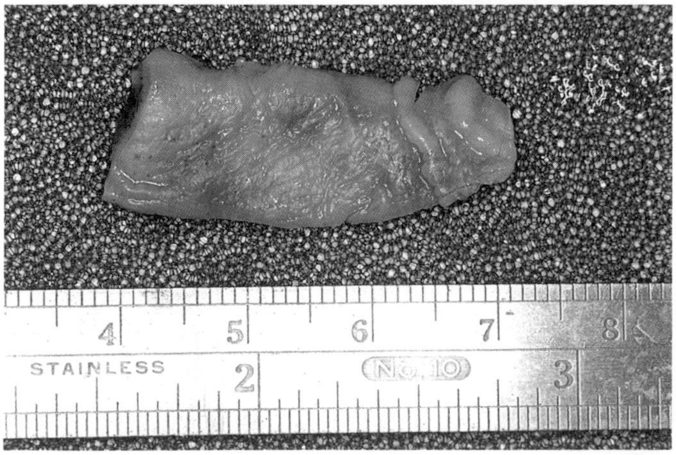

FIGURE 26–28

Grafting of Hard Palate Mucosa

Figure 26–29. A horizontal infratarsal conjunctival incision is made through conjunctiva and lower eyelid retractors, extending from the punctum to the lateral canthus. A Westcott scissors is used to dissect between the orbicularis and the orbital septum, so that maximum recession of the conjunctiva, retractors, and septum can be achieved. A forceps is shown grasping the edge of the conjunctiva and retractors. The pointer is directed at the orbital septum. When a hard palate graft is used as a "spacer," it is unnecessary to extirpate the retractors en bloc.

Figure 26–30. Prolapsing orbital fat can be removed and the stump cauterized. The recipient bed is now ready to receive the interpositional graft.

Figure 26–31. The hard palate graft is then trimmed to conform to the configuration of the recipient bed. The graft is usually elliptical in shape, but wider over the lateral portion to lessen the temporal "flair" of the lower lid. The portion of the graft containing rugae is oriented toward the fornix or laterally, away from the cornea. The mucosal surface of the graft is facing the globe; the rough submucosal surface is in apposition with the preseptal orbicularis.

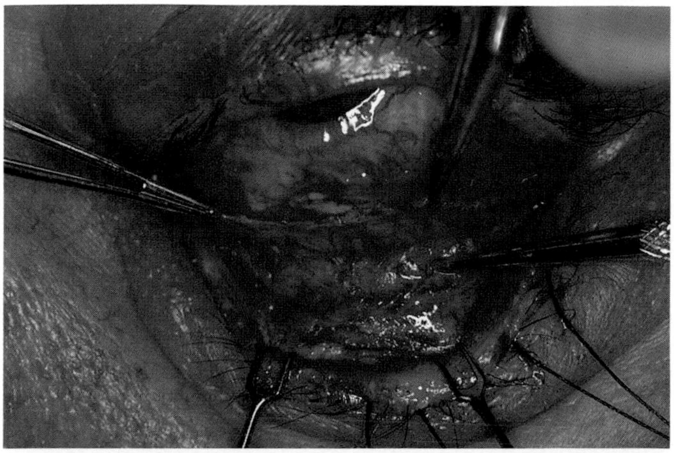

FIGURE 26–29

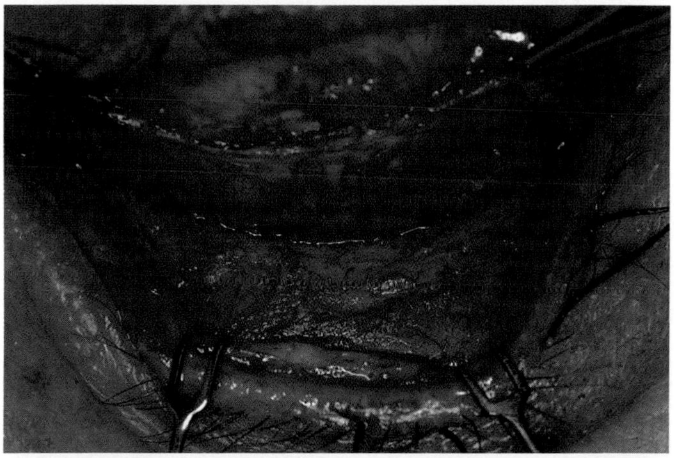

FIGURE 26–30

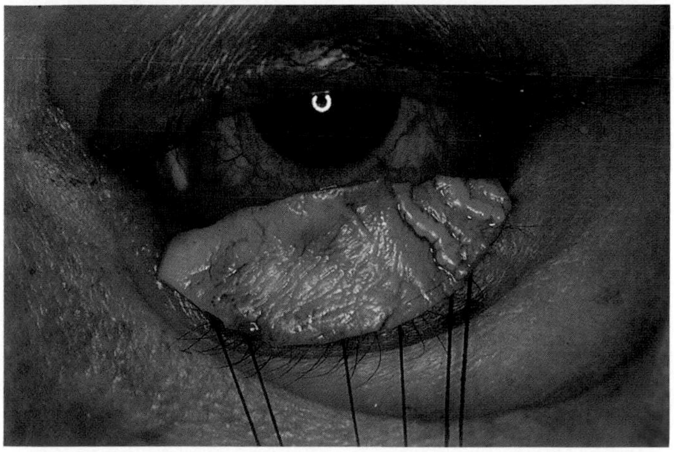

FIGURE 26–31

Figure 26–32A. The inferior border of the graft is sutured to the edge of the recessed retractors and conjunctiva with a 7–0 chromic suture in a running fashion.

Figure 26–32B. The graft is ready to be fitted under the inferior margin of the tarsal plate. The submucosal surface is in apposition with the preseptal orbicularis muscle.

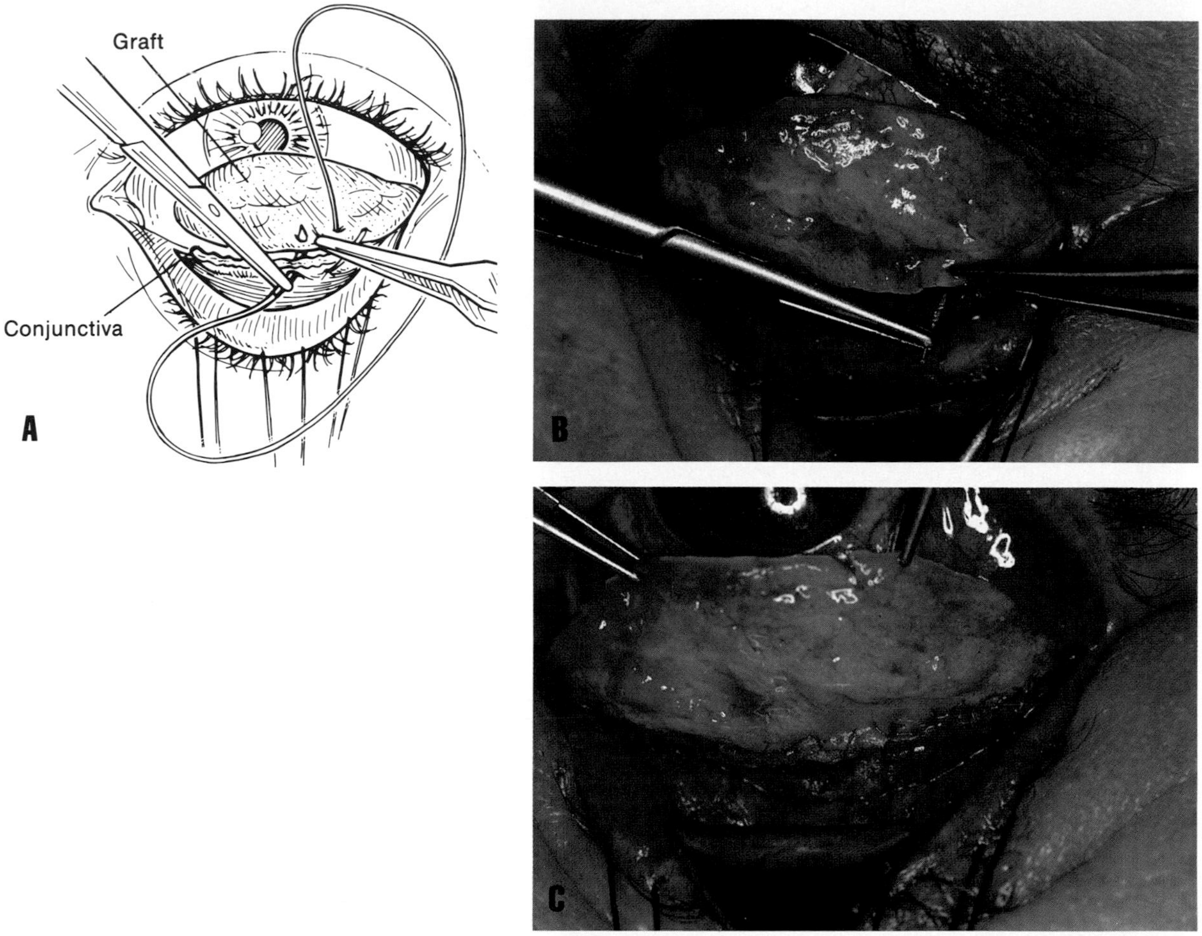

FIGURE 26–32

Figure 26–33A, B. The superior edge of the graft is sutured to the inferior border of the tarsus (**A**) with a 7–0 chromic suture in a running horizontal mattress manner (**B**). Suture knots are buried at both ends of the graft.

Figure 26–33C. A sagittal view illustrates graft placement. Antibiotic ointment is applied to the inferior fornix, and modified Frost sutures are taped to the forehead to elevate the lower eyelid.

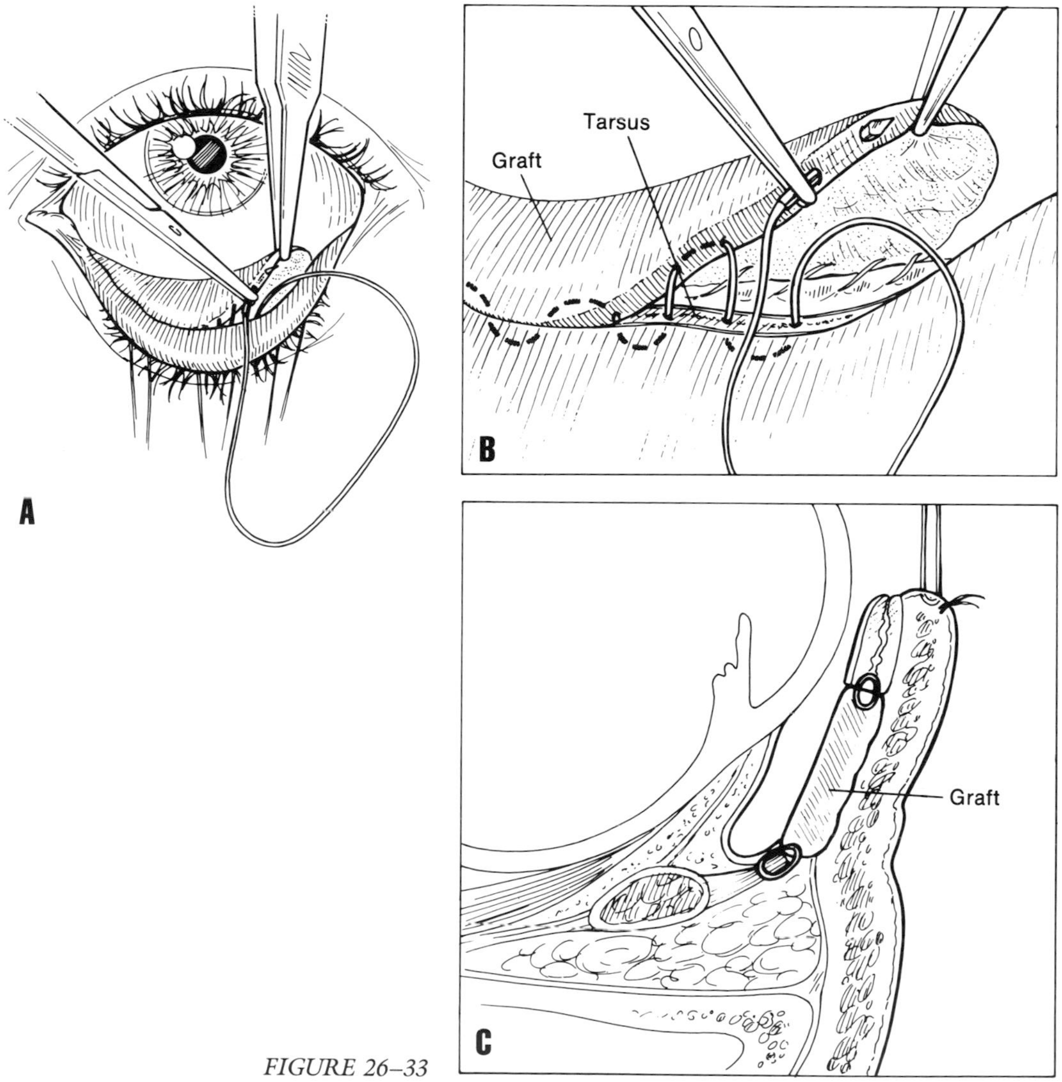

FIGURE 26–33

Chapter Twenty-Seven

ORBITAL DECOMPRESSION

John V. Linberg
William K. Blaylock

SURGICAL INDICATIONS

Orbital Graves' Disease

The majority of orbital decompression procedures are performed for the treatment of dysthyroid orbital Graves' disease. Most patients with orbital Graves' disease have exophthalmos caused by orbital edema and enlargement of extraocular muscles. Spontaneous anterior displacement of the globe is usually sufficient to decompress the orbit and maintain normal optic nerve function. However, in 2% to 5% of patients, the extraocular muscles enlarge within the confines of the bony orbit and compress the optic nerve, causing dysfunction. Muscular enlargement in orbital Graves' disease is often most pronounced in the posterior one-third of the muscles, creating pressure in the orbital apex. The extraocular muscles in the apex are not only much closer to the nerve, but they are also fixed in position by the annulus of Zinn.

Systemic steroid therapy is the preferred medical treatment for compressive optic neuropathy (CON). Unfortunately, not all patients respond to these medications, and there are frequent recurrences when steroids are withdrawn. Many patients cannot tolerate the high dosage required, and the complications of long-term steroids are well known. Beneficial effects usually occur within the first 2 weeks of treatment, and no further improvement can be expected after 6 to 8 weeks. When neuropathy is unresponsive to steroids, or recurs when steroids are withdrawn, surgical decompression is usually recommended.

In addition to visual loss from CON, potential indications for surgical decompression in orbital Graves' disease include corneal exposure, strabismus, pain, choroidal folds, recurrent globe luxation, and cosmesis. Eyelid surgery is usually adequate for the management of corneal exposure. Strabismus, when stable, is best corrected with prisms or muscle surgery. In recent years, decompressions have been performed more frequently for cosmetic reasons. However, because of the serious potential complications of orbital decompression, we usually reserve decompression surgery for the preservation of vision in cases of CON.

Trauma

Direct trauma to the orbit can produce expansion of orbital contents from hemorrhage, edema, or emphysema. Proptosis relieves orbital pressure, but if this spontaneous anterior decompression is inadequate, then compression of the globe may cause an elevated intraocular pressure, with risk of central retinal artery occlusion. Pressure elevations within the orbit can also compromise blood flow to the eye or optic nerve, resulting in an ischemic optic neuropathy. The probable site of optic nerve compression in trauma is again the orbital apex, a rigidly confined space filled with vital structures.

Posttraumatic orbital hemorrhage and edema may occasionally require surgical treatment if proptosis is very severe and there are clinical signs of optic nerve dysfunction. Vision that is initially intact and subsequently deteriorates suggests reversible compression. Lateral canthotomy and cantholysis will decompress the anterior orbit, but posterior surgical decompression may be necessary in rare cases. Needle aspiration should be reserved for orbital emphysema.

Traumatic optic nerve injury usually results from mechanisms other than orbital compression. A history of immediate visual loss after trauma suggests optic nerve transection at the moment of impact. Visual loss from nerve edema within the osseous canal can occur without significant proptosis. Recognition of these other mechanisms for traumatic optic neuropathy can prevent unnecessary decompression surgery. Only patients with *massive* hemorrhage and extremely firm orbits should even be considered for decompression, as most cases of traumatic optic neuropathy are related to other mechanisms.

EVALUATION OF PATIENTS

Clinical Evaluation

Patients followed for orbital Graves' disease require repeated ophthalmic examinations, with special emphasis on optic nerve function. Examinations should be more frequent during active phases of the disease. Optic nerve dysfunction may occur at any time, even while the patient is receiving anti-inflammatory therapy. The degree of proptosis is not an accurate indication of risk for optic neuropathy. In fact, most patients with compressive optic neuropathy have only moderate exophthalmos. Patients with an initial diagnosis of orbital Graves' disease also require evaluation of thyroid function by an endocrinologist.

Visual acuity is only a gross indication of optic nerve function. Examinations must also include evaluation of the pupils, visual fields, color vision, and dilated examinations of the optic disc (looking for pallor or edema). Motility examinations reveal extraocular muscle involvement. Slit-lamp examinations may disclose signs of corneal exposure. The same examination should be performed for trauma patients with suspected optic nerve injury.

Further Diagnostic Tests

If optic neuropathy is diagnosed, then a computerized tomography (CT) scan of the orbit provides the best image of the optic nerve and adjacent structures. Axial sections may demonstrate contact between the optic nerve and the enlarged extraocular muscles. Coronal sections are especially useful for evaluation of the orbital apex. In orbital Graves' disease, the enlarged extraocular muscles may displace orbital fat, eliminating any perceivable space between themselves and the nerve. This CT scan image in association with clinical signs of optic neuropathy suggests the need for surgical orbital decompression, when medical therapy fails.

The diagnosis of orbital Graves' disease with CON must be carefully documented before surgery. Most patients have classic eye findings of Graves' disease and a past history of thyroid dysfunction. There may be other orbital disorders that mimic Graves' disease, especially when the findings are asymmetric. A careful neuro-ophthalmic examination is needed to rule out other causes of visual loss or optic neuropathy. High-quality CT scans or magnetic resonance imaging (MRI) are necessary to confirm the diagnosis of orbital Graves' disease with optic nerve compression and to eliminate the possibility of other disorders.

SURGERY

Surgical Anatomy of the Orbit

The most important anatomic consideration during surgical decompression is adequate expansion of the orbital apex. Decompression of this area, near the optic foramen, relieves pressure on the nerve. This can be accomplished only by bone removal from the posterior medial wall or the orbital roof. A simple lateral wall or orbital floor decompression does not adequately decompress the apex. Laterally, the temporal lobe of the brain prevents posterior access to the orbital apex. Expansion is further limited by the temporalis muscle. An inferior decompression also fails to achieve the necessary apical decompression because the floor does not extend as far posterior as the optic canal.

Figure 27–1. Although removal of the orbital roof by a subfrontal approach decompresses the orbital apex, this neurosurgical technique subjects the patient to greater risks. For these reasons, resection of the orbital floor and medial wall have been widely accepted as the best approach to orbital decompression for optic nerve dysfunction. Orbital tissues can expand into the ethmoid compartment once the lamina papyracea and ethmoid air cells have been removed.

A floor and medial wall decompression can be performed using either a transantral (Caldwell–Luc) approach, lower eyelid incision, or inferior conjunctival fornix incision, combined with lateral cantholysis.

Preparations for Surgery

Immediately before surgery, routine sinus films should be examined to rule out the possibility of sinusitis. Since most patients have a history of thyroid dysfunction, an endocrinologic consultation just before surgery reduces the risk of anesthetic complications related to thyroid storm or arrhythmia. The patient should be cross-matched and typed for 2 units of blood, although they will rarely be needed.

Surgery is routinely performed under general anesthesia. A cuffed endotracheal tube is needed because significant quantities of blood may accumulate in the pharynx. The patient is placed in a moderate reverse Trendelenburg's position. Cottonoid strips moistened with a 4% cocaine solution are packed in the nasal cavity to minimize mucosal bleeding. If a rolled blanket is placed under the shoulders, and the neck is extended, exposure of the orbital floor and medial wall will be easier during the operation.

Description of Operative Procedure

The inferior conjunctival fornix incision provides excellent exposure and avoids the need for a lower eyelid skin incision (see Chapter 4).

A 4–0 silk traction suture is placed through the lower eyelid margin, with care to avoid the marginal artery. A piece of Gelfoam is sutured over the cornea with a 6–0 silk suture to prevent epithelial loss during the procedure. A short skin incision is marked at the lateral canthus and the orbital floor as far laterally as the inferior orbital fissure. This periorbital elevation is then extended up the medial orbital wall. Orbital tissues may be retracted with malleable ribbon retractors or Ferris–Smith blade retractors.

For the remainder of the procedure, it is imperative that the surgeon have loupes for magnification and a high-quality fiberoptic headlight. An assistant is necessary to provide gentle retraction of the orbital tissues, but care must be taken not to apply excessive pressure on the globe. The surgeon may wish to hold a Frazier suction tip in the nondominant hand while using the dominant hand to remove bone with appropriate rongeurs.

It is virtually impossible to photograph the deep orbital procedure. Therefore, the remainder of the operation is demonstrated using photographs of a skull.

Figure 27–2. A number of landmarks critical during the operative procedure may be identified on this skull. The entire orbital floor and medial wall will be removed to achieve adequate decompression, but care must be taken to avoid adjacent structures. Injury to the lacrimal drainage system is avoided by not removing bone from the lacrimal sac fossa (*LF*). The suture between the frontal bone and ethmoid bone is an important landmark (*open arrow*) on the upper edge of the medial wall. The bone resection stops at this level, and care must be taken not to injure the ethmoid arteries that exit from the anterior ethmoid foramen (*AF*) and posterior ethmoid foramen (*PF*). The inferior orbital fissure (*IOF*) limits the lateral extent of the bone resection along the floor. Care is also taken to avoid injury to the infraorbital neurovascular bundle that passes along the orbital floor and exits at the infraorbital foramen (*IF*).

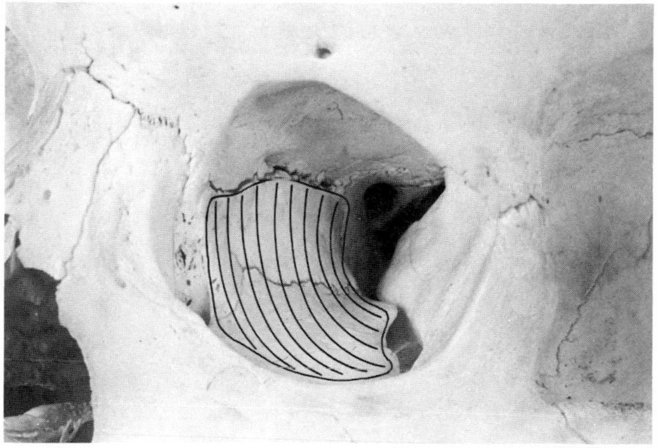

FIGURE 27–1

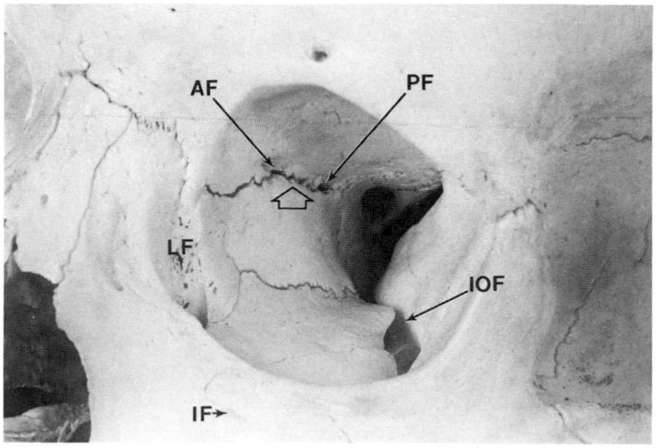

FIGURE 27–2

Figure 27–3. After adequate exposure, the sharp end of a Freer elevator is used to gently shave an opening in the medial aspect of the orbital floor. With care, it is possible to open the bone without lacerating the underlying mucosa of the maxillary sinus. If the mucosa can be left intact, then there is less bacterial contamination of the orbit and also less bleeding.

Figure 27–4. The orbital floor is removed in pieces, using rongeurs. A Takahashi ethmoidectomy rongeur (shown here) is useful. Kerrison rongeurs may be used for removing bone near the anterior rim.

Figure 27–5. Bone is removed as far back as the posterior wall of the maxillary sinus. This important landmark may be palpated with a finger or instrument.

Bone is now removed from the lateral orbital floor, carefully working around the infraorbital neurovascular bundle. It is possible to gently remove this bone piecemeal, without tearing the nerve. The lateral orbital floor is usually resected as far as the inferior orbital fissure.

The medial orbital wall is perforated through the thin lamina papyracea of the ethmoid bone. Ethmoidectomy rongeurs are also used for this part of the procedure. Brisk bleeding is sometimes encountered from the ethmoid air cells, and this is best controlled by completing the exenteration of ethmoid air cells. Intermittent packing with cottonoid pledgets moistened in 4% cocaine solution or epinephrine solution 1:200,000 may be helpful.

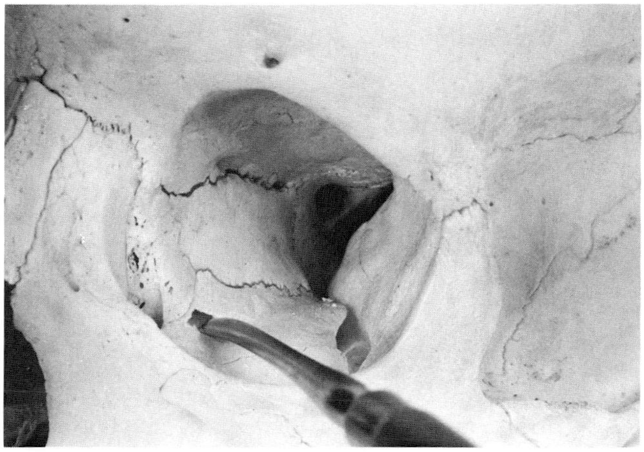

FIGURE 27–3

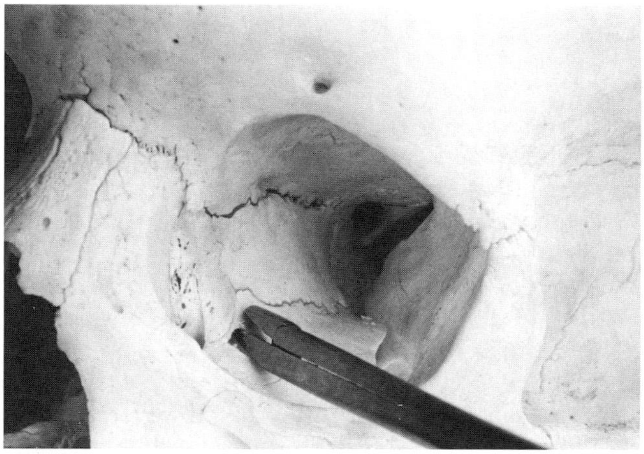

FIGURE 27–4

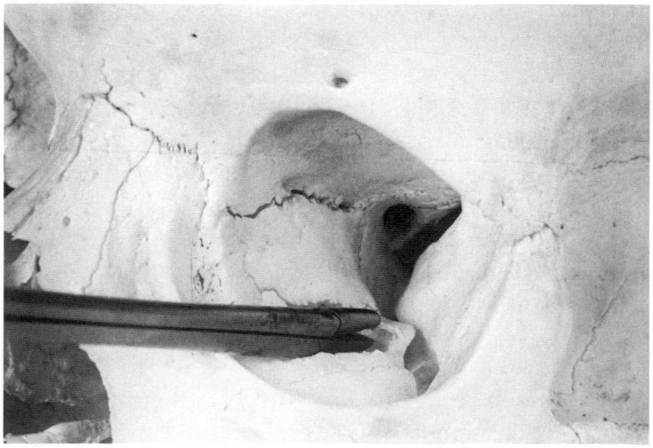

FIGURE 27–5

Figure 27–6. Bone is removed from the medial orbital wall up to the suture between the frontal bone and ethmoid plate. This suture (which is usually palpable) is a useful landmark. Bone removal should stop at this suture to avoid fractures of the cribiform plate and cerebrospinal fluid leaks. The suture is also the location of the anterior and posterior ethmoid arteries, and care should be taken to avoid these vessels.

Figure 27–7. Bone is removed from the medial wall as far posterior as the optic foramen. The posterior extent of this bone removal is difficult to judge, but crucial to the orbital decompression. Near the optic canal, the bone of the medial wall thickens and resists further removal. This change in the character of the bone is a reliable and useful anatomic landmark. The posterior wall of the maxillary sinus may also be used to judge the depth of the medial wall resection. The most posterior edge of the medial wall resection should normally be about 40 mm from the orbital rim.

Figure 27–8. At the end of bone removal, the entire floor and medial wall have been resected. The anterior edge of the medial wall resection is just posterior to the posterior lacrimal crest. If the posterior lacrimal crest has not been damaged, then injury to the lacrimal sac can be avoided. Notice that the bone removal extends into the orbital apex adjacent to the optic canal.

Once the bone removal has been completed, and the ethmoid air cells exenterated, bleeding should be minimal. Residual bleeding may be controlled by packing the area with cottonoid strips. Because the orbit is widely decompressed into the adjacent sinuses, optic nerve compression by an orbital hematoma is very unlikely. However, there is risk of significant blood loss from a lacerated ethmoid artery, and the wound should not be closed until all bleeding has been controlled.

Attention is now directed to the condition of the periorbita. This fascia is often quite thin and may have ruptured during the bone removal. If the periorbita is still intact, it should be incised superficially with Westcott scissors to release the orbital fat. Unless the periorbita is widely open, orbital fat may not prolapse into the area of decompression, even though bone removal has been adequate.

A good decompressive effect should be observable at the end of the procedure. Gentle palpation of the globe should disclose that the firm preoperative resistance to retroplacement has been replaced by a soft orbit. If the change is not obvious, the completeness of bone removal should be examined. Further openings in the periorbita should also be considered. The surgical field is again inspected for hemostasis.

At the end of the procedure, the inferior conjunctiva is sutured with three or four interrupted 5–0 chromic sutures. The lateral canthal tendon is sutured to the inner aspect of the lateral orbital rim with 4–0 Vicryl sutures.

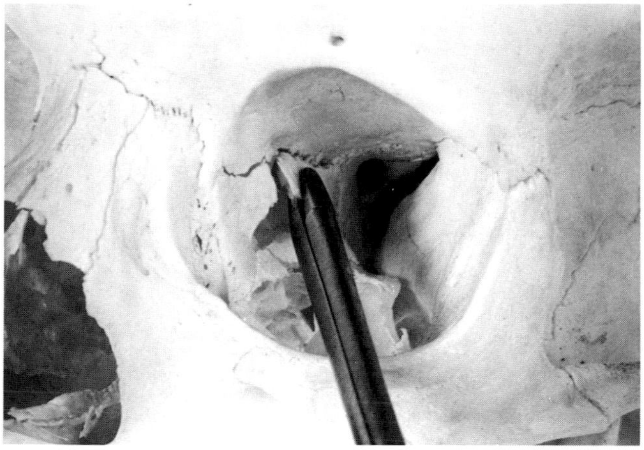

FIGURE 27–6

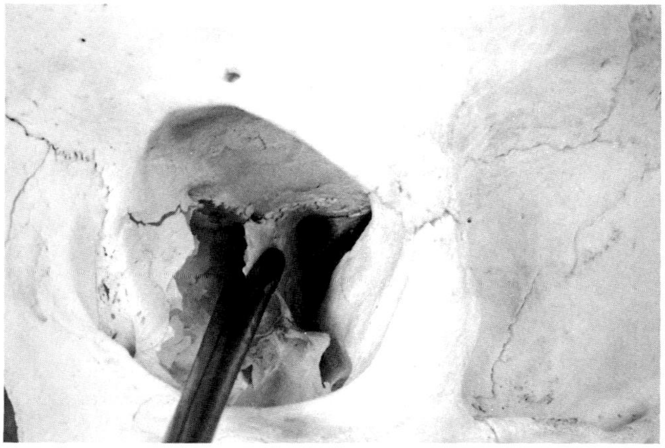

FIGURE 27–7

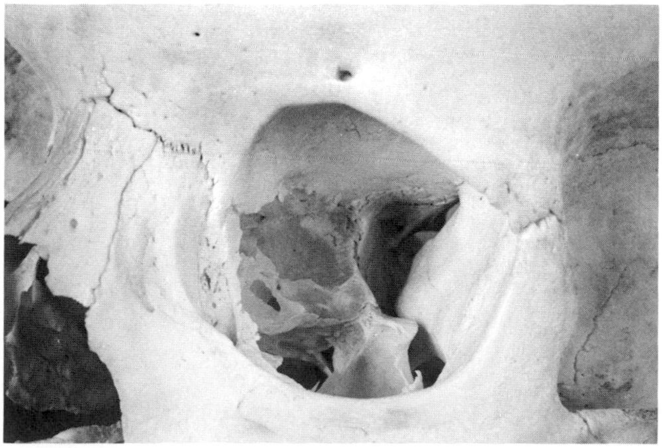

FIGURE 27–8

RESULTS AND POSTOPERATIVE CARE

Successful orbital decompression for neuropathy often produces an immediate improvement in visual function. Visual acuity may even improve during the first few hours after surgery. If optic nerve injury has been long-standing, visual acuity and visual fields improve slowly. Preoperative optic atrophy suggests irreversible damage, but even in this situation, remarkable improvement may occur after decompression.

Comparison of pre- and postoperative CT scans is valuable.

Figure 27–9. Preoperative CT scan of patient with compressive optic neuropathy caused by orbital Graves' disease.

Figure 27–10. The same patient as in Figure 27–9, following bilateral orbital floor and medial wall decompression. Orbital contents have expanded into the ethmoid compartment after removal of the air cells. Note that the ethmoid air cells have been removed as far posterior as the sphenoid sinus, to decompress the orbital apex. Complete removal of the ethmoid air cells and expansion of orbital tissues into the ethmoid compartment may be documented, confirming the adequacy of decompression surgery. It is especially important to observe removal of the posterior ethmoid air cells (just anterior to the sphenoid sinus).

Reduction in exophthalmos ranges between 2 and 10 mm, but an average of 4.5 mm should be achieved after a floor and medial wall decompression.

Intravenous antibiotics are administered during surgery to decrease the risk of orbital infection from sinus pathogens. Perioperative steroids (usually 20 mg of dexamethasone sodium, intravenously) enhance the effect of decompression by reducing orbital edema related to surgery.

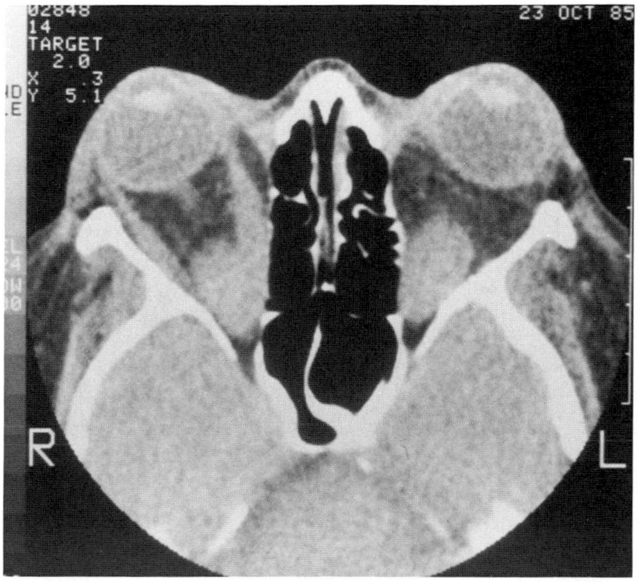

FIGURE 27–9

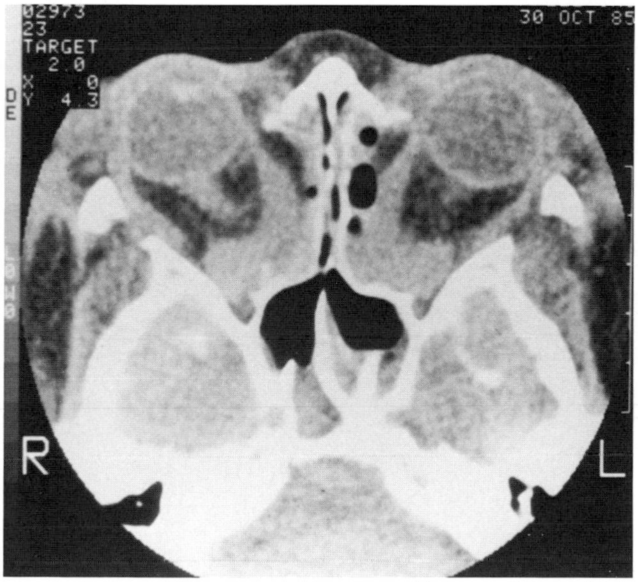

FIGURE 27–10

POTENTIAL COMPLICATIONS

By far the most common complication of orbital decompression surgery is strabismus. Correction of diplopia may require a secondary strabismus procedure, often using adjustable sutures.

Upper eyelid retraction may also be exaggerated after decompression because the globe and orbital tissues shift downward into the maxillary sinus. Patients will often need a separate procedure for correction of lid retraction, such as recession of the levator aponeurosis and Muller's muscle extirpation (see Chapter 26).

Visual loss is the most serious complication of decompression surgery. Compared with other types of orbital surgery, decompression carries an increased risk because of the necessary manipulation in the orbital apex (adjacent to the optic nerve). Injury to the optic nerve from postoperative orbital hemorrhage is of less concern because the orbit is widely decompressed into the sinuses. Other rare complications include orbital infection, infraorbital anesthesia, cerebrospinal fluid leaks, and nasolacrimal duct obstruction.

Chapter Twenty-Eight

ANTERIOR ORBITOTOMIES

Myron Tanenbaum

There are important fundamental prerequisites to successful orbital surgery. The surgeon must have a thorough working knowledge of orbital anatomy, orbital diagnosis and diseases, and orbital diagnostic-imaging techniques, including computed tomography (CT) scan, ultrasound (echography), and magnetic resonance imaging (MRI).

Modern orbital surgery is deliberate meticulous microsurgery performed in a bloodless field. Preoperative localization and assessment combined with excellent intraoperative exposure and direct visualization will be emphasized as the key elements toward safe and successful orbital surgery.

PREOPERATIVE DECISIONS

Figure 28–1. Localization will generally determine which surgical approach is used. Lesions palpated anteriorly in the orbit are usually approached through a *transseptal* (translid) orbitotomy. If CT scan, ultrasound, or MRI demonstrate the lesion to be in the posterior orbit, an *extraperiosteal* approach is chosen to safely gain access to the deep orbit. Intraconal lesions located between the medial rectus muscle and optic nerve are approached through a *transconjunctival* medial orbitotomy.

Assessment of the nature of the lesion will modify the surgical approach that has been chosen, based on localization only. Proper preoperative assessment is critical toward formulating the correct surgical plan. Thus, the "goals" of orbital surgery are determined preoperatively (Table 28–1). The surgeon must assess whether the lesion represents a localized or diffuse process. A plan for total excision is formulated if a localized tumor is present. Diffuse infiltrative tumors are approached for diagnostic biopsy only.

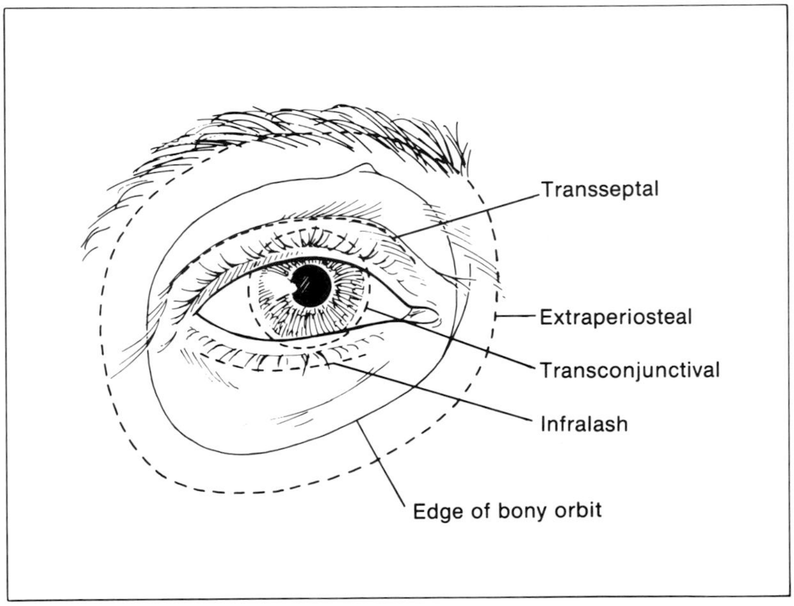

FIGURE 28–1

TABLE 28–1
Overview of the Anterior Orbitotomies

LOCATION IN ORBIT	NATURE OF LESION	GOAL OF SURGERY	SURGICAL APPROACH
Anterior	localized (e.g., dermoid)	total excision	trans-septal (translid)
Anterior	diffuse (e.g., lymphoma, inflammatory pseudotumor, metastatic tumor)	diagnostic biopsy	trans-septal
Anterior	infectious abscess	drainage	trans-septal
Medial, Anterior	localized (e.g., varix, hemangioma, tumor of medial rectus muscle)	biopsy/excision	transconjunctival
Medial, Anterior	infectious abscess	drainage/excision	transconjunctival
Optic Nerve	localized tumor (e.g., glioma, meningioma)	excisional biopsy	transconjunctival, medial
Optic Nerve	enlarged optic nerve sheath with compression of O.N. (e.g., hematoma, increased CSF pressure)	optic nerve sheath decompression	transconjunctival, medial
Medial, Posterior	localized tumor (e.g., intraconal neurilemmoma or cavernous hemangioma)	total excision	transconjunctival, medial
Medial, Posterior	infectious abscess	drainage/excision	extraperiosteal, medial
Superior or Inferior, Posterior	localized (e.g., hemangioma, neurilemmoma, foreign body)	total excision	extraperiosteal, superior, or inferior
Superior Nasal	localized (e.g., frontal-orbital mucocele)	excision/drainage	extraperiosteal, superior nasal

PREOPERATIVE MANAGEMENT

The patient is instructed to discontinue aspirin products 10 to 14 days preoperatively. Control of hypertension is very important, and general medical evaluation is sought when necessary. Patients are asked not to drink alcohol within 2 days of the surgery. Oral corticosteroids are commonly given to the patient the night before surgery to help reduce the postoperative swelling and inflammation.

SURGICAL TECHNIQUE

Transseptal Anterior Orbitotomy

The transseptal, or translid orbitotomy is perhaps the simplest of the anterior orbitotomies. The transseptal approach may be performed in the upper eyelid or the lower eyelid. The transseptal anterior orbitotomy is most commonly used to treat lesions that are visible within the substance of the eyelid or palpable within the anterior orbital space.

This surgical approach is commonly used for excision if the lesion is well demarcated (e.g., dermoid cyst or cavernous hemangioma), for diagnostic biopsy if the lesion is diffuse and infiltrative (e.g., inflammatory pseudotumor or metastatic carcinoma), and for drainage (e.g., infectious abscesses within the anterior orbit).

The transseptal anterior orbitotomy may be performed under local or general anesthesia. The more localized anterior tumors are most amenable to excision under local anesthesia. Straight local anesthesia may fail to achieve the desired effect in patients with larger infiltrative tumors of the orbit. The surgical site is infiltrated with lidocaine 2% with 1:100,000 epinephrine. Adequate time is allowed for the hemostatic effect of epinephrine to begin before any incisions are made. The mixture of lidocaine 2% with epinephrine is infiltrated locally, even in cases in which general anesthesia is used. The addition of 150 units of hyaluronidase into the mixture of local anesthetic allows the rapid dissolution of the mixture and prevents the local anesthetic from causing any undue distortion of the tissues.

In the upper eyelid, the transseptal orbitotomy incision line is concealed within the upper eyelid crease. After marking the lid crease incision, the skin incision is made with a size 15 blade. A hard corneal protector is used. With the lid held under tension, the orbicularis muscle layer is incised across the width of the lid. Meticulous hemostasis is maintained during all phases of the procedure. Gentle pressure placed on the globe will prolapse the orbital fat forward and bulge the orbital septum forward. Sharp dissection is used to open the orbital septum across the entire width of the upper eyelid. One may take a biopsy of the lesion, excise the entire lesion, or drain an abscess if present. Closure of the transseptal anterior orbitotomy involves re-formation of the upper eyelid crease. This re-formation is accomplished by suturing the pretarsal skin muscle edge to the levator aponeurosis. Three cardinal sutures are adequate to form a good eyelid crease. The remainder of the myocutaneous incision is closed with running or interrupted sutures. In situations during which a moderate amount of postoperative oozing of blood is anticipated, interrupted sutures are selected. In procedures for which drainage of an orbital abscess was involved, a postoperative drain is left in place for 24 to 48 hours.

The lower eyelid transseptal anterior orbitotomy is very similar, in principle, to the upper eyelid procedure. The surgical site is infiltrated with lidocaine 2% with epinephrine and hyaluronidase (Wydase), allowing adequate time for onset of the hemostatic effect. The translid incision is made within 1 to 2 mm of the lower eyelid lashes. Following the skin incision, the orbicularis muscle is incised across the width of the eyelid.

Figure 28–2. The entire lower eyelid myocutaneous flap is then elevated using sharp and blunt dissection and retracted downward with multiple rake retractors. The anterior orbital lesion is either palpated or visualized at this point.

Figure 28–3. The orbital septum is "tented" with fine forceps. It is then opened widely with Westcott scissors to expose the lesion.

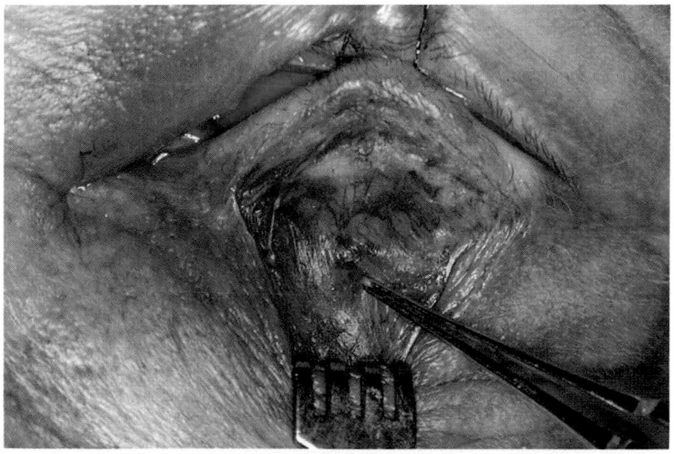

FIGURE 28–2

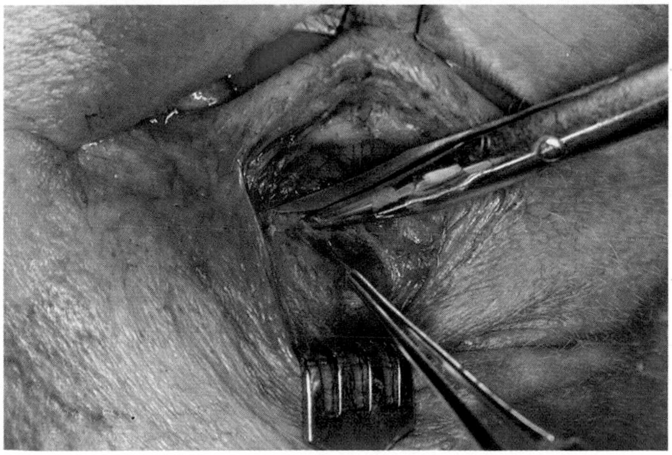

FIGURE 28–3

Figure 28–4. Surgical retractors or traction sutures are used as is necessary to achieve good exposure. A large tumor mass is exposed in the anteroinferior orbital space. As with the upper eyelid transseptal orbitotomy, the lesion at this point is either biopsied, excised, or drained. The lower lid incision is closed with running or interrupted sutures. Some patients are susceptible to developing postoperative lower eyelid ectropions following this simple transseptal orbitotomy. Such patients include those with significant horizontal laxity of the eyelid and patients with long-standing infiltrative tumors in whom extensive biopsies are performed. In these patients, the use of postoperative temporary tarsorrhaphy sutures or upward traction sutures through the lower lid margin may help avert postoperative ectropion.

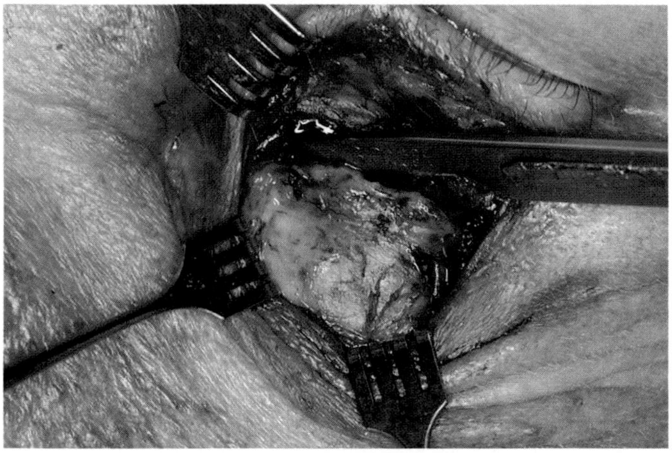

FIGURE 28–4

The Orbital Biopsy Specimen

Tumor biopsy for purpose of diagnosis is among the most common indications for anterior orbitotomy. Although the technical aspects of the surgery are of utmost importance, the surgeon should discuss the diagnostic possibilities with the pathologist and a mutual understanding should be reached before surgery concerning proper tissue handling for the specific case.

In many circumstances, standard formalin tissue fixation is adequate. Alternatively, if a lymphocytic tumor is suspected, fresh (nonfixated) tissue must be sent to the pathologist for immunologic marker studies. With lymphomas, it is important to obtain a deep incisional biopsy into the tumor as well as to obtain a large biopsy specimen. Lymphomatous tumors may be composite, and sampling errors may occur if smaller biopsy specimens are submitted for cell surface immunoglobulin studies. Fresh tissue is also necessary for all immunofluorescent, immunoperoxidase, and immunohistochemical enzyme studies. Estrogen receptor assays are similarly performed on unfixed tissue; this assay is important if metastatic breast carcinoma is known or suspected. It is important that the surgeon know the minimum volume of tissue required to perform the estrogen receptor assay. This information is gained by contacting the appropriate pathologist preoperatively. With orbital tumor biopsy specimens, obtaining an adequate volume of tissue can be difficult.

If the orbital tumor is a metastasis of unknown primary source, consider fixing a tissue specimen in glutaraldehyde for transmission electron microscopy. A 2 × 2 × 2-mm biopsy is adequate for electron microscopy. It is a common error to place too large a biopsy specimen in glutaraldehyde; the end result of this may be uneven or poor tissue fixation. The electron microscopy findings "may" elucidate the source of the primary tumor in many situations, including neuroblastoma (neurosecretory dense-core vesicles and neurotubules), breast carcinoma (mucin-producing cells or secretory granules), renal cell carcinoma (glycogen granules or lipid inclusions), oat cell carcinoma or carcinoid tumor (electron-dense granules), metastatic melanoma (cytoplasmic premelanosomes), colon carcinoma (elaborate cellular brush border), and bronchogenic carcinoma (Clara cells of alveolae).

The ongoing advances in tissue diagnosis occur rapidly, and a careful review of the subject is warranted each time the situation arises.

Transconjunctival Anterior Orbitotomy

The transconjunctival surgical approach allows the simplest and most direct access to lesions located in the subconjunctival space and lesions in the anterior portion of the orbit located outside the muscle cone. This approach can be applied to any quadrant of the globe. The transconjunctival orbitotomy can be used to gain access to the intraconal space by disinserting the appropriate rectus muscle. This approach to the intraconal space is most commonly performed medially.

The transconjunctival orbitotomy remaining outside the muscle cone is commonly performed to drain a localized abscess, to partially resect a benign tumor, and to biopsy a malignant tumor. Indications for the intraconal transconjunctival orbitotomy with disinsertion of the medial rectus muscle include excision of localized tumors (e.g., cavernous hemangioma or neurilemmoma), excision or biopsy of primary optic nerve tumor (e.g., glioma or meningioma), and decompression of the optic nerve sheath.

The transconjunctival orbitotomy for an extraconal lesion is performed under local or general anesthesia, when appropriate. An adequate conjunctival peritomy is made for good exposure in the appropriate quadrant. Relaxing incisions are made in the conjunctiva at each end of the peritomy. Biopsies are taken of infiltrative tumors, with appropriate handling of the specimen. Localized abscesses are drained. Other benign tumors, such as lipodermoids, are partially resected. It is important to limit the resection of these lesions to the proximal portion overlying the epibulbar surface. Overzealous excision of such lesions carried up under the eyelid or into the posterior orbit can result in significant complications. These complications include difficult to control hemorrhages, severe symblepharon formation, and ptosis of the upper eyelid, either because of levator damage or cicatrization. The conjunctiva is closed with loose interrupted sutures to permit postoperative drainage. In treating orbital abscesses, the use of a thin transconjunctival Penrose drain as well as appropriate subconjunctival antibiotic injections is indicated.

The medial transconjunctival orbitotomy is among the most difficult of the orbital surgeries. The complications of optic nerve damage and visual loss are real. Although good exposure is important for all orbital surgery, it is especially important for medial orbitotomy of the intraconal space. It is critically important to recognize important anatomic landmarks. The vortex veins number between four and eight and lie 5 to 8 mm posterior to the equator of the globe. They are close to the vertical meridian and are most commonly seen in the temporal quadrants. The short posterior ciliary arteries branch from the ophthalmic artery to encircle the optic nerve. The paired long posterior ciliary arteries also course on either side of the optic nerve.

Violation of any of these vascular structures can lead to serious hemorrhaging, which could jeopardize the surgical procedure or visual function of the eye. The surgeon must remain patient and meticulous in all phases of this orbitotomy, always maintaining good exposure and direct visualization.

The medial transconjunctival orbitotomy is most commonly performed under general anesthesia. The surgeon will, nonetheless, infiltrate the subconjunctival space with local anesthetic containing epinephrine. As with other orbitotomies, the head of the bed is elevated 15° to 20° to decrease venous congestion of the head and orbit. The medial conjunctival peritomy should be a "full" 180°.

Figure 28–5. A transconjunctival medial orbitotomy incision line has been outlined in methylene blue. A Westcott scissors has been introduced to undermine the conjunctiva and begin the peritomy. Smaller conjunctival incisions may limit the exposure. A conjunctival relaxing incision is made superiorly and inferiorly and the edges of the conjunctiva tagged with suture. Gentle blunt and sharp dissection of Tenon's fascia is performed to expose the medial rectus tendon. The tendon is gathered on a muscle hook and good exposure of the medial rectus is obtained. The medial rectus muscle is traced posteriorly to its point of penetration through Tenon's capsule.

Figure 28–6. The globe is rotated laterally with a silk traction suture. A double-armed 6–0 Vicryl suture is used to secure the medial rectus muscle with locking stitches placed on the superior and inferior edges of the muscle. A fine scissors is used to disinsert the muscle from the globe. It is important to leave a large stump of the medial rectus tendon attached to the globe to be used for traction during the remainder of the procedure. The tendon stump of the medial rectus is secured with a lock-stitched 4–0 silk suture. The globe is abducted with the 4–0 silk traction suture and the medial rectus muscle, which has been detached from the globe, is retracted medially. At this point, the surgeon typically visualizes orbital fat billowing around the posterior aspects of the medial rectus muscle and the globe.

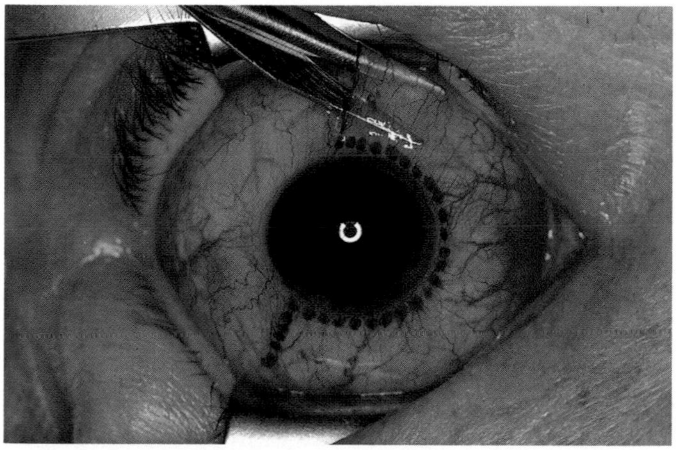

FIGURE 28–5

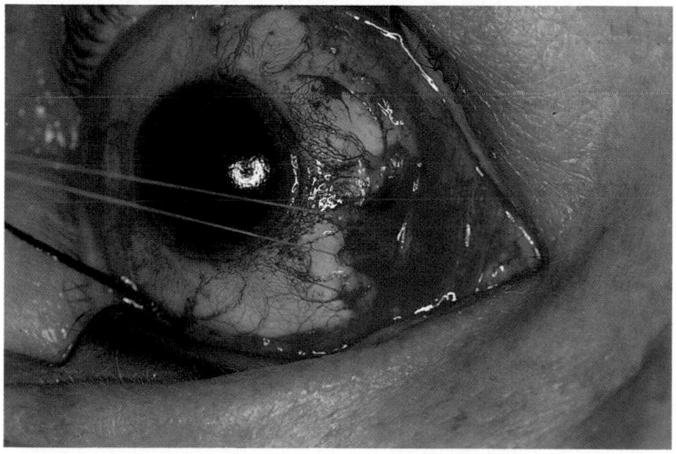

FIGURE 28–6

Figure 28–7. Thin malleable ribbon retractors are placed superiorly and inferiorly to hold back prolapsing orbital fat. An additional retractor may be used to further retract the medial rectus muscle medially. Moist cottonoid sponges are carefully packed between or behind the malleable retractors. The dissection proceeds posteriorly in a very cautious manner. The posterior extent of the globe and the optic nerve will eventually come under direct visualization. Occasional small vessels within the orbital fat will ooze blood into the surgical field. The surgeon must never blindly cauterize areas of bleeding. It is most helpful to lavage iced saline solution into the orbit to maintain hemostasis. A Frazier suction tip with a cottonoid sponge held over the opening of the tip is used to aspirate the iced saline solution. Keeping the Frazier tip behind a cottonoid sponge will prevent accidental aspiration of any of the delicate intraorbital structures.

Figure 28–8. If a localized tumor is visualized, such as the illustrated tumor of the medial posterior intraconal orbit, it may now be excised. The cryoprobe is very helpful in engaging a localized cavernous hemangioma and extracting it. If significant bleeding is encountered with tumor extraction (e.g., neurilemmoma), the surgeon should continually irrigate the field with iced saline solution. Extreme caution must be exercised when using cautery instruments around the optic nerve. The neurosurgical bipolar cautery forceps are helpful for cauterizing vessels in the posterior orbit. The medial surgical exposure is used to excise the intraorbital portion of an optic nerve tumor. In such instances, the surgeon should first transect the optic nerve tumor flush with the posterior aspect of the globe. It is important to have adequate exposure to prevent having the tumor retract posteriorly and be difficult to retrieve. A traction suture may be placed through the cut stump of the optic nerve tumor. Gentle blunt dissection should continue posteriorly to expose as much of the lesion as possible. An enucleation snare is then threaded down the length of the optic nerve and optic nerve tumor toward the orbital apex. The snare is then slowly tightened until the distal-most portion of the optic nerve and tumor is transsected. The specimen is submitted for pathologic examination, with the 4–0 silk traction suture tagging the portion of the tumor closest to the globe. The transconjunctival medial orbitotomy provides direct exposure of the optic nerve sheath for purposes of decompression. The most common indication for this procedure being in cases of pseudotumor cerebri, with increased intracranial pressure, optic nerve sheath distention, papilledema, and visual loss. It is appropriate to use the operating microscope for optic nerve sheath decompression to maximize magnification and illumination. The key to the optic nerve sheath decompression is to maintain excellent exposure to allow maximum visualization and control. Although the medial transconjunctival orbitotomy is the most direct approach to the optic nerve, other sur-

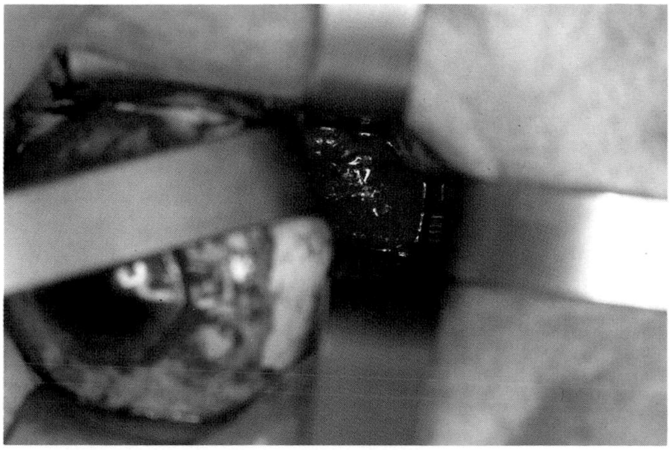

FIGURE 28–7

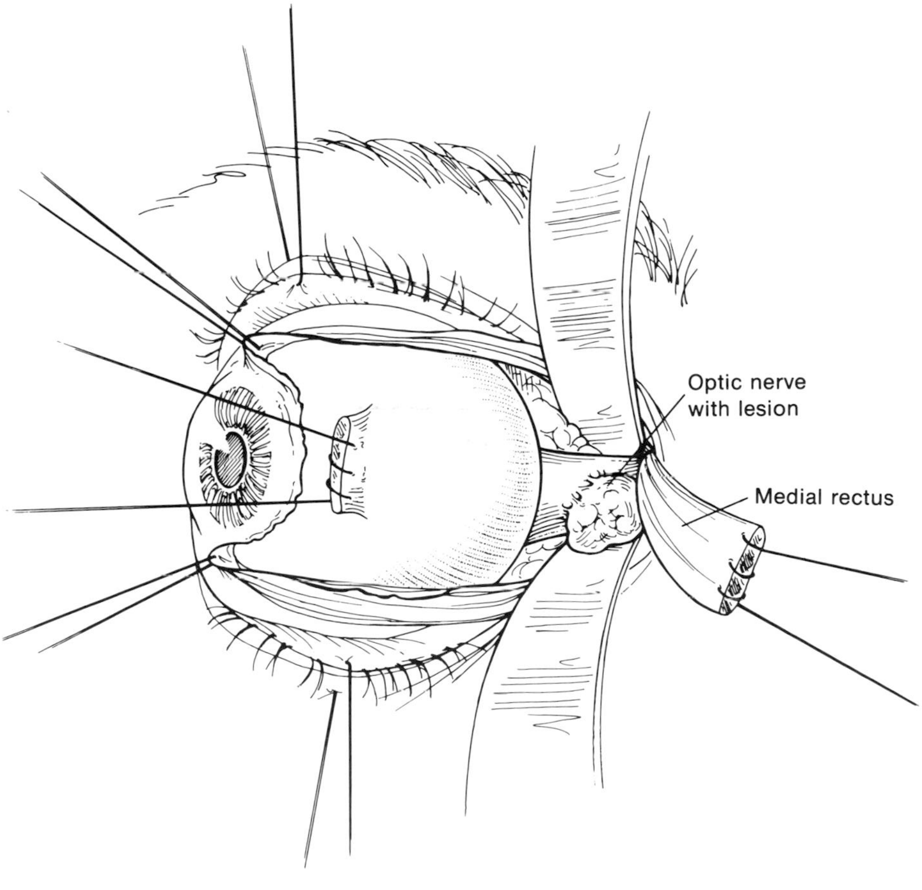

FIGURE 28–8

geons prefer the lateral approach to enhance exposure. The medial transconjunctival orbitotomy can be combined with a lateral orbitotomy with outfracturing of the lateral orbital wall. This combined orbitotomy allows the globe to be displaced farther temporally to enhance the medial exposure. Other surgeons prefer a full lateral orbitotomy with intraconal dissection from the lateral approach alone. The surgeon must traverse a greater distance into the orbit with this method, although a greater length of the optic nerve is ultimately exposed.

With the intraconal dissection completed, the medial rectus muscle is reattached to the tendon stump. The conjunctiva is closed loosely with interrupted 6–0 plain sutures.

Extraperiosteal Anterior Orbitotomy

The extraperiosteal anterior orbitotomy is an excellent surgical approach to gain access to the posterior aspects of the orbit. The key principle here is for the surgeon to remain in an extraperiosteal plane as long as possible during the procedure. This important principle of surgery allows safe access to the deep orbit while avoiding delicate intraorbital structures.

This section will concentrate on the superior, superior nasal, and inferior extraperiosteal orbitotomies. Indications include excision of a localized lesion from the posterior orbit (e.g., cavernous hemangioma, neurilemmoma), or a retained intraorbital foreign body. The superior nasal extraperiosteal orbitotomy is often the surgical approach of choice for excision and drainage of frontal or ethmoidal mucoceles or related orbital abscesses. The superior nasal approach may also be used for transethmoidal decompression of the bony optic canal.

The periosteum of the orbit (periorbita) serves as a barrier against the spread of intraorbital malignant tumors. The presence of a nonresectable, intraorbital malignant tumor (e.g., lymphoma), or a metastatic carcinoma is a contraindication to using an extraperiosteal surgical approach that would violate the periosteal barrier. Whenever possible, biopsies of malignant intraorbital tumors should be taken through an anterior transseptal orbitotomy.

Superior and Superior Nasal Extraperiosteal Orbitotomy

The superior surgical approach to the orbit is most commonly performed with a general anesthesia. The patient is positioned supine, with the head of the bed elevated approximately 15°. The subcutaneous tissues of the brow, upper eyelid, and inner canthus are infiltrated with local anesthetic solution with epinephrine. Additionally, the local anesthetic is cautiously infiltrated along the superior orbital roof.

The skin incision is marked in methylene blue in a manner that would allow the necessary exposure. Certain lesions of the superior orbit can be approached through an infrabrow incision in the superior quadrant only. An orbital abscess and frontoethmoidal sinus mucoceles are approached through a curvilinear incision spanning the medial one-half of the brow and curving over the inner canthal angle down to a level of the medial canthal tendon. The skin incision is made with a size 15 blade, and the dissection is carried down to the level of periosteum. The periosteum is incised about 5 mm outside the orbital rim. The surgeon will typically encounter the supraorbital neurovascular bundle in the superior or superior nasal portion of the orbit. Meticulous hemostasis must be achieved as the neurovascular bundle is incised. Number 4–0 silk sutures are sewn into the subcutaneous tissues and used for traction to spread the incision widely. The typical orbitotomy incision involves at least six to eight of these traction sutures. Multiple hemostat clamps are used to attach these traction sutures to the sterile drape, thereby achieving excellent exposure while keeping the hands of the surgeon, assistant, and scrub nurse free.

A periosteal elevator is used to elevate the periosteum down toward the arcus marginalis and the orbital rim. The periosteum will initially be tightly adherent to bone. As the surgeon "turns the corner" of the orbital rim and proceeds posteriorly into the orbit, the periorbita is very loosely adherent to bone. It is here that the surgeon must proceed with care and caution. In many patients, especially the elderly, the periorbita is quite attenuated. Careless or hasty dissection can create rents in the periorbita through which orbital fat will billow. This will obscure the surgeon's visualization of the surgical field and possibly prevent further access to the posterior orbit. Superiorly, the surgeon must be careful while working along the bony roof of the orbit. This may be thin or attenuated in elderly patients, and inadvertent injury to the dura can be made. In the superior nasal quadrant, special attention must be paid to the attachment of the trochlea to the fovea centralis of the bony orbit. The surgeon must maintain the integrity of the trochlea–periorbita as a unit, such that final closure at the end of the procedure will restore and maintain proper extraocular muscle balance. In the medial extension of the extraperiosteal orbitotomy, it is typical to encounter first the anterior and then the posterior ethmoidal arteries. The ethmoidal arteries are branches of the ophthalmic artery, and they exit and orbit at the level of the frontal ethmoidal bony suture line. This suture line and the ethmoidal arteries are important anatomic landmarks and are present at the approximate level of the cribiform plate. The surgeon must isolate and cauterize each of these arteries before proceeding posteriorly.

The surgeon should palpate the intraorbital contents through the thin periorbita. Firm lesions, such as a neurilemmoma, can be best localized by this method. Thin malleable retractors help hold the periorbita and orbital contents downward to maintain good exposure. A trapdoor opening is made in the periorbita overlying the area of interest. This localized opening in the periorbita is most effective for lesions in the posterior peripheral orbit (outside of the muscle cone).

Figure 28–9. A sagittal view illustrates a superior extraperiorbital orbitotomy. An opening has been made in the periorbita. A forceps is shown removing a tumor from the peripheral (extraconal) posterior orbital space.

For intraconal lesions in the inferior or superior nasal orbit, the periorbital opening is strategically placed between the levator muscle and the superior oblique muscle. This opening should be large enough that it does not limit the visualization or maneuverability of the intraconal lesion. Cotton umbilical tape can be placed around the belly of the extraocular muscles or the levator muscle to enhance exposure.

Careful blunt dissection generally works best with well-encapsulated tumors, for example, a neurilemmoma or cavernous hemangioma. A fine-tipped cryoprobe helps to engage these tumors for extraction. If the lesion is a very large cavernous hemangioma, the surgeon should not hesitate to decompress the vascular tumor to facilitate total removal. Forcing an "intact" cavernous hemangioma beyond the normal limits of the extraperiosteal surgical exposure has a far greater morbidity than removal of a decompressed lesion. If the deep orbital lesion is an iron foreign body, a long-tipped electromagnet may be helpful for its removal.

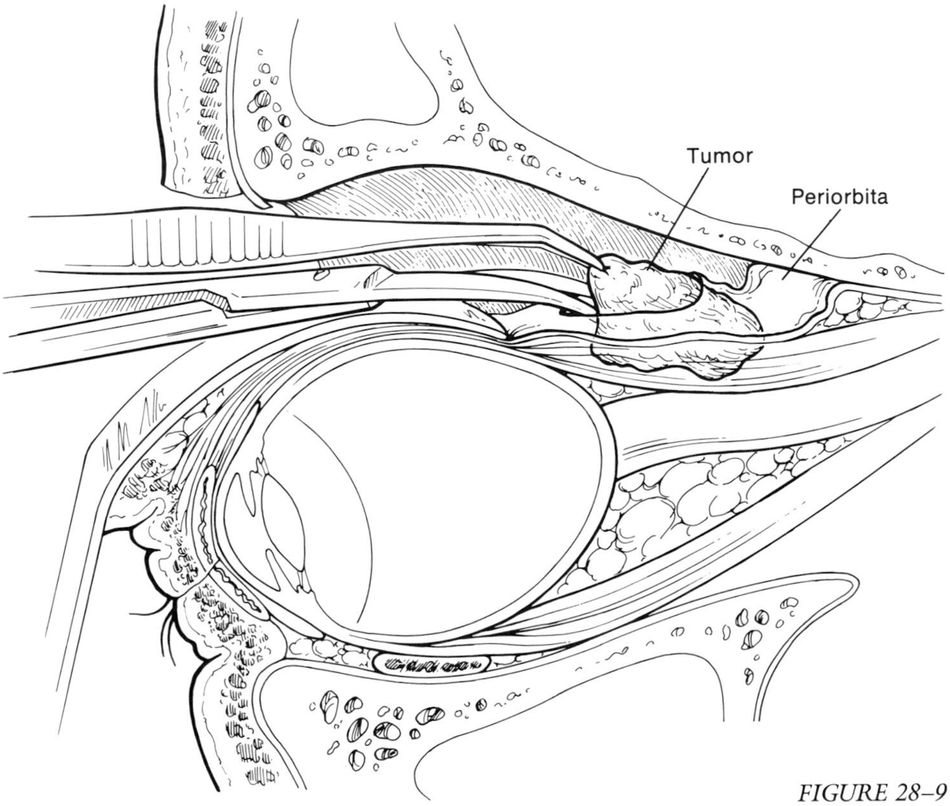

FIGURE 28–9

Figure 28–10. A superior extraperiosteal orbitotomy is shown. The trochlea–periorbita complex is reflected downward to expose the mucocele. The entire mucocele lining and contents are removed. The superior nasal extraperiosteal orbitotomy is an excellent approach for frontoorbital mucoceles. The main principles of treatment involve total obliteration of the mucocele lining and reestablishment of proper sinus drainage. The mucocele is first punctured and decompressed with appropriate material taken for culture. The roof of the bony orbit is typically eroded, and this bone is removed in piecemeal fashion with rongeurs. With adequate exposure achieved, the entire lining of the mucocele and frontal sinus is removed by curettage. Drainage for the frontal sinus must be reestablished through the ethmoid sinuses or through the nasofrontal duct itself. A catheter is maintained in place postoperative for a minimum of 2 to 3 weeks. Recurrent mucoceles or larger mucoceles with posterior erosion are treated by sinus obliteration with an osteoplastic flap technique. The osteoplastic flap technique is not an extraperiosteal orbitotomy, but rather, a midforehead procedure. This approach allows the surgeon to have an "open sky" view into the frontal sinus for the purpose of complete exenteration of the mucocele and sinus lining, followed by obliteration of the sinus with autogenous adipose tissue. This surgical approach now has the highest percentage success rate for treatment of frontal orbital mucoceles. Some surgeons favor this approach for all frontal sinus mucoceles, not simply the larger or recurrent ones.

It is common to use a postoperative drain for 24 to 48 hours after an extraperiosteal orbitotomy. Generally, the trapdoor opening in the

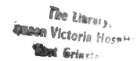

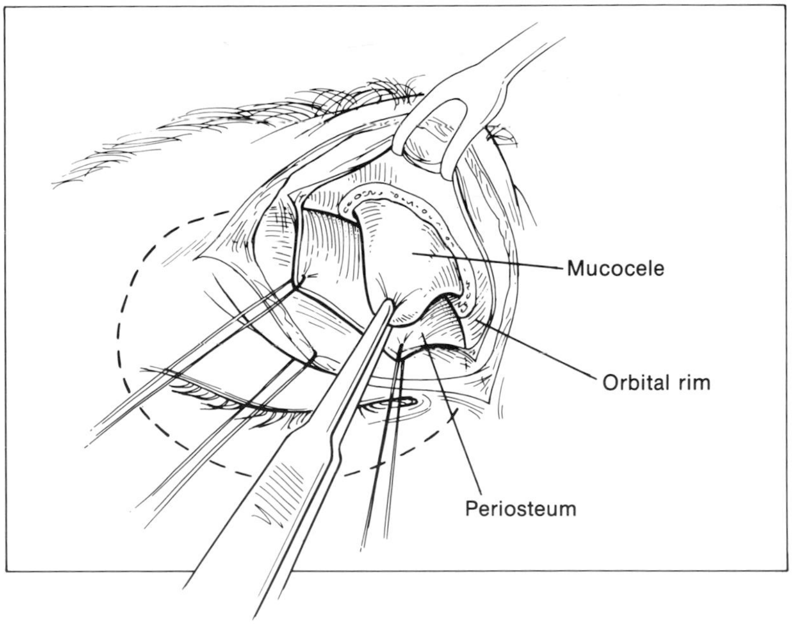

FIGURE 28–10

periorbita is left open, and the drain is placed in the extraperiosteal space. The periosteum outside the orbital rim is closed with interrupted absorbable sutures. Meticulous layered closure of the deep and subcutaneous tissues of the brow area is performed. Cutaneous sutures may be placed in running or interrupted fashion.

To avoid direct facial incisions, which may be conspicuous, the surgeon can use the bicoronal forehead flap to achieve excellent exposure for the extraperiosteal orbitotomy. The bicoronal forehead flap is readily applicable to the superior, superolateral, and superior nasal extraperiosteal orbitotomies.

Inferior Extraperiosteal Orbitotomy

The inferior extraperiosteal orbitotomy is analogous to the superior approach. Both the transconjunctival and the transcutaneous lower lid approaches can give excellent exposure for removal of inferior orbital tumors, biopsy of tumors arising from the maxillary sinus, repair of blow-out fractures of the orbital floor, and decompression of the bony orbit for thyroid-related orbitopathy (antral–ethmoidal decompression).

The surgical procedure is most commonly performed under general anesthesia. The surgeon should infiltrate the lateral canthal tendon and inferior fornix conjunctiva with lidocaine 2% with epinephrine, and hyaluranidase.

The initial step is a small lateral canthotomy incision and inferior cantholysis. This permits the lower lid to swing downward and offers broad exposure of the inferior conjunctival fornix. The inferior fornix conjunctival incision is made from the lateral canthotomy to approximately the level of the puncta medially. A hard corneal protector along with malleable ribbon retractors are used to protect the globe. The needle-tip Bovie unit makes a clean incision while maintaining a dry surgical field. The surgeon must be experienced in the use of this instrument and exercise caution at all times. The surgeon directs the dissection toward the inferior orbital rim. Small Blair retractors and, eventually, larger Senn retractors are helpful in reflecting the lower eyelid downward. The surgeon must incise the capuslopalpebral fascia of the lower lid and typically the orbital septum to reach the bony rim. In the occasional patient, the surgeon must excise some of the protuberant lower lid fatty tissue to maintain good visualization and exposure of the surgical field. The periosteum is incised outside of the arcus marginalis. A periosteal elevator is used to carefully elevate the periosteum up over the inferior orbital rim and to elevate the more loosely adherent periorbita. The surgeon should continue to palpate the orbital contents through the periorbita as the dissection continues posteriorly. Once the lesion is localized, an opening is made in the periorbita through which the tumor is excised.

POSTOPERATIVE MANAGEMENT

Heavy Valsalva maneuvers must be avoided. Crushed ice compresses are lightly applied to the orbit for 48 hours postoperatively, or longer if indicated. Drains may be left in place for 24 to 48 hours. Postoperative pain and nausea can be profound following major orbital surgery. Parenteral analgesics and antiemetics should be used when necessary. Although patients are typically hospitalized for major orbital procedures, minor transseptal tumor biopsies, with local anesthesia, can be performed on an outpatient basis. A brief anti-inflammatory course of oral corticosteroids may be tapered over a 3- to 5-day period postoperatively. Decisions concerning use of antibiotics are made on an individualized basis.

COMPLICATIONS

Blindness is a risk of any orbital surgery. Careful handling of the patient preoperatively, intraoperatively, and postoperatively will help minimize this risk. Preoperatively, the patient's general medical status should be evaluated. Clotting abnormalities and bleeding tendencies are corrected whenever possible; hypertension and diabetes are controlled. Intraoperatively, the blood supply to the optic nerve or the optic nerve itself may be injured. This risk is perhaps greatest during intraconal dissection in the medial orbit. The surgeon must maximize exposure and maintain meticulous hemostasis to avoid traumatizing the optic nerve or its blood supply. Optic nerve decompression must be performed in a most delicate manner with microscopic control. Large hemangiomas of the orbit should be decompressed or "deflated" before removal to avoid damage to the optic nerve. After tumor removal, bleeding in the orbit must be dealt with. Lavage and iced saline is helpful when direct cautery cannot be applied. Postoperative orbital hemorrhage, with increased intraorbital pressure, can compromise the optic nerve. Hemorrhaging can be exacerbated during "vigorous" awakening and extubation from general anesthesia. The anesthesiologist should be alerted to extubate the patient in an especially atraumatic fashion following orbital surgery. Drains can be used, if necessary, for any of the anterior orbitotomies. Postoperatively, the drains allow egress of blood and fluid. Compressive bandages are specifically avoided. Such pressure dressings could cause a hazardous buildup of intraorbital pressure. Lightly applied crushed ice compresses are preferred and help minimize postoperative hemorrhage and edema.

Cerebrospinal fluid (CSF) leakage is a potential complication of the superior and superior nasal extraperiosteal orbitotomies. Superior tumors and frontal mucoceles commonly erode bone, bringing dura into direct contact with the orbit. Preoperative radiologic studies (e.g., CT scan) will often reveal this situation and preclude difficult intraoperative "surprises." The orbital surgeon should plan to work with the neurosurgeon preoperatively and intraoperatively when indicated. When unexpected cerebrospinal fluid leaks occur, they must be dealt with individually. Decisions must be made for the specific situation concerning closure of the leak (e.g., suturing dura); tissue graft to plug the leak, versus no intervention for small cerebrospinal fluid leaks; and broad-spectrum antibiotic prophylaxis, versus no antibiotic use. The specifics of each case must be analyzed. The complications of CSF leaks include meningitis, brain abscesses, and death.

Many patients experience transient postoperative diplopia. This can certainly be expected following the superior nasal extraperiosteal orbitotomy. Permanent superior oblique muscle dysfunction is usually avoided if the trochlea–periorbita unit is maintained intact and the periorbita–periosteum is carefully repositioned during closure. The medial rectus muscle is disinserted from the globe during the transconjunctival medial orbitotomy with intraconal dissection. Reapproximation of the medial rectus muscle must be precise. There is a tendency to shorten (resect) the medial rectus muscle slightly, which induces an esotropia. All other extraocular muscles encountered during orbital surgery should be handled gently. Soft cotton umbilical tape can be used to atraumatically retract the muscles when necessary for exposure.

Severe orbital hemorrhage may lead to serious blood loss. Select high-risk patients and those with vascular orbital tumors should be prepared preoperatively for possible blood transfusion. Death secondary to exsanguination is very rare.

Ptosis can follow orbital surgery from a variety of mechanisms. Severe postoperative edema and swelling can result in levator stretching and aponeurosis dehiscence. Inadvertent injury can occur to the levator during the transseptal upper eyelid orbitotomy. The surgeon should avoid overly aggressive biopsies of infiltrative preaponeurotic tumors. Dissection at the superior orbital apex can injure the superior division of the third cranial nerve. This can result in severe ptosis combined with a difficult motility disturbance.

Rarely, the globe itself can be injured during orbital surgery. Hard-shell corneal protectors and malleable ribbon retractors should be used to shield the globe during appropriate phases of the orbitotomy.

Orbital surgery is generally safe and effective. Modern techniques have minimized the once common morbidity and mortality of orbitotomies. Nonetheless, the surgeon and patient must be aware of the very serious potential complications.

Figure 28–11. An inferior extraperiosteal orbitotomy has been performed through the inferior conjunctival fornix. As the periorbita is reflected superiorly, a large tumor mass is encountered in the extraperiosteal space. Following tumor biopsy or excision, meticulous hemostasis should be achieved.

For closure, the conjunctiva and lower eyelid retractors are reapproximated with a running absorbable suture, such as a 6–0 plain or 6–0 Vicryl suture. The lateral canthal tendon is restored with a single suture. A 4–0 Vicryl or Prolene suture may be used to reattach the tarsal elements to the periosteum of the lateral orbital rim. It is important to refixate the eyelid to the periorbita overlying the natural lateral orbital tubercle (approximately 4 mm inside the lateral orbital rim). It is necessary to fixate the eyelid inside of the orbital rim such that the lower lid follows the natural curvature of the globe. The upper and lower lid margins are brought into correct apposition with a single placement suture. The lateral canthal skin incision is closed with interrupted sutures.

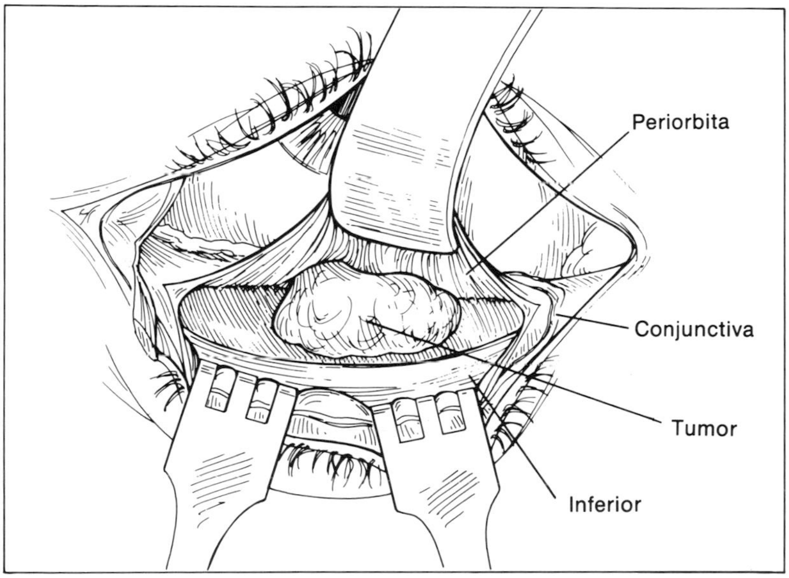

FIGURE 28–11

Chapter Twenty-Nine

LATERAL ORBITOTOMY

David T. Tse

The surgical procedure utilized for the excision of an orbital lesion will depend on the lesion's location, size, and suspected pathology. In addition, the biological behavior of the suspected lesion may influence the approach. Thus, a lacrimal gland lesion may be approached through a transseptal anterior orbitotomy if biopsy of a suspected inflammatory or malignant process is anticipated. However, if a benign mixed tumor of the lacrimal gland is the working diagnosis, a lateral orbitotomy is necessary for total removal. Some disease processes that involve only the subperiosteal space, such as subperiosteal hematoma or abscess, floor fracture, and mucocele, are best approached through a transperiosteal route that does not violate the periorbita. The lateral approach provides the best access to the retrobulbar compartments inside and outside the muscle cone. It is especially useful for lesions in the lacrimal gland fossa, but may be inadequate for some lesions at the orbital apex. The key for any successful and atraumatic surgical exploration is adequate exposure. This is especially true in the orbit because of the many important structures confined within this tight space. To minimize operative morbidity, the surgeon must have a thorough understanding of the orbital anatomy as well as a complete familiarity with the chosen surgical technique.

PREOPERATIVE MANAGEMENT

It is usually unnecessary to type and crossmatch blood in preparation for orbital surgery. However, it should be considered in patients with low hemoglobin or hematocrit values, or in whom significant intraoperative bleeding is anticipated, such as in resecting an arteriovenous malformation. Patients taking anticoagulants, such as warfarin sodium (Coumadin), or inhibitors of platelet aggregation, such as aspirin, should have these drugs discontinued at least 2 weeks before surgery, if possible. The surgeon should also inquire about the intake of any over-the-counter drugs containing aspirin, such as Alka-Seltzer, Sine-Off, and Midol. Fish oil, a product sold for prevention of heart disease, is frequently not regarded as medication by patients; hence, their use is often not disclosed to the surgeon. Fish oil, when taken in large quantity, can interfere with platelet function and prolong bleeding time.

ANESTHESIA

General endotracheal anesthesia is preferred when the retrobulbar area is explored. Induced intraoperative hypotensive anesthesia, although usually not required, may be considered, to improve hemostasis and to facilitate tissue dissection in some cases. This technique should be employed only in patients in good physical health and in conjunction with an anesthesiologist who is acquainted with its application.

MAGNIFICATION AND ILLUMINATION

A fiberoptic headlight and magnifying loupes are essential to provide illumination and magnification of fine orbital structures during lateral orbitotomy. A binocular operating microscope with coaxial illumination is particularly useful when surgery, such as sheath fenestration, is performed on the optic nerve. By choosing an objective lens between 200 and 250 mm, adequate room can be obtained between the surgical field and the microscope for instrument manipulation. An improvement in visualization, combined with proper microsurgical techniques and working knowledge of the deep orbital anatomy, adds a new dimension to the safety of orbital surgery.

OPERATIVE PROCEDURE

The patient is placed in a slight reverse Trendelenburg's position to reduce orbital venous pressure. The face is turned slightly away from the operative site. The primary surgeon is seated on the side of the orbit on which surgery is to be performed, and the assistant is seated at the head of the table. The cornea may be protected by a small piece of moistened Gelfoam during surgery, particularly for eyes that are proptotic. One should refrain from placing a suture tarsorrhaph on the lids, as it will prevent forward displacement of the globe and preclude monitoring pupillary reactions during orbital manipulation.

An S-shaped Stallard skin incision is preferred because it gives excellent exposure and eliminates the necessity to reconstruct the lateral canthal angle at the end of the procedure.

Figure 29–1. After the surgical site has been prepared, the S-shaped skin outline is marked with a marking pen. The marking begins beneath the inferior cilia of the lateral one-third of the eyebrow, extending inferolaterally along the superior and lateral bony orbital rim, past the level of the lateral commissure to terminate over the zygomatic arch. The tail end of the marking may be camouflaged within a laugh line. The lateral canthal region and the temporalis muscle are infiltrated with lidocaine 2% with 1 : 100,000 dilution of epinephrine before draping and scrubbing of hands. This allows the vasoconstrictive effect of epinephrine to work before an incision is made.

The initial incision is carried down to, but not through the periosteum.

Figure 29–2. Subcutaneous tissues and orbicularis oculi muscle are bluntly dissected away with a Freer periosteal elevator to expose the periosteum and fascia of the temporalis muscle. Bleeding from orbicularis muscle is controlled by bipolar cautery. Traction sutures of 4–0 black silk are positioned in both sides of the skin–muscle flaps and secured to the surgical drapes with hemostats.

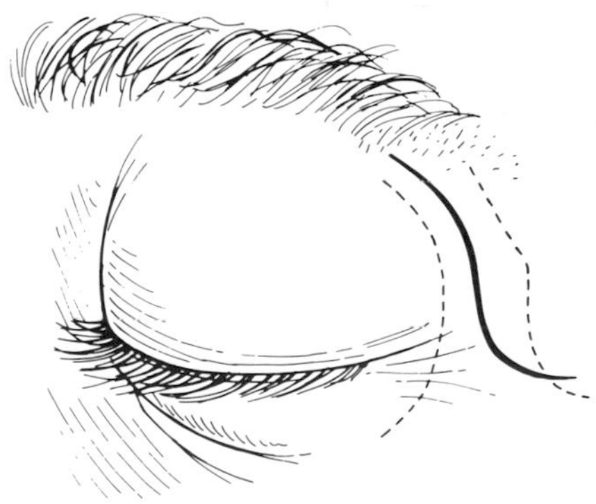

FIGURE 29–1

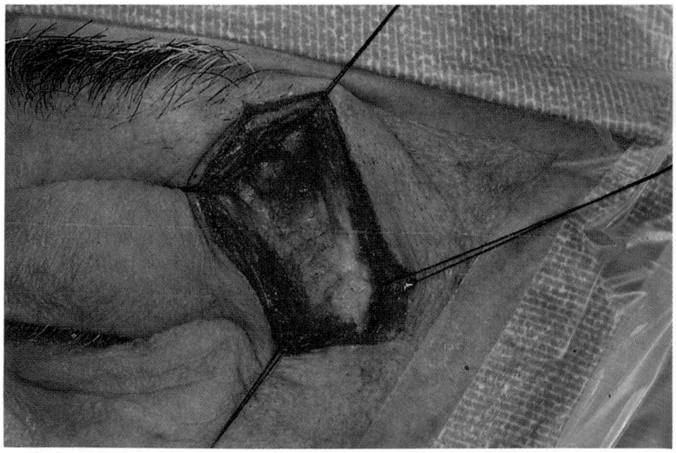

FIGURE 29–2

Figure 29–3. The periosteum is then incised with a size 15 Bard–Parker blade parallel to and approximately 2 mm lateral to the orbital rim. The periosteal incision is carried superiorly above the zygomatico-frontal suture line and inferiorly past the superior aspect of the zygomatic arch. Periosteal relaxing incisions are made at the superior and inferior ends of the incision.

Figure 29–4. The periosteum and temporalis muscle are reflected from the zygomatic process of the frontal bone and the frontal processes of the zygomatic bone. This maneuver is accomplished by using either a Woodson or Freer periosteal elevator.

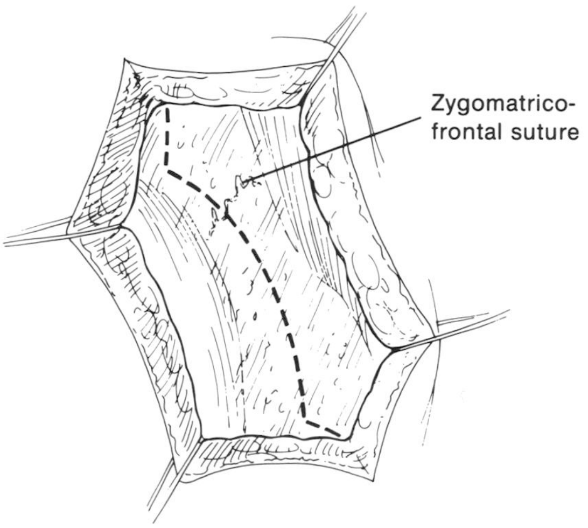

FIGURE 29–3

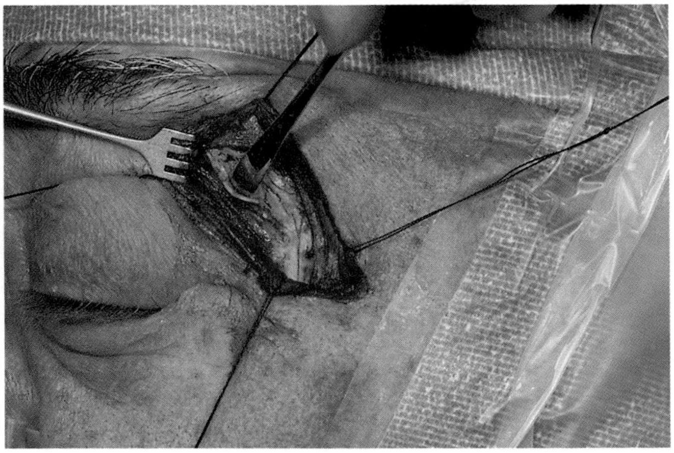

FIGURE 29–4

Figure 29–5A, B. Once the dissection is carried into the temporalis fossa, the separation of the periosteum and temporalis muscle is facilitated by forcing an opened 4 × 4 gauze into the dissection plane, with a Freer elevator, to just behind the sphenozygomatic suture line. By bluntly dissecting the temporalis muscle off its bony attachment with a gauze, shredding of the muscle by the sharp tip of the periosteal elevator can be avoided. Brisk bleeding may be encountered in the bed of the temporalis muscle or from avulsion of the zygomaticotemporal artery. This can be controlled either by pressure or with bipolar cautery. Oozing from the bony surface can be stopped with bone wax.

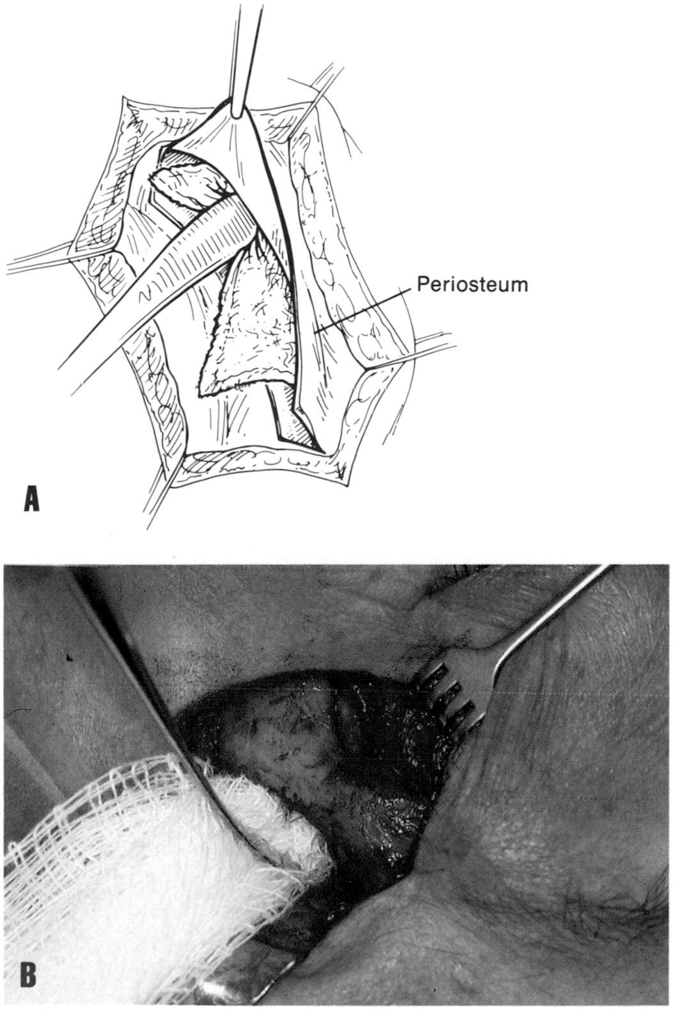

FIGURE 29–5

Figure 29–6. After the periosteum and temporalis muscle have been separated from the external aspect of the lateral orbital wall, the periorbita is gently reflected away from the inner aspect of the lateral wall with a Freer periosteal elevator. Within the orbit, the periorbita is loosely adherent and can be easily separated from the bone. Care should be taken to maintain the integrity of the periorbita. The zygomaticotemporal and zygomaticofacial arteries may be seen as they penetrate the lateral wall from within the orbit. These should be cauterized before dissecting further posteriorly. It is unnecessary to dissect beyond the sphenofrontal suture line, since removal of the lateral wall often stops short of this landmark.

Figure 29–7. The lateral orbital rim and wall are fully exposed.

Figure 29–8. Once the full dimension of the lateral orbital wall has been delineated and hemostasis assured, the proposed bony incisions are determined, as shown outlined. The superior bone incision is positioned about 5 mm above the zygomaticofrontal suture line, and the inferior bone cut is made above the upper margin of the zygomatic arch. If the inferior bone cut is made too low, there is a potential hazard of fracturing into the inferior orbital fissure during bone removal. The distance between the two cuts is usually 3 to 3.5 cm.

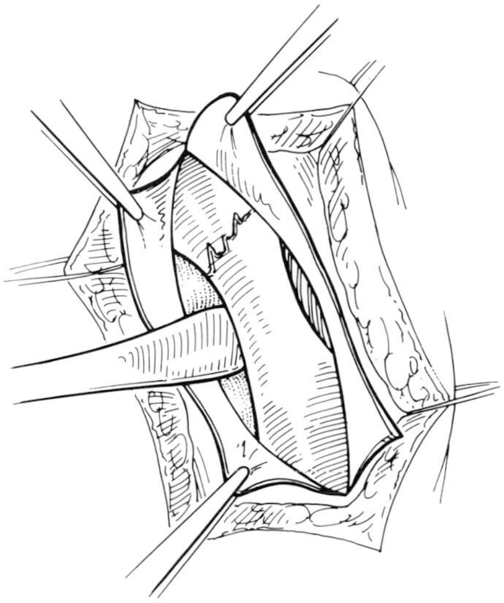

FIGURE 29–6

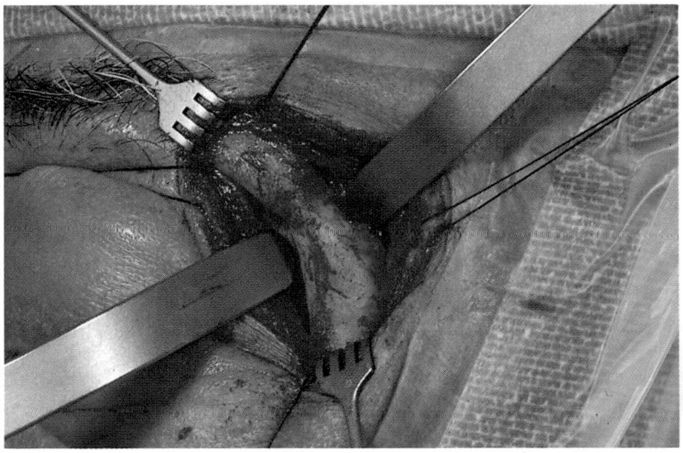

FIGURE 29–7

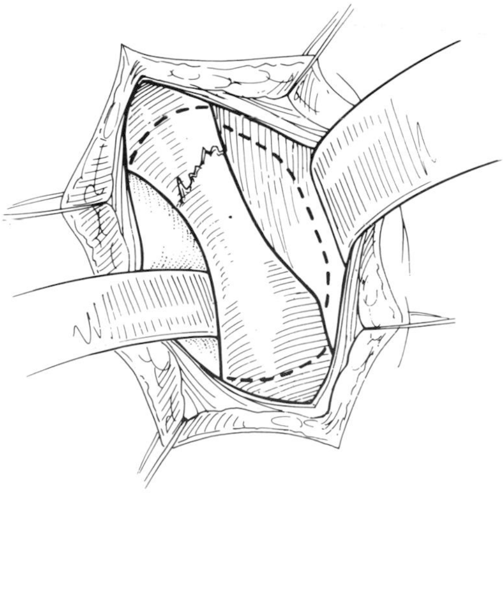

FIGURE 29–8

Figure 29–9A, B. Bone incisions are made with an oscillating saw. During the entire bone cutting process, a broad metal malleable retractor is positioned in the orbit along the lateral wall to protect the periorbita and globe. Another malleable retractor is placed in the temporalis fossa to protect the temporalis muscle. The surgeon should hold the oscillating saw like holding a pen in writing, with the hand resting firmly over the temporalis fossa for stabilization. The blade is held parallel to the plane of the orbital floor. Irrigating fluid is dripped into the bony incision throughout the cutting process to prevent heat necrosis of the bone. A suction tip is positioned within the temporalis fossa to evacuate blood and fluid from obscuring the line of incision.

Figure 29–10. The superior and inferior incisions should be parallel and the depth of incision usually does not exceed 1.5 cm. For the superior incision, the depth of the cut should terminate anterior to the sphenofrontal suture line.

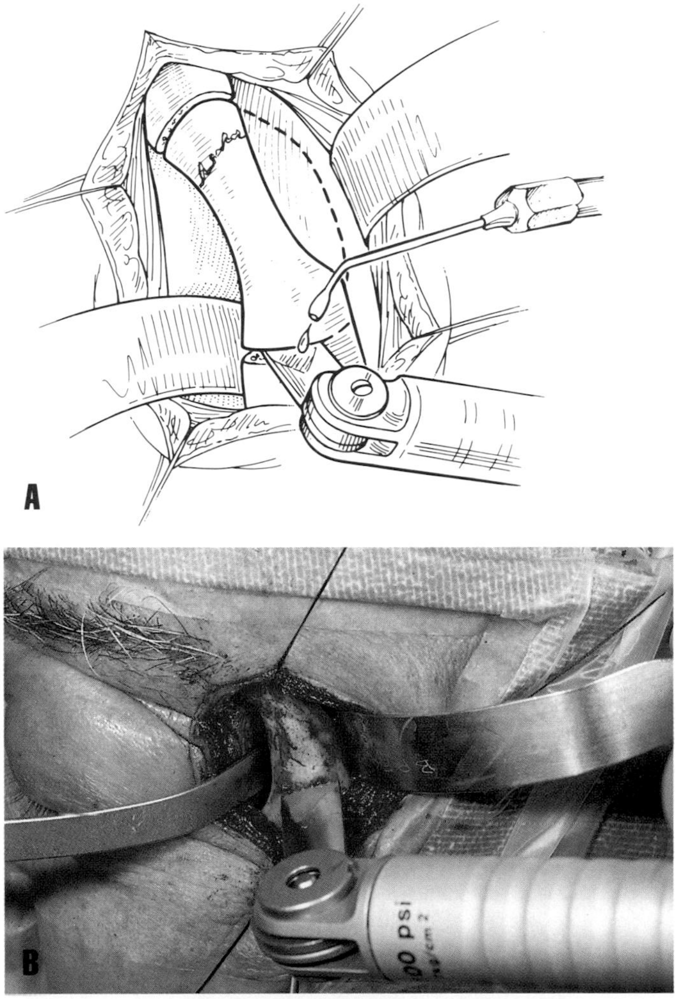

FIGURE 29–9

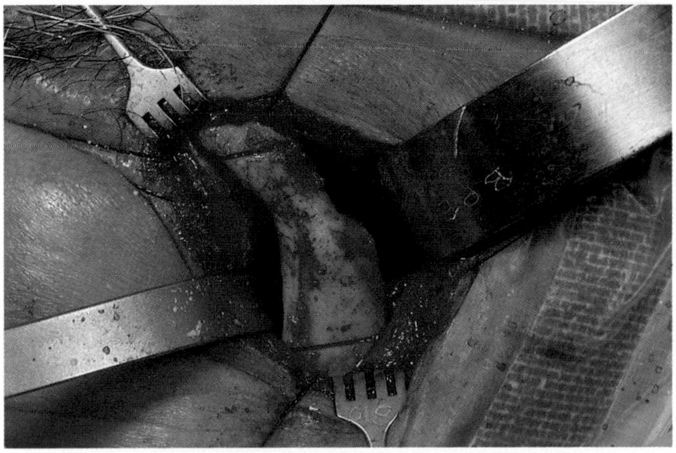

FIGURE 29–10

Figure 29–11A, B. Holes are made with a pneumatic drill to either side of the bone incision to allow fixation with sutures when the bone fragment is returned to its original position at the conclusion of the procedure.

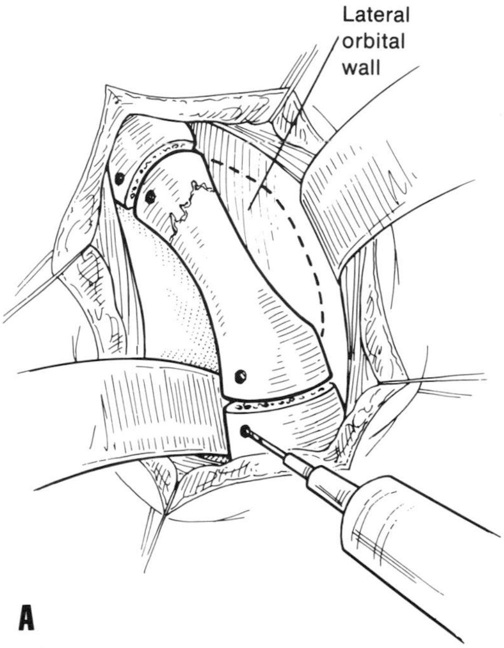

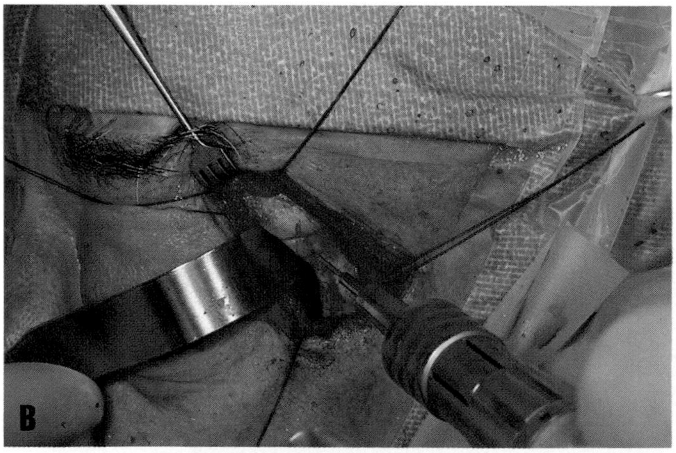

FIGURE 29–11

Figure 29–12. The lateral orbital wall is then grasped at the rim with a large double-action bone rongeur.

Figure 29–13. It is gently rocked outward until it fractures posteriorly and can be removed. The bony fragment is then wrapped in a saline-soaked gauze and saved for later replacement.

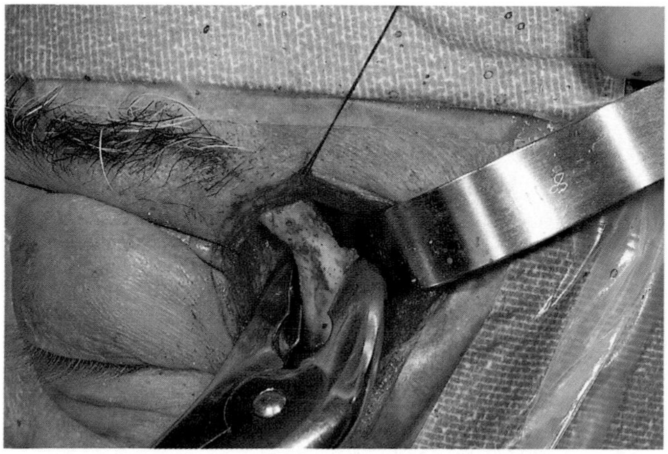

FIGURE 29–12

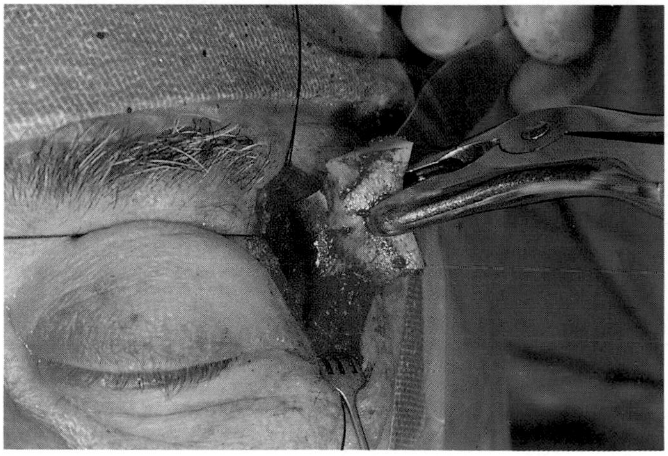

FIGURE 29–13

Figure 29–14. Further bony resection in the depth of the temporalis fossa may be accomplished in a piecemeal fashion by using a bone rongeur until the thick cancellous bone of the sphenoid is reached. This is the most posterior extent of bony resection before entering the middle cranial fossa. Bleeding from the cancellous bone can be controlled with bone wax. Hemostasis must be assured before opening the periorbita.

Figure 29–15. The intact periorbita is now visualized. A T-shaped periorbital incision is made. The anteroposterior incision is made just to one side of the lateral rectus muscle, and it is carried posteriorly as far as possible. The vertical incision is made beginning at the level of the lacrimal gland and extending inferiorly to below the lateral rectus. The incision can be started with a Bard–Parker blade, but is completed with a Westcott scissors to prevent injury to orbital tissues. The edge of the periorbital incision is grasped with a forceps and gently reflected away from the orbital content with a Freer elevator.

Figure 29–16. With the periorbita opened, the perimuscular fascial sheaths are bluntly dissected open with periosteal elevators to locate the lateral rectus muscle. It is preferable to retract the lateral rectus away with a malleable retractor, rather than dissecting it free from the surrounding fat and looping it with a suture or a vascular band. Overmanipulation of the lateral rectus muscle may result in transient postoperative motility dysfunction.

At this point, gentle finger palpation can usually locate the position of the orbital mass. For deeper exploration within the central surgical compartment, two malleable retractors are used to spread the orbital fat away in a hand-over-hand fashion. Perhaps the most difficult feature of this dissection is the tendency of orbital fat to obscure normal anatomic landmarks. The fat is divided into lobules by fine connective tissue septae; these lobules often billow over the edges of the retractors, obscuring the plane of dissection. This problem can be minimized by using moistened ½-in. neurosurgical cottonoids to which the orbital fat will adhere slightly, preventing it from billowing over the edges. By gradually removing and reinserting the orbital retractor blades over the cottonoids, the fat can be kept away from the plane of dissection. Care should be taken not to traumatize the vortex vein that passes through the orbital fat.

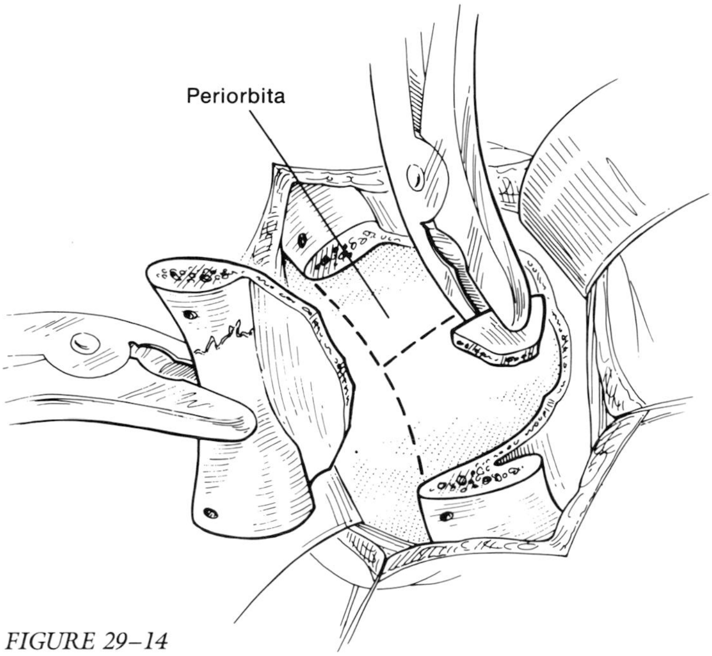

FIGURE 29–14

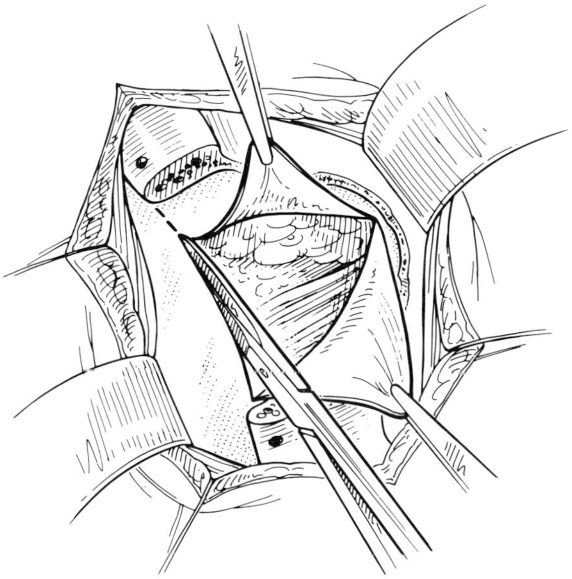

FIGURE 29–15

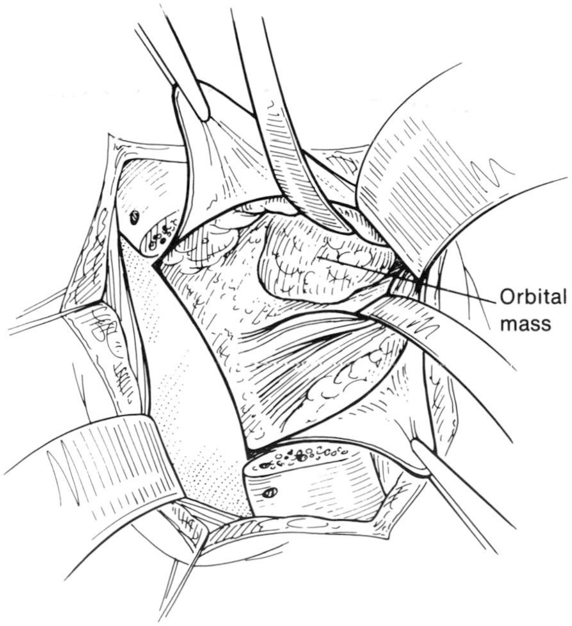

FIGURE 29–16

Figure 29–17. Once the lesion is located, gentle traction is applied and a Freer periosteal elevator is used to bluntly dissect the orbital tissues away from the surface of the tumor. If the lesion is encapsulated, it may be engaged with a retinal cryoprobe while blunt dissection is continued around the capsule with the periosteal elevator. Dissection should be blunt and in the plane of the tumor or capsule. Under no circumstances should there be blind cutting with scissors. If the lesion is infiltrative and adherent to vital structures, frozen-section examination of the tissue will determine whether intraconal dissection should continue. If tissue planes are not clearly defined, it may be wise to leave some of the lesion behind, rather than risking ocular dysfunction by overaggressive extirpation.

Once the lesion has been removed, hemostasis should be obtained. Hemostasis must be meticulous and can be accomplished by using pinpoint bipolar cautery with fine-tipped forceps. The use of a unipolar Bovie cautery within the orbit is discouraged, as is the use of suction within the periorbita, as undue suction on orbital fat may cause bleeding from avulsion of fine blood vessels. Closure of an orbitotomy should not commence until complete hemostasis is assured. The use of microfibrillar collagen hemostat (Avitene) to stop bleeding within the orbit is discouraged, as it can cause tissue scarring. Regenerated oxidized cellulose hemostat (Surgicel) may be helpful in controlling slow ooze, but should be removed completely from within the orbit after hemostasis has been achieved. This material induces hemostasis in the surgical wound, but it swells and takes on a gelatinous consistency when in contact with blood. Within an enclosed space, it can exert considerable compressive force, and at least one case of compressive optic neuropathy has been reported with its use around the orbital apex.

Following removal or biopsy of an intraorbital tumor, the periorbita is closed with interrupted 5–0 chromic catgut or 5–0 polygalactin 910 (Vicryl) sutures.

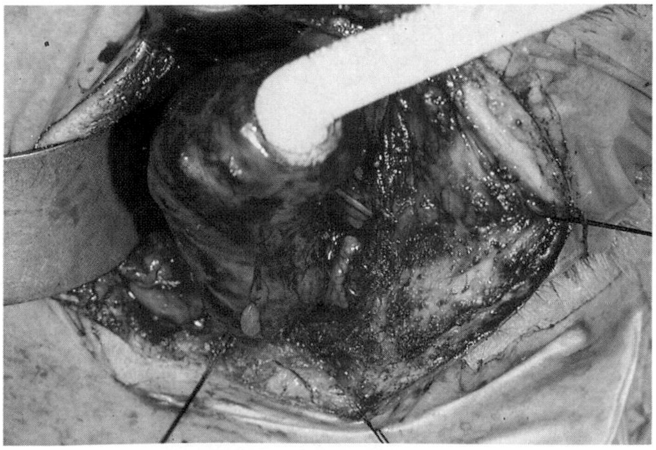

FIGURE 29–17

Figure 29–18A, B. The lateral orbital wall bone fragment is returned to its original position and anchored with a 2–0 Prolene suture through the preplaced drill holes. The suture knots are then rotated and buried into a drill hole on the external surface of the bony rim.

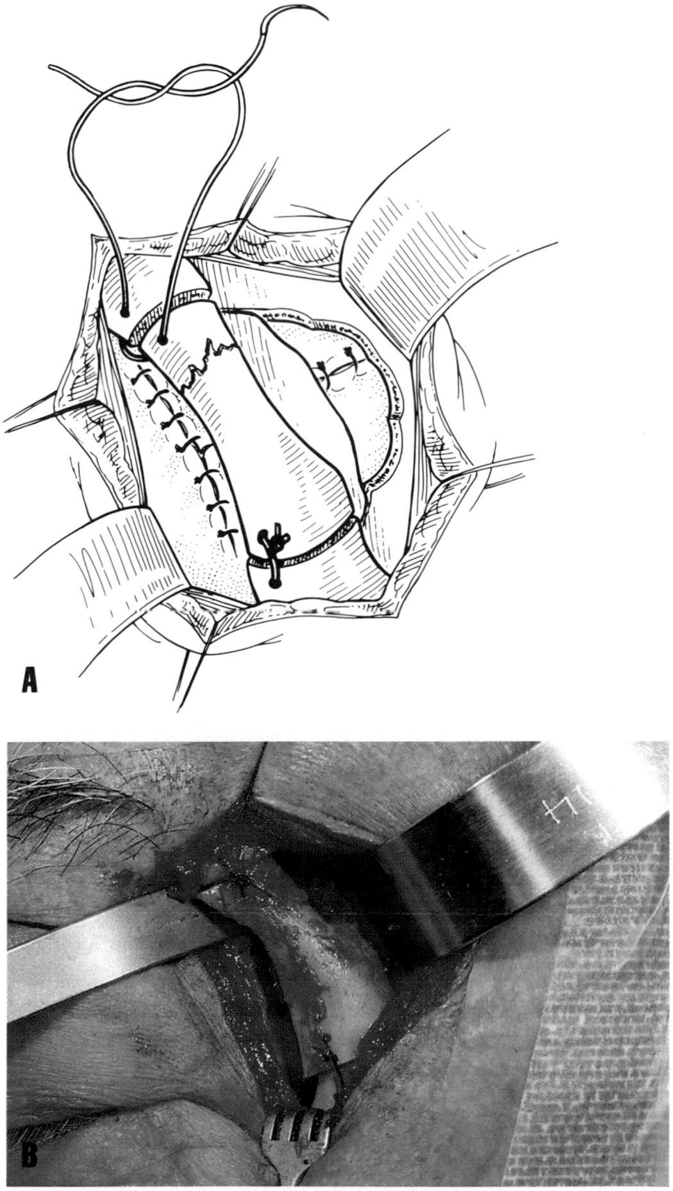

FIGURE 29–18

Figure 29–19. The periosteum and anterior temporalis fascia are reapproximated with 4–0 Vicryl sutures. Traction sutures are removed. Orbicularis muscle and subcutaneous tissues are reapproximated with 5–0 chromic sutures in an interrupted fashion.

Figure 29–20A, B. The skin incision is closed with multiple interrupted vertical mattress sutures of 6–0 nylon.

I usually ask the anesthesiologist to extubate the patient while the patient is still in a slightly "deeper" plane of anesthesia. This will minimize the chance of bucking and the potential development of retrobulbar hemorrhage from acute increase in venous and intraorbital pressures.

An antibiotic ointment is applied onto the incision site. An orbital drain is not routinely used. A firm pressure dressing is placed over the wound. One should not place a patch over the eye, so that the physician and nursing staff can watch for signs of progressive proptosis in the event of postoperative retrobulbar hemorrhage. Additionally, this will enable the patient to help monitor vision and to alert the physician to any sudden change in acuity.

POSTOPERATIVE MANAGEMENT

After the patient awakes from anesthesia in the recovery room, visual acuity and pupillary reaction are checked. The skin incision is also inspected for any oozing. The head of the bed is elevated to a 45° position, and the patient is cautioned to report any deep orbital pain that might signal the development of an orbital hemorrhage.

In the immediate postoperative period, an analgesic is given only for incisional pain. Any complaints of deep orbital pain should be investigated. A stool softener is given and Valsalva is discouraged. An ice pack is applied onto the periorbital region.

Systemic corticosteroids are given if a biopsy has been taken from any inflammatory lesion, or if the optic nerve was traumatized or manipulated during surgery. Intravenous antibiotic is used in the immediate postoperative period and is then switched to oral intake for 7 days. The dressing is removed in 24 hours. An antibiotic ointment is applied onto the incision three times daily for 1 week. Sutures are removed after 7 days and the wound reinforced with Steri-strip.

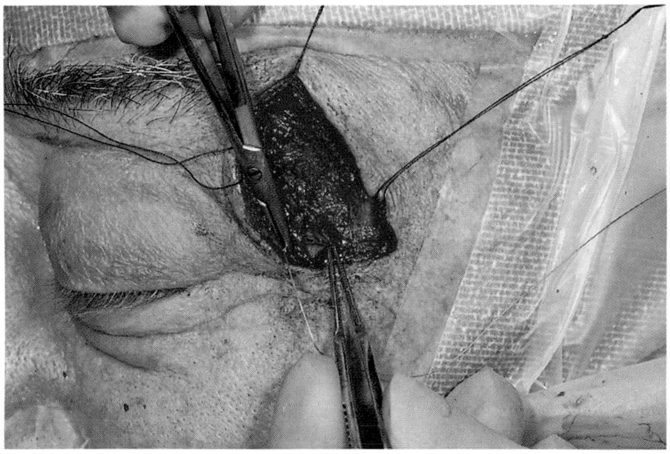

FIGURE 29–19

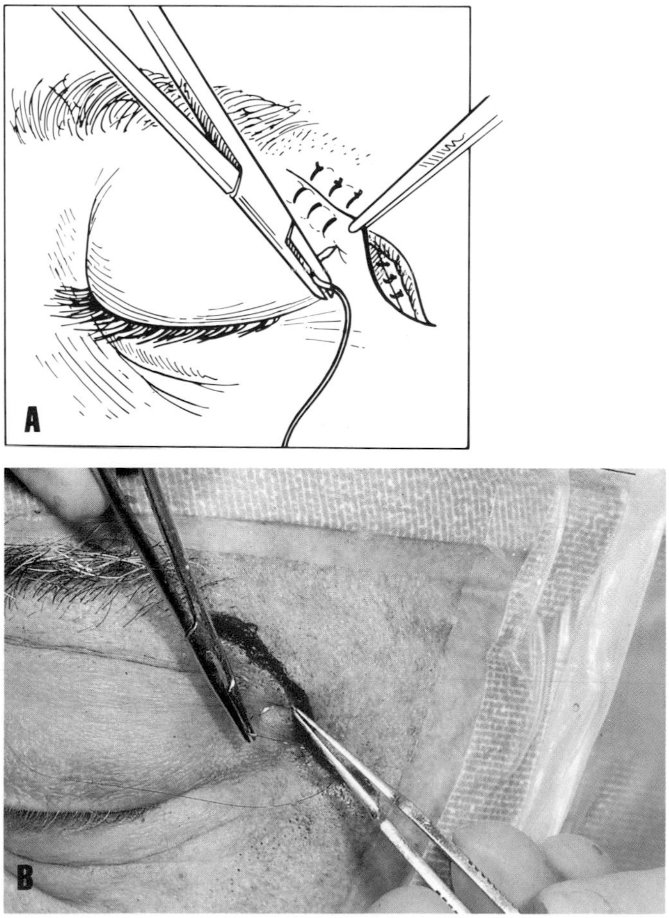

FIGURE 29–20

POSTOPERATIVE COMPLICATIONS

One of the most dreaded complications of orbital surgery is orbital hemorrhage, with visual loss. Visual loss from retrobulbar hemorrhage is most likely due to an interruption of ocular perfusion and resultant ischemia of the eye. As orbital pressure approaches the systolic blood pressure, central retinal artery flow may be compromised, resulting in decreased retinal perfusion. Occlusion of the posterior ciliary arteries that supply the optic nerve also has been proposed as the cause of visual loss in orbital hemorrhage. Concomitantly, elevated intraocular pressure may contribute to retinal and optic nerve ischemia. Increased intraocular pressure may result from direct transmission of elevated orbital pressure or from acute angle closure. As the intraocular pressure rises, obstruction of blood flow within the capillaries of the optic disc, followed by central retinal artery occlusion, may occur. Recovery of vision is unlikely if retinal ischemia persists for more than 100 minutes. Therefore, maximum effort should be directed at restoring retinal and optic nerve perfusion within this vulnerable period. The main sources of bleeding are from the temporalis muscle, bone incisions, and small vessels traversing the orbital fat lobules.

Treatment of an expanding orbital hematoma must be initiated without delay. The patient is returned to the operating room immediately, and the wound is explored. Blood clots are evacuated and the source of bleeding identified and cauterized. In the interim, the patient's intraocular pressure and retinal perfusion should be monitored. In the presence of elevated intraocular pressure, medical therapy should be given. Topical timolol (Timoptic, 0.5%), intravenous acetazolamide (500 mg), and mannitol (1–2 g/kg of a 20% solution infused over 20 minutes) may be administered to decrease the intraocular pressure and enhance retinal perfusion. Intravenous corticosteroids should also be given to reduce orbital swelling, to decrease vascular permeability, and to protect the optic nerve from ischemic damage.

Chapter Thirty

TEMPORAL ARTERY BIOPSY

Kevin R. Scott
David T. Tse

Temporal arteritis is a systemic disorder affecting medium and large arteries, primarily within the region of the head and neck. It is a disease of the elderly, and rarely occurs in individuals younger than 50 years of age. Temporal arteritis is twice as common in women and is most frequently seen in Caucasians.

Classically, patients present with temporal headaches, visual symptoms, jaw claudication, and temporal artery tenderness. Constitutional complaints of fever, anorexia, weight loss, and fatigue are also common. Polymyalgia rheumatica is frequently associated with temporal arteritis, and most now believe that these two disorders represent a spectrum of disease.

In temporal arteritis, the erythrocyte sedimentation rate (ESR) is usually higher than 50 mm/h and commonly exceeds 100 mm/h. A normal ESR, however, does not rule out temporal arteritis. The Westergren method of performing the sedimentation rate is preferred to the Wintrobe method, because of its increased accuracy at the higher test values.

The term *cranial arteritis* has been used to describe this disorder because of the frequent involvement of the superficial temporal, vertebral, ophthalmic, and posterior ciliary arteries. Temporal arteritis has also been referred to as granulomatous arteritis and giant cell arteritis, as a result of the characteristic granulomatous inflammation with giant cells seen on histopathologic examination.

The exact etiology of temporal arteritis is unknown. It is believed, however, to be related to an autoimmune reaction directed against the elastic tissue within the media and adventitia of the arteries of the head and neck.

The superficial temporal artery is chosen for biopsy almost exclusively, because of its readily accessible location and its high frequency of involvement. The rich arterial anastomosis within the forehead allows the anterior branch of the superficial temporal artery to be excised without a significant risk of vascular compromise. Additionally, "skip" areas of involvement have been demonstrated within a single arterial specimen; therefore, a large biopsy (more than 2 cm) is recommended. A positive arterial biopsy is required to conclusively establish the diagnosis of temporal arteritis.

The surgical technique presented here is based on the common anatomic branching patterns of the superficial temporal artery, the various fascial layers, and the location of the temporal branches of the facial nerve. Proper surgical technique combined with a working knowledge of the anatomy of the temporalis region, adds a new dimension to the safety of the temporal artery biopsy procedure.

SURGICAL ANATOMY

Superficial Temporal Artery

The superficial temporal and maxillary arteries are the two terminal branches of the external carotid artery. The superficial temporal artery (STA) arises from within the parotid gland and ascends superiorly to cross the zygomatic process of the temporal bone, approximately 1 cm anterior to the tragus.

Figure 30–1A. The proximal STA gives off four main branches: the transverse facial, middle temporal, parietal, and frontal.

The transverse facial artery (zygomaticomalar) runs in a medial direction either along the surface, or immediately inferior to the zygomatic arch. The middle temporal artery arises from the undersurface of the superficial temporal artery and travels superiorly over the anterior surface of the zygomatic arch. The artery then penetrates the superficial fascial planes to supply the underlying deep temporalis fascia.

The distal STA divides into an anterior frontal and a posterior parietal branch. There are five major branching patterns described for the distal STA; however, in 80% of cases the bifurcation of the frontal and parietal branches occurs above the zygomatic arch. The frontal and parietal branches, along with the transverse facial, supraorbital, and supratrochlear arteries, arborize extensively to form a rich arterial plexus within this region. Collectively, these vessels supply the superficial temporal fascia and the overlying skin.

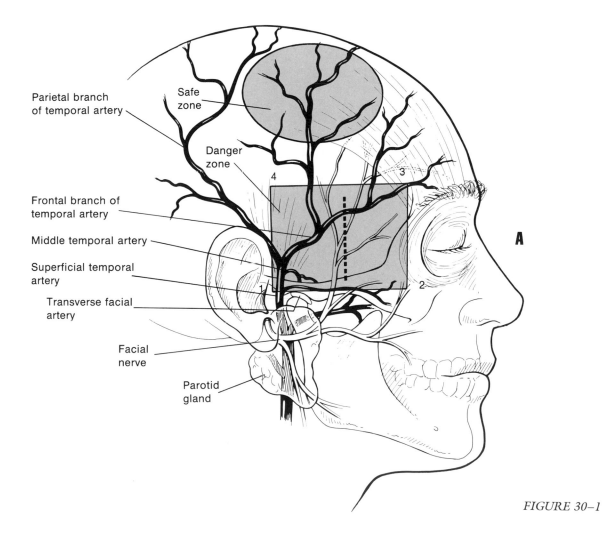

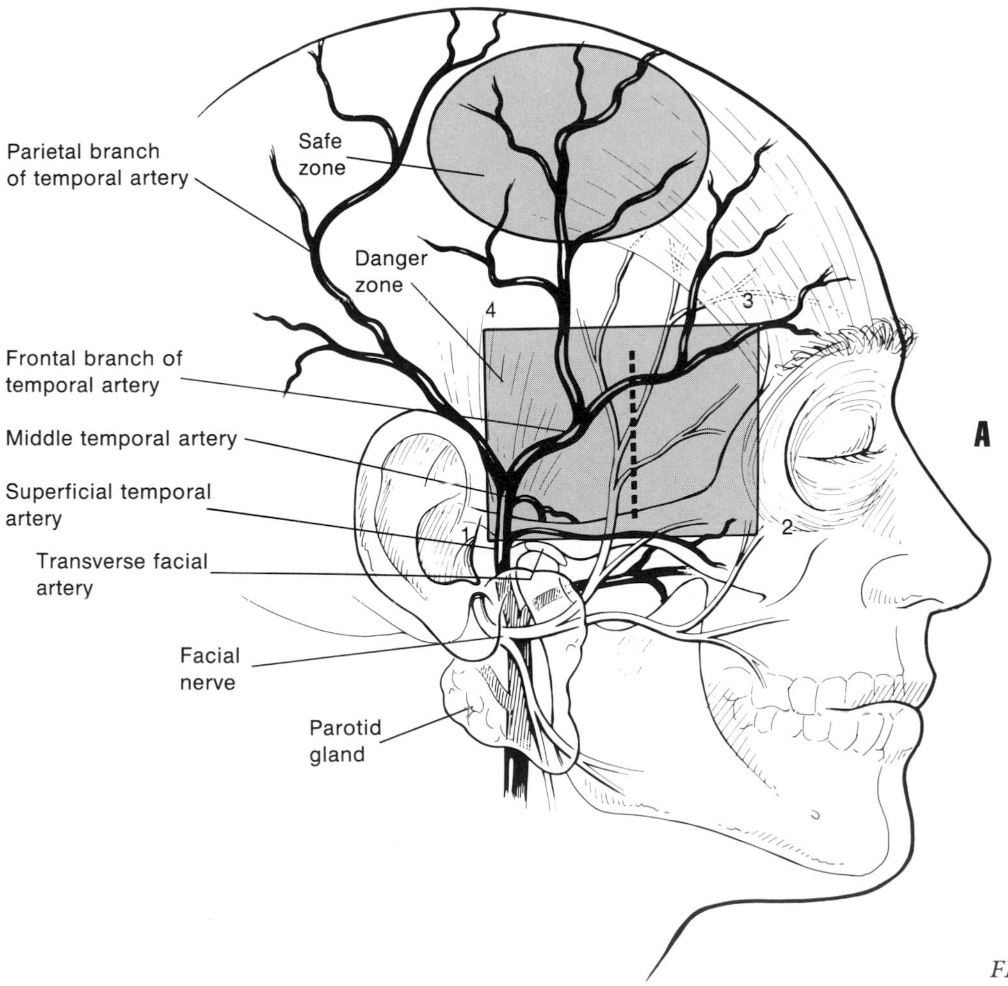
Parietal branch
of temporal artery
Safe
zone
Danger
zone
4
3
Frontal branch of
temporal artery
Middle temporal artery
Superficial temporal
artery
1
2
Transverse facial
artery
Facial
nerve
Parotid
gland
A

FIGURE 30–1

Fascial Planes

Figure 30–1B. As the STA crosses the zygomatic process of the temporal bone (zygomatic arch), it enters and ascends within the superficial temporal fascia (STF). The STF lies directly below the subdermal fatty layer and hair follicles. The STF is loosely adherent to the overlying subdermal fatty layer just superior to the zygomatic arch. In a cephalad direction, the adherence between these layers increases gradually from the zygomatic arch to the galea aponeurotica.

The STF is also referred to as the temporoparietal fascia and epicranial aponeurosis. The STF is bounded by and contiguous with the galea superiorly, the frontalis anteriorly, and occipitalis posteriorly, and the subcutaneous musculoaponeurotic system inferiorly. As such, there are no clearly defined boundaries to this fascial plane.

Immediately deep to the STF is a loose avascular areolar layer, separating the STF from the deep temporalis fascia (DTF). The DTF covers the temporalis muscle superiorly and splits into a superficial and deep layer below the level of the superior orbital rim. The point at which the deep temporal fascial layers unite together as a single unit has been referred to as the temporal line of fusion. The superficial and deep temporal fat pads are separated by the superficial and deep layers of the DTF, respectively. The DTF vasculature is supplied by the middle temporal artery without contributions from the frontal or parietal branches of the STA. The intervening loose avascular areolar layer separates the vasculature of the STF and the DTF.

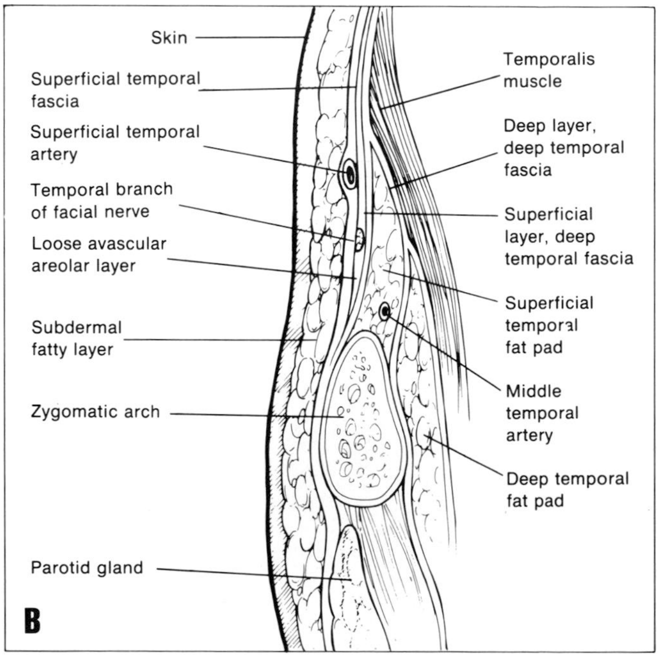

FIGURE 30–1 (Continued)

Facial Nerve

The temporal branches of the facial nerve supply motor innervation to the frontalis, upper half of the orbicularis oculi, and corrugator supercilii. These branches initially emerge from the parotid gland just above the zygomatic arch and arborize extensively. Despite variable branching patterns, all nerve fibers travel within the same plane as they traverse the zygomatic arch. Branches of this nerve run along the undersurface of the STF just within the loose avascular areolar layer (Figure 30–1B). While maintaining this constant position immediately below the STF, these branches proceed in a superomedial direction to innervate the facial musculature from the undersurface. The zone where the temporal branches of the facial nerve are most vulnerable to injury during a temporal artery biopsy is outlined by the following anatomic landmarks: (*1*) the tragus of the ear, (*2*) the junction of the zygomatic arch and the lateral orbital rim, (*3*) 2 cm above the level of the superior orbital rim and in a line directly superior to (*2*), (*4*) superior to the tragus and in horizontal alignment with (*3*) (Figure 30–1A). [The vertical dotted line defines the site of the cross-sectional diagram (Figure 30–1B) and is not an incision line]. This "danger zone" delineates the area where the facial nerve is superficial in location and in close proximity to the frontal branch of the STA.

Biopsy Site Selection

The frontal branch of the superficial temporal artery usually can be palpated throughout its course. It can be detected by its arterial pulsation or a cordlike sensation. The site selected for vessel biopsy is individualized and is based on several factors: the ability to precisely outline the arterial path, evidence of localized clinical signs of involvement, and the location of the palpable vessel relative to the danger zone.

Clinical signs of temporal arteritis include temporal artery tenderness, absent pulsations, overlying skin erythema, and arterial nodularity or swelling. When present, these localized clinical signs of arterial involvement determine the actual site selected for biopsy. If only the parietal branch of the STA is clinically involved, then it should be biopsied rather than a random biopsy of the frontal branch.

If localized clinical signs of arterial involvement are confined solely to the danger zone, then the biopsy should be obtained in this area. When surgery is performed within this zone, one should take extra care to remain in a superficial dissection plane, above the superficial temporal fascia, to avoid injuring the underlying branches of the facial nerve. In patients without localized clinical signs of involvement, a distal segment of the frontal branch should be selected for temporal artery biopsy (see safe zone in Figure 30–1A).

OPERATIVE PROCEDURE

Arterial Mapping

Once the actual site to be biopsied is determined, a small amount of hair may need to be shaved from the temporal region. This facilitates marking the arterial path and skin closure. The skin surrounding the biopsy site is cleaned with isopropyl alcohol, which removes excess oil and debris and allows easier outlining with a marker pen. The palpation and initial marking of the artery are critical to the planning of an appropriate incision line and to the harvesting of the vessel. Occasionally, vessel localization on both sides may be difficult. In this situation, a Doppler may aid in the detection of arteries with reduced blood flow and faint pulsations.

Incision Line

Figure 30–2. After the arterial mapping is completed, an incision line (*dotted line*) of approximately 3 cm in length is marked along the frontal branch of the superficial temporal artery (*solid line*). The proposed incision line should be in general alignment with the artery, but without running directly along the path of the vessel. This allows a large arterial biopsy to be harvested through a small incision. A skin incision made directly along the arterial marking may risk an accidental longitudinal laceration of the underlying vessel. In addition, the artery may be difficult to identify if the arterial skin marking is not precisely over the vessel, but instead is aligned on either side of the vessel. This may result in the surgeon dissecting through the superficial temporal fascia into the deeper layers before identifying the STA, thereby risking injury to the underlying branches of the facial nerve. However, if the incision line is made to cross the arterial path at some point, vessel identification is facilitated by this crossing. The incision line should also be oriented to follow the relaxed skin tension lines (*RSTL*) of the face to help camouflage the wound and to obtain the most aesthetic closure. Within this region, forehead creases (*three arrows*) approximate the RSTL and can be used to determine the orientation of the incision line.

If clinical signs of arterial involvement necessitate a biopsy within the danger zone, the incision is made in a more vertical orientation, to remain in alignment with the RSTL. If the artery to be biopsied travels in a path nearly perpendicular to the RSTL of the face, the incision line is oriented obliquely.

For patients in whom the artery is difficult to palpate, this process may take 10 to 15 minutes and is best completed before prepping the patient. Following the arterial outlining, the surgical field is prepared with povidone–iodine (Betadine) in the usual sterile manner. Care is taken not to wash off the arterial and incisional markings. A sterile self-adherent plastic drape is used to isolate the surgical field.

Biopsy Technique

Lidocaine 2% with 1:100,000 epinephrine is injected subcutaneously along the proposed incision line. After allowing 10 minutes for the vasoconstrictive effect of epinephrine to occur, the skin is incised with a scalpel blade. The incision should be superficial, no deeper than the subdermal fatty layer. As one can see from the cross-section of the temporal region (see Figure 30–1B), an incision deeper than the subdermal fatty layer will place the surgeon in an incorrect tissue plane, rendering STA identification more difficult.

Figure 30–3. The skin is grasped with a forceps on each side of the incision centrally and lifted anteriorly to tent up the subdermal fatty layer from the underlying STF. An incision is made centrally through the subdermal fatty layer (*arrow*) with a blunt Westcott scissors. As the snip incision is made, the tissue plane between the subdermal fatty layer and STF (*asterisk*) can be identified. One blade of the scissors is passed along the undersurface of the subdermal fatty layer and the full length of the incision is opened.

With a combination of sharp and blunt dissection, the wound is undermined on both sides of the incision line following the direction of the arterial skin markings (*arrowhead*). The dissection should hug

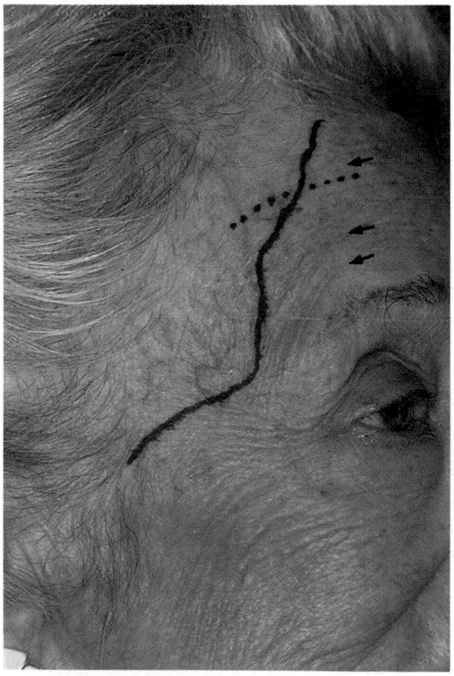

FIGURE 30–2

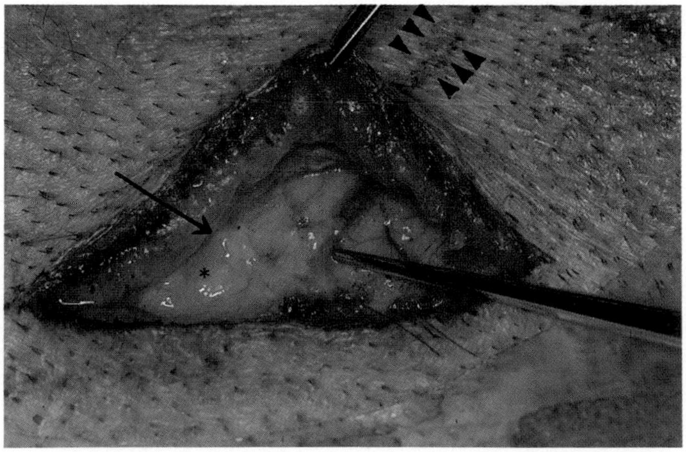

FIGURE 30–3

the undersurface of the subdermal fatty layer, which helps to avoid inadvertent trauma to the STA. Once a dissection plane is developed, a cotton-tipped applicator may be used to bluntly separate the subdermal fatty layer from the STF. Meticulous hemostasis during this maneuver enables immediate identification of the underlying branch of the STA (*pointer*) traveling within the STF.

On rare occasions, a branch of the superficial temporal vein may be adjacent to the artery. The vein, however, is often superficial to the artery and travels on the surface, instead of within, the STF. The vein may be seen to cross over the artery. These anatomic features help to differentiate a vein from an artery intraoperatively. Infrequently, it may be necessary to use direct palpation to identify the proper vessel for biopsy.

Figure 30–4. When a biopsy of the STA (*arrowhead*) is obtained in the most superior aspect of the temporalis region or overlying the frontalis muscle, the branches of the STA lie superficial to the STF and the frontalis, respectively. Within this same area, vertically oriented sensory branches of the supraorbital nerve (*arrows*) may be encountered and should be avoided. In addition to severing these nerves, extensive manipulation or stretching of the nerve branches may result in postoperative hypesthesia. In these two areas, a very superficial dissection is essential to avoid incising the artery or damaging sensory nerve fibers. This is especially important in thin patients in whom the subdermal fatty layer is not prominent.

Following the arterial path, the dissection along the undersurface of the subdermal fatty layer is continued until at least 3 cm of artery has been uncovered.

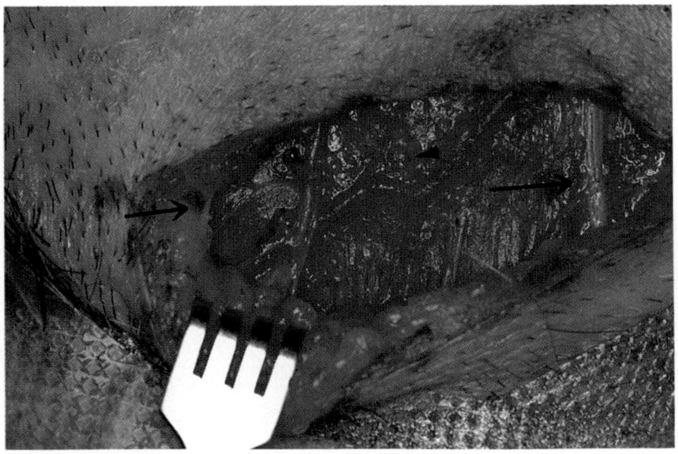

FIGURE 30–4

Figure 30–5A. At the most proximal end of the arterial dissection, a round-tipped Westcott scissors is used to bluntly dissect along both sides of the artery. Blunt dissection minimizes the chance of avulsing any small feeder vessels emanating from the main arterial trunk. Notably, the feeder vessels travel within the plane of the STF and do not extend directly out from the anterior arterial surface.

Figure 30–5B. A Westcott scissors is gently inserted under the vessel at the most proximal point of dissection.

Figure 30–5C. A 4–0 silk suture is passed under the artery in a reverse fashion (holding the tip of the needle) to avoid accidental puncturing of the artery. The suture is tied and this proximal ligature must be tight enough to close off the arterial flow. A second ligature may be placed more proximal than the first suture to ensure hemostasis.

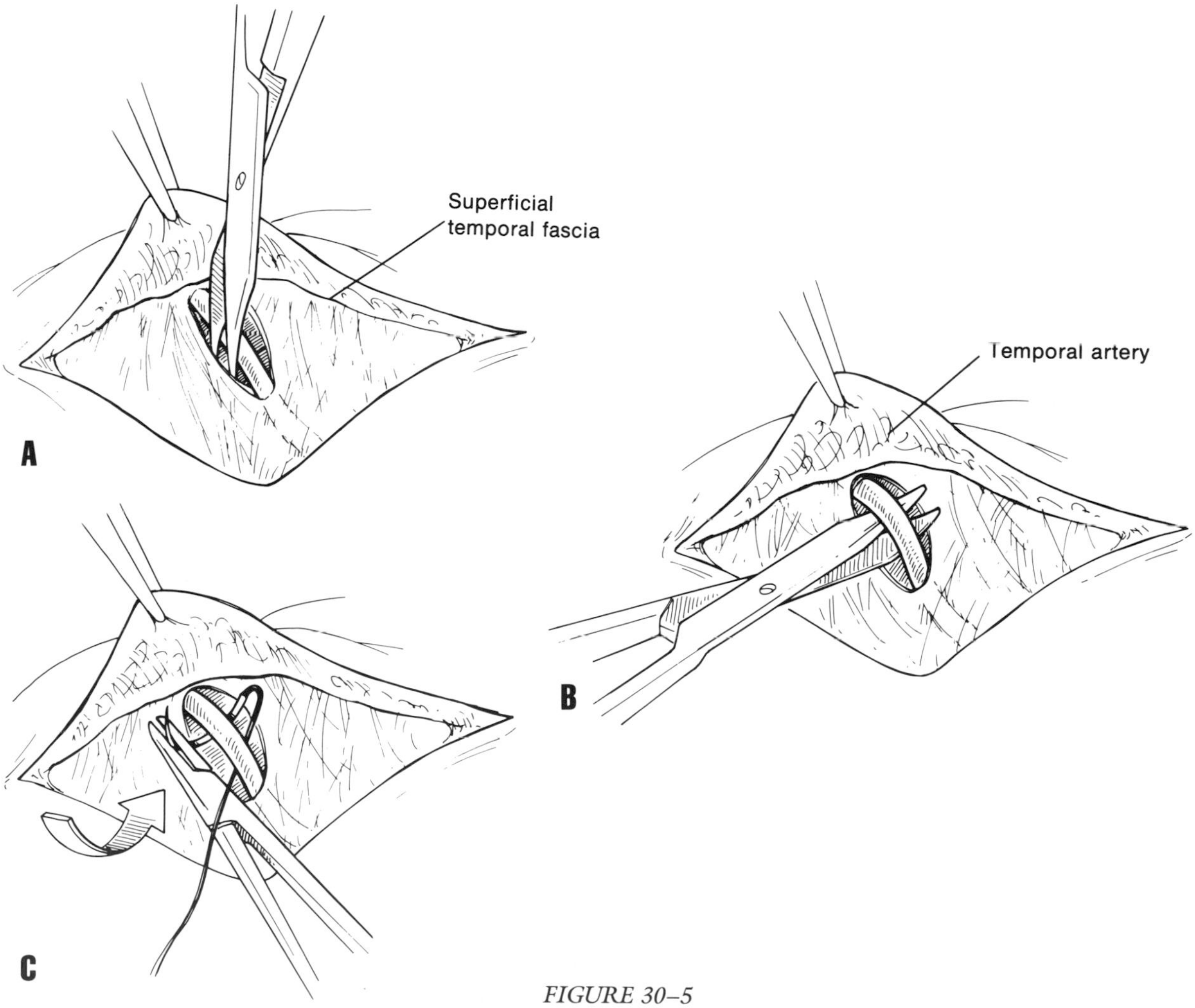

FIGURE 30–5

The distal end of the artery is dissected free in a similar fashion and ligated with a single 4–0 silk suture. To reduce the risk of damage to the branches of the facial nerve, dissection should not extend beyond the depth of the STF. If there are no additional large branches to be ligated, the artery is cut 1 to 2 mm distal to the two proximal 4–0 silk suture ligatures. The cut end of the arterial specimen is gently grasped with a 0.3 forceps and lifted away from the STF. A Westcott scissors is used to bluntly dissect out any small feeder vessels, which are then cauterized and cut close to the main arterial specimen. After reaching the distal ligature, the artery is again cut leaving a 1- to 2-mm stump to avoid slippage of the suture. The cut ends of the artery adjacent to the silk sutures are then cauterized as an added safety measure against bleeding. Gentle handling of the arterial specimen is essential to avoid creating crush artifact, which could alter the histopathologic interpretation of the internal elastic lamina.

The wound closure is best completed as two separate layers. The dermal and subdermal fatty layer are first approximated with buried interrupted 5–0 Vicryl sutures. The skin is then closed with interrupted vertical mattress sutures using 6–0 nylon. After applying bacitracin ointment, a Telfa pad and a folded 2 × 2 cotton gauze are placed over the wound. Benzoin solution is used on the skin surrounding the wound to allow placement of a small, tight pressure dressing.

The dressing is removed after 24 hours and bacitracin ointment applied to the wound three times a day. The skin sutures are removed at 5 to 7 days, and the ointment is continued for several additional days.

BIBLIOGRAPHY

CHAPTER 1

Anderson RL. Medial canthal tendon branches out. Arch Ophthalmol 1977;95: 2051.

Anderson RL, Beard C. The levator aponeurosis: attachments and their clinical significance. Arch Ophthalmol 1977;95:1437.

Anderson RL, Dixon RS. The role of Whitnall's ligament in ptosis surgery. Arch Ophthalmol 1979;97:705.

Doxanas MT, Anderson RL. Oriental eyelids: An anatomic study. Arch Ophthalmol 1984;102:1232.

Gioio VM, Linberg JV, McCormick SA. The anatomy of the lateral canthal tendon. Arch Ophthalmol 1987;105:529.

Hawes MJ, Dortzbach RK. The microscopic anatomy of the lower eyelid retractors. Arch Ophthalmol 1982;100:1313.

Hayreh SS, Dass R. The ophthalmic artery. II Intraorbital course. Br J Ophthalmol 1962;46:165.

Jones LT, Wobig JL. Surgery of the Eyelids and Lacrimal Systems. Birmingham: Aesculapius Publishing, 1976.

Koornneef L. Spatial aspects of orbital musculo-fibrous tissue in man. Amsterdam: Swets & Zeitlinger, 1977.

Lemke BN, Stasior, OG. The anatomy of eyebrow ptosis. Arch Ophthalmol 1982; 100:981.

CHAPTER 2

Borges AF. Relaxed skin tension lines (RSTL) versus other lines. Plast Reconstruc Surg 1984;73:144.

Doxanas MT. Orbicularis mobilization in eyelid reconstruction. Arch Opthalmol 1986;104:910.

Leibsohn J, Bullock J, Waller R. Full thickness eyelid biopsy for presumed carcinoma in situ of the palpebral conjunctiva. Ophthalmol Surg 1982;13:840.

Liu D, Stasior OG. Thermal orbital injuries from disposable cauteries. Plast Reconstr Surg 1984;74:1.

Putterman AM. Conjunctival map biopsy to determine pagetoid spread. Am J Ophthalmol 1986;102:87.

Wilkins RB, Kulwin DR, McCord DD, Tanenbaum M. Skin and tissue techniques. In: McCord CD, Tanenbaum M, eds. Oculoplastic surgery. New York: Raven Press, 1989:10.

CHAPTER 3

Divine RD, Anderson RL. Techniques in eyelid wound closure. Ophthalmic Surg 1982;13:283.

Dortzbach RK, Angrist RA. Silicone intubation for lacerated lacrimal canaliculi. Ophthalmic Surg 1985;16:639.

Harris GJ, Fuerste FH. Lacrimal intubation in the primary repair of midfacial fractures. Ophthalmology 1987;94:242.

CHAPTER 5

Busse H, Steinkogler FJ, Fries J. Ring intubation of lacerated canaliculi lacrimales. Orbit 1985;4:73.

Hecht SD. Evaluation of the lacrimal drainage system. Ophthalmology 1978;85: 1250.

Jones LT, Wobig JL. The lacrimal system. In: Surgery of the eyelids and lacrimal system. Birmingham: Aesculapius, 1976:57.

Jordan DR, Nerad JA, Tse DT. The pigtail probe revisited. Ophthalmology 1990; 97:512.

Kartch MC. French eye pigtail probe for lacrimal canaliculus repair. Am J Ophthalmol 1971;72:1145.

Worst JG. Method for reconstructing torn lacrimal canaliculus. Am J Ophthalmol 1962;53:520.

CHAPTER 6

Harris GJ, Diclementi D. Congenital dacryocystocele. Arch Ophthalmol 1982; 100:1763.

Havins WE, Wilkins RB. A useful alternative to silicone intubation in congenital nasolacrimal duct obstructions. Ophthalmic Surg 1983;14:666.

Katowitz JA, Welsh MG. Timing of initial probing and irrigation in congenital nasolacrimal duct obstruction. Ophthalmology 1987;94:698.

Kushner BJ. Congenital nasolacrimal system obstruction. Arch Ophthalmol 1982;100:597.

Nelson LB, Calhoun JH, Menduke H. Medical management of congenital nasolacrimal duct obstruction. Ophthalmology 1985;92:1187.

Peterson RA, Robb RM. The natural course of congenital obstruction of the nasolacrimal duct. J Pediatr Ophthalmol Strabismus 1978;15:246.

Robb RM. Probing and irrigation for congenital nasolacrimal duct obstruction. Arch Ophthalmol 1986;104:378.

Tse DT, Anderson RL. A new modification of the standard lacrimal groove director for nasolacrimal intubation. Arch Ophthalmol 1983;101:1938.

Welsh MG, Katowitz JA. Timing of silastic tubing removal after intubation for congenital nasolacrimal duct obstruction. Ophthalmic Plast Reconstr Surg 1989; 5:43.

Wesley RE. Interior turbinate fracture in the treatment of congenital nasolacrimal duct obstruction and congenital nasolacrimal duct anomaly. Ophthalmic Surg 1985;16:368.

CHAPTER 9

Ballen PH. A simple procedure for the relief of trichiasis and entropion of the upper lid. Arch Ophthalmol 1964;72:239.

Jones LT, Reeh MJ, Wobig JL. Senile entropion: a new concept. Am J Ophthalmol 1972;74:327.

Nowinski T, Anderson RL. Advances in eyelid malpositions. Ophthalmic Plast Reconstr Surg 1985;1:145.

Quickert MH, Rathbun E. Suture repair of entropion. Arch Ophthalmol 1971;85: 304.

Wies FA. Spastic entropion. Trans Am Acad Ophthalmol Otolaryngol 1955;59: 503.

CHAPTER 10

Anderson RL, Gordy DD. The tarsal strip procedure. Arch Ophthalmol 1979;97: 2192.

Frueh BR, Schoengarth LD. Evaluation and treatment of the patient with ectropion. Ophthalmology 1982;89:1049.

Hawes MJ, Dortzbach RK. The microscopic anatomy of the lower eyelid retractors. Arch Ophthalmol 1982;100:1313.

Putterman AM. Ectropion of the lower eyelid secondary to Muller's muscle—capsulopalpebral fascia attachment. Am J Ophthalmol 1978;85:814.

Tse DT. Surgical correction of punctal malposition. Am J Ophthalmol 1985;100: 339.

Wesley RE. Tarsal ectropion from detachment of the lower eyelid retractors. Am J Ophthalmol 1982;93:491.

CHAPTER 11

Dutton JJ, Anderson RL, Tse DT. Combined surgery and cryotherapy for scleral invasion of epithelial malignancies. Ophthalmic Surg 1984;15:289.

Jakobiec FA, Brownstein S, Albert W, Schwarz F, Anderson RL. Cryotherapy of conjunctival melanoma. Am J Ophthalmol 1982;89:502.

Peksayar G, Soyturk MK, Demiryont M. Long-term results of cryotherapy on malignant epithelial tumors of the conjunctiva. Am J Ophthalmol 1989;107:337.

Sullivan JH. The use of cryotherapy for trichiasis. Trans Am Acad Ophthalmol Otolaryngol 1977;83:708.

Sullivan JH, Beard C, Bullock JD: Cryosurgery for treatment of trichiasis. Am J Ophthalmol 1976;82:117.

Wood JR, Anderson RL. Complications of cryosurgery. Arch Ophthalmol 1981; 99:460.

CHAPTER 12

Anderson RL. The aponeurotic approach to ptosis surgery. Adv Ophthalmic Plast Reconstr Surg 1982;1:145.

Anderson RL, Dixon RS. The aponeurotic approach to ptosis surgery. Arch Ophthalmol 1979;97:1123.

Anderson RL, Dixon RS. Neuromyopathic ptosis: a new surgical approach. Arch Ophthalmol 1979;97:1129.

Anderson RL, Dixon RS. The role of Whitnall's ligament in ptosis surgery. Arch Ophthalmol 1979;97:705.

Anderson RL, Gordy DD. Aponeurotic defects in congenital ptosis. Ophthalmology 1979;86:1493.

Beard C. Ptosis, 3rd ed. St Louis: CV Mosby, 1981.

Dillman DB, Anderson RL. Levator myectomy in synkinetic ptosis. Arch Ophthalmol 1984;102:422.

Jordan DR, Anderson RL. Obtaining fascia lata. Arch Ophthalmol 1987;105:1139.

Patrinely JR, Anderson RL. The septal pulley in frontalis suspension. Arch Ophthalmol 1986;104:1707.

CHAPTER 13

Baker TJ. Upper blepharoplasty. In Rees TD, ed. Modern trends in blepharoplasty. Clin Plast Surg 1981;8:635.

Courtiss EH. Selection of alternatives in esthetic blepharoplasty. In: Rees TD, ed. Modern trends in blepharoplasty. Clin Plast Surg 1981;9:739.

Doxanas MT, Anderson RL. Oriental eyelids: an anatomic study. Arch Ophthalmol 1984;102:1232.

Flowers RS. Blepharoplasty. In: Courtiss EH, ed. Male aesthetic surgery. St Louis: CV Mosby, 1982:207.

Gavaris PT. The eyelid crease. In: Hornblass A, ed. Oculoplastic, orbital and reconstructive surgery, vol 1. Baltimore: Williams & Wilkins, 1988:505.

Gradinger GP. Cosmetic upper blepharoplasty. In: Jelks GW, ed. Oculoplastic surgery. Clin Plast Surg 1988;15:289.

Hisatomi C, Fujino T. Anatomic considerations concerning blepharoplasty in the Oriental patient. In: Smith B, Bosniak S, eds. The aging face. Adv Ophthalmic Plast Reconstr Surg 1983;2:151.

Hornblass H. Ptosis and pseudoptosis and blepharoplasty. In: Rees TD, ed. Modern trends in blepharoplasty. Clin Plast Surg 1981;8:811.

Liu D. Oriental eyelids: anatomic difference and surgical consideration. In: Hornblass A, ed. Oculoplastic, orbital and reconstructive surgery, vol 1. Baltimore: Williams & Wilkins, 1988:513.

Putterman AM. Upper eyelid blepharoplasty. In: Hornblass A, ed. Oculoplastic, orbital and reconstructive surgery, vol 1. Baltimore: Williams & Wilkins, 1988: 474.

Rees TD. Blepharoplasty. In Rees TD, ed. Aesthetic Plastic Surgery. Philadelphia: WB Saunders, 1980:459.

Shorr N, Seiff SR. Cosmetic blepharoplasty, an illustrated surgical guide. Thorofare, NJ: Slack, 1986.

Siegel R. Surgical anatomy of the upper eyelid fascia. Ann Plast Surg 1984;13:263.

Smith B, Petrelli R. Surgical repair of prolapsed lacrimal glands. Arch Ophthalmol 1978;96:113.

Sutcliffe T, Baylis H, Fett D. Bleeding in cosmetic blepharoplasty: an anatomic approach. Ophthalmic Plast Reconstr Surg 1985;1:107.

Zide BM. Anatomy of the eyelids. In: Rees TD, ed. Modern trends in blepharoplasty. Clin Plast Surg 1981;8:623.

CHAPTER 18

Arion HG. Dynamic closure of the lids in paralysis of the orbicularis muscle. Int Surg 1972;57:48.

Chapman P, Lamberty BGH. Results of upper lid loading in the treatment of lagophthalmos caused by facial palsy. Br J Plast Surg 1988;41:369.

Frueh BR. Exposure keratitis. In: Surgery of the eye. New York: Churchill-Livingstone, 1988:563.

May M. Gold weight and wire spring implants as alternatives to tarsorrhaphy. Arch Otolaryngol Head Neck Surg 1987;113:656.

Morel-Fatio D, Lalardrie JP. Palliative surgical treatment of facial paralysis: the palpebral spring. Plast Reconstr Surg 1964;33:446.

Neuman AR, Weinberg A, Sela M, et al. The correction of seventh nerve palsy lagophthalmos with gold lid load (16 years experience). Ann Plast Surg 1989;22:142.

Seiff SR, Sullivan JH, Freeman LN, Ahn J. Pretarsal fixation of gold weights in facial nerve palsy. Ophthalmic Plast Reconstr Surg 1989;5:104.

Sheehan JE. Progress in correction of facial palsy with tantalum wire and mesh. Surgery 1950;27:122.

Smellie GD. Restoration of the blinking reflex in facial palsy by a simple lid load operation. Br J Plast Surg 1966;19:279.

CHAPTER 19

Jobe RP. A technique for lid-loading in the management of lagophthalmos in facial paralysis. Plast Reconstr Surg 1974;53:29.

Levine RE. Management of lagophthalmos with palpebral spring and silastic elastic prosthesis. In: Hornblass A, ed. Ophthalmic and orbital plastic reconstructive surgery, vol. 1. Baltimore: Williams & Wilkins, 1989.

Levine RE, House WF, Hitselberger WE. Ocular complications of seventh nerve paralysis and management with the palpebral spring. Am J Ophthalmol 1972;73:219.

Morel-Fatio D, Lalardrie JP. Palliative surgical treatment of facial paralysis: the palpebral spring. Plast Reconstr Surg 1964;33:446.

CHAPTER 20

Anderson RL, Ceilley RI. A multispecialty approach to the excision and reconstruction of eyelid tumors. Ophthalmology 1978;85:1150.

Caro WA, Bronstein BR. Basal cell epithelial (basal cell carcinoma). In: Moschella SL, Hurley HJ, ed. Dermatology. Philadelphia: WB Saunders, 1985:1564.

Cottel WI, Proper S: Mohs surgery, fresh tissue technique. J Dermatol Surg Oncol 1982;8:576.

Folberg R, Whitaker DC, Tse DT, et al. Recurrent and residual sebaceous carcinoma after Mohs excision of the primary lesion. Am J Ophthalmol 1987;103:817.

Lang PG, Osguthorpe JD. Indications and limitations of Mohs micrographic surgery. Dermatol Clin 1989;7:627.

Lever WF, Schaumberg-Lever G. Histopathology of the skin, 6th ed. Philadelphia: JB Lippincott, 1983:562.

Panje WR, Ceilley RI. The influence of embryology of the mid-face on the spread of epithelial malignancies. Laryngoscope 1979;89:1914.

Whitaker DC, et al. Postoperative techniques for corneal protection in Mohs micrographic surgery. J Dermatol Surg Oncol 1988;14:951.

Zitelli JA. Mohs surgery: concepts and misconceptions. Int J Dermatol 1985;24:541.

CHAPTER 21

Anderson RL, Edwards JJ. Reconstruction by myocutaneous eyelid flaps. Arch Ophthalmol 1979;97:2358.

Borges AF. The rhombic flap. Plast Reconstr Surg 1981;67:458.

Carrol RP. Entropion following the Cutler–Beard procedure. Ophthalmology 1983;90:1052.

Cutler N, Beard C. A method for partial and total upper lid reconstruction. Am J Ophthalmol 1955;39:1.

Dortzbach RK, Hawes MJ. Midline forehead flap in reconstructive procedures of the eyelids and exenterated socket. Ophthalmic Surg 1981;12:257.

Hughes WH. Total lower lid reconstruction: technical details. Trans Am Ophthalmol Soc 1976;74:321.

Leone CR. Lateral canthal reconstruction. Ophthalmology 1987;94:238.

McCord CD, Nunery WR. Reconstruction of the lower eyelid and outer canthus. In: McCord CD, Tanenbaum M, eds. Oculoplastic surgery, 2nd ed. New York: Raven Press, 1987:93.

McCord CD, Wesley R. Reconstruction of the upper eyelid and medial canthus. In: McCord CD, Tanenbaum M, eds. Oculoplastic surgery, 2nd ed. New York: Raven Press, 1987:73.

Miller EA, Boynton JR. Complications of eyelid reconstruction using a semicircle flap. Ophthalmic Surg 1987;18:807.

Patrinely JR, Marines HM, Anderson RL. Skin flaps in periorbital reconstruction. Surv Ophthalmol 1987;31:249.

Shotton FT. Optimal closure of medial canthal surgical defects with rhomboid flaps: "rules of thumb" for flap and and rhomboid defect orientations. Ophthalmic Surg 1983;14:46.

Stephenson CM, Brown BZ. The use of tarsus as a free autogenous graft in eyelid surgery. Ophthalmic Plast Reconstr Surg 1985;1:43.

Tenzel RR. Reconstruction of the central one half of an eyelid. Arch Ophthalmol 1975;93:125.

Weinstein GS, Anderson RL, Tse DT, et al. The use of a periosteal strip for eyelid reconstruction. Arch Ophthalmol 1985;103:357.

CHAPTER 22

Aguilar GL, Shannon GM, Flanagan JC. Experience with dermis–fat grafting: an analysis of early postoperative complications and methods of prevention. Ophthalmic Surg 1982;13:204.

Dortzbach RK. Socket reconstruction: what really happens. Ophthalmology 1976;81:583.

Dortzbach RK, Callahan A. Advances in socket reconstruction. Am J Ophthalmol 1970;70:800.

McCord CD. The extruding implant. Ophthalmology 1976;81:287.

Meltzer MA. Reconstruction of lower fornix: a new approach. Arch Ophthalmol 1977;95:1031.

Mustarde JC. General principles in the management of the contracted socket. Orbit 1986;5:77.

Neuhaus RW, Baylis HI, Shorr N. Complications at mucous membrane donor sites. Am J Ophthalmol 1982;93:643.

Putterman AM. Deep ocular socket reconstruction. Arch Ophthalmol 1977;95:1221.

Shore JW, McCord CD, Bergin DJ. Management of complications following dermis–fat grafting for anophthalmic socket reconstruction. Ophthalmology 1985;92:1342.

Smith B, Petrellia R. Dermis–fat graft as a movable implant within the muscle cone. Am J Ophthalmol 1978;85:62.

Soll DB. Insertion of secondary intraorbital implants. Arch Ophthalmol 1973;89:214.

Soll DB. The use of sclera in surgical management of extruding implants. Ophthalmology 1978;85:863.

Soll DB. The anophthalmic socket. Ophthalmology 1982;89:407.

Spivey BE, Stewart W, Allen L. Surgical correction of superior sulcus deformity occurring after enucleation. Am J Ophthalmol 1976;82:365.

Stewart WB, Gratiot JB, Soll DB. Surgical management of orbital implant extrusion by implant placement posterior to Tenon's fascia. Ophthalmic Surg 1982;13:807.

Tse DT: Cyanoacrylate tissue adhesive in securing orbital implants. Ophthalmic Surg 1986;17:577.

Vistnes LM, Paris GL. Uses of RTV silicone in orbital reconstruction. Am J Ophthalmol 1977;83:577.

CHAPTER 23

Bayliss H, Schoor N, McCord C, Tanenbaum M. Evisceration, enucleation, and exenteration. In: McCord C, Tanenbaum M, eds. Oculoplastic surgery. New York: Raven Press, 1987:407.

Dortzbach R, Woog J. Choice of procedure. Enucleation, evisceration, or prosthesis fitting over globes. Ophthalmology 1985;92:1249.

Frueh BR, Felker GV. Baseball implant: a method of secondary insertion of an intraorbital implant. Arch Ophthalmol 1976;94:429.

Jordan D, Anderson R, Nerad J, Allen L. A preliminary report on the Universal implant. Arch Ophthalmol 1987;105:1726.

Nunery WR, Hetzler KJ. Improved prosthetic motility following enucleation. Ophthalmology 1983;90:1110.

Perry AC. Development of integrated orbital implant [Abstract]. Presented at the 10th Annual Scientific Symposium of the American Society of Ophthalmic Plastic and Reconstructive Surgery, New Orleans, October 28, 1989.

Raflo G. Enucleation and evisceration. In: Duane T, Jaeger E, eds. Clinical ophthalmology. Philadelphia: JB Lippincott, 1988.

Schaefer D, Della Rocca R. Enucleation. In Della Rocca R, Nesi F, Lisman R, eds. Ophthalmic plastic and reconstructive surgery. St Louis: CV Mosby, 1987: 1278.

Soll DB. Donor sclera in enucleation surgery. Arch Ophthalmol 1974;92:494.

Walter WL. Update on enucleation and evisceration surgery. Ophthalmic Plast Reconstr Surg 1985;1:243.

CHAPTER 24

Bayliss H, Schorr N, McCord C, Tanenbaum M. Evisceration, enucleation, and exenteration. In: McCord C, Tanenbaum M, eds. Oculoplastic surgery. New York: Raven Press, 1987:407.

Dortzbach R, Woog J. Choice of procedure. Enucleation, evisceration, or prosthetic fitting over globes. Ophthalmology 1985;92:1249.

Green R, Maumenee A, Sanders T, Smith M. Sympathetic uveitis following evisceration. J Am Acad Ophthalmol Otolaryngol 1972;76:625.

Green W, Maumenee A, Sanders T, Smith M. Sympathetic uveitis following evisceration. Trans Am Acad Ophthalmol Otolaryngol 1972;76:625.

Meltzer M, Schaefer D, Della Rocca R. Evisceration. In: Della Rocca R, Nesi F, Lisman E, eds. Ophthalmic plastic and reconstructive surgery. St Louis: CV Mosby, 1987:1300.

CHAPTER 25

Buus D, Tse D. The use of enucleation snare during orbital exenteration. Arch Ophthalmol 1990;108:636.

deConciliis C, Bonavolonta G. Incidence and treatment of dural exposure and CSF leak during orbital exenteration. Ophthalmic Plast Reconstr Surg 1987;3:61.

Kennedy R. Indications and surgical techniques for orbital exenteration. Ophthalmology 1979;86:967.

Kersten R, Tse D, Anderson R, Blodi F. The role of orbital exenteration in choroidal melanoma with extrascleral extension. Ophthalmology 1985;92:436.

Small R. Exenteration of the orbit: indications and techniques. In: Della Rocca R, Nesi F, Lisman R, eds. Ophthalmic plastic and reconstructive surgery. St Louis: CV Mosby, 1987:1151.

Small R, LaFuente H. Exenteration of the orbit in selected cases of severe orbital contracture. Ophthalmology 1983;90:236.

Stewart W. Exenteration: an overview of the operation and its role. In: Della Rocca R, Nesi F, Lisman R, eds. Ophthalmic plastic and reconstructive surgery. St Louis: CV Mosby, 1987:1148.

Tse D, Bumstead R. A two-layer closure of sino-orbital fistulas. Ophthalmology 1989;96:1673.

Tse D, Panje W, Anderson R. Cyanoacrylate adhesive use to stop CSF leaks during orbital surgery. Arch Ophthalmol 1984;102:1337.

CHAPTER 26

Bartley GB, Kay PP. Posterior lamellar eyelid reconstruction with a hard palate mucosal graft. Am J Ophthalmol 1989;107:609.

Harvey JT, Anderson RL. The aponeurotic approach to eyelid retraction. Ophthalmology 1981;88:513.

Kersten RC, Kulwin DR, Levartovsky S, et al. Management of lower lid retraction with hard palate mucosa grafting. Arch Ophthalmol 1990;108:1339–1343.

Siegel R. Palate grafts for eyelid reconstruction. Plast Reconstr Surg 1985;76:411.

CHAPTER 27

Anderson RL, Linberg JV. Transorbital approach to decompression in Graves' disease. Arch Ophthalmol 1981;99:120.

Linberg JV, Anderson RL. Transorbital decompression: indications and results. Arch Ophthalmol 1981;99:113.

McCord CD. Current trends in orbital decompression. Ophthalmology 1985;92: 21.

McCord DC, Moses JL. Exposure of the inferior orbit with fornix incision and lateral canthotomy. Ophthalmic Surg 1979;10:53.

Seiff SR, Shorr N. Nasolacrimal drainage system obstruction after orbital decompression. Am J Ophthalmol 1988;106:204.

Shorr N, Seiff SR. The four stages of surgical rehabilitation of the patient with dysthyroid ophthalmopathy. Ophthalmology 1986;93:476.

Trobe TD, Glaser JS, Laflamme P. Dysthyroid optic neuropathy: clinical profile and rationale for management. Arch Ophthalmol 1981;99:120.

CHAPTER 28

Furado Y. Results in 400 cases of surgical decompression of the optic nerve. Mod Probl Ophthalmol 1975;14:474.

Galbraith JEK, Sullivan JH. Decompression of the perioptic meninges for relief of papilledema. Am J Ophthalmol 1973;76:687.

Kronish JW, Dortzbach RK. Upper eyelid crease surgical approach to dermoid and epidermoid cysts in children. Arch Ophthalmol 1988;106:1625.

Linberg JV, Orcutt JC, Van Dyk HJL. Orbital Surgery. In: Duane TD, Jaeger EA, eds. Clinical ophthalmology, vol 5. Philadelphia: JB Lippincott, 1985;1.

McCord CD. A combined lateral and medial orbitotomy for exposure of the optic nerve and orbital apex. Ophthalmic Surg 1978;9:58.

McCord CD, Moses JL. Exposure of the inferior orbit with fornix incision and lateral canthotomy. Ophthalmic Surg 1979;10:59.

Montgomery WW. Surgery of the frontal sinuses. Otolaryngol Clin North Am 1971;4:97.

Rootman J. Orbital surgery. In: Rootman J, ed. Diseases of the orbit. A multidisciplinary approach. Philadelphia: JB Lippincott, 1988:579.

CHAPTER 30

Abul-Hassan HS, Ascher GVD, Acland RD. Surgical anatomy and blood supply of the fascial layers of the temporal region. Plast Reconstr Surg 1986;77:17.

Albert DM, Ruchman MC, Keltner JL. Skip areas in temporal arteritis. Arch Ophthalmol 1976;94:2072.

De Castro Correia PC, Zani R. Surgical anatomy of the facial nerve as related to ancillary operations in rhytidoplasty. Plast Reconstr Surg 1973;52:549.

Kelley JS. Doppler ultrasound flow detector used in temporal artery biopsy. Arch Ophthalmol 1978;96:845.

Keltner JL. Giant cell arteritis: signs and symptoms. Ophthalmology 1982;89:1101.

Liebman EP, Webster RC, Berger AS, Della Vecchia M. The frontalis nerve in the temporal brow lift. Arch Otolaryngol 1982;108:232.

McDonnell PJ, Moore GW, Miller NR, ct al. Temporal arteritis: a clinicopathologic study. Ophthalmology 1986;93:518.

Slavin ML. Brow droop after superficial temporal artery biopsy. Arch Ophthalmol 1986;104:1127.

Stuzin JM, Wagstrom L, Kawamoto HK, Wolfe SA. Anatomy of the frontal branch of the facial nerve: the significance of the temporal fat pad. Plast Reconstr Surg 1989;83:265.

Wilkinson IMS, Russell RWR. Arteries of the head and neck in giant cell arteritis: a pathological study to show the pattern of arterial involvement. Arch Neurol 1972;27:378.

INDEX

D

E

N

O

T